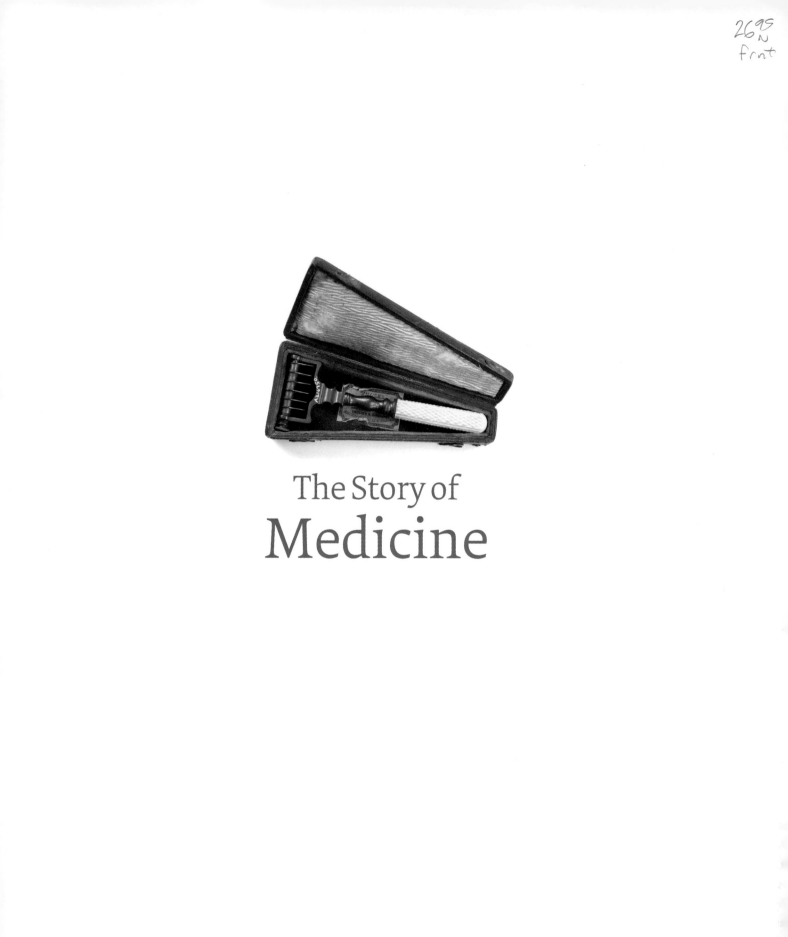

The Story of
Medicine

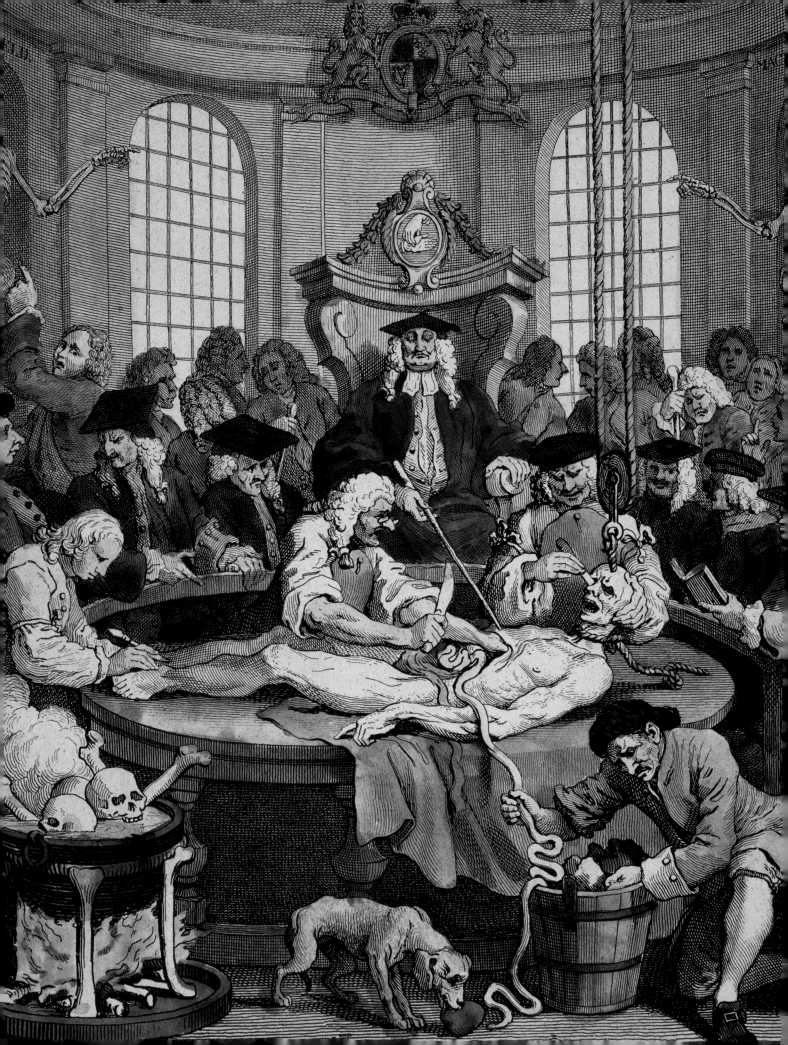

The Story of
Medicine

From Bloodletting to Biotechnology

Mary Dobson

Quercus

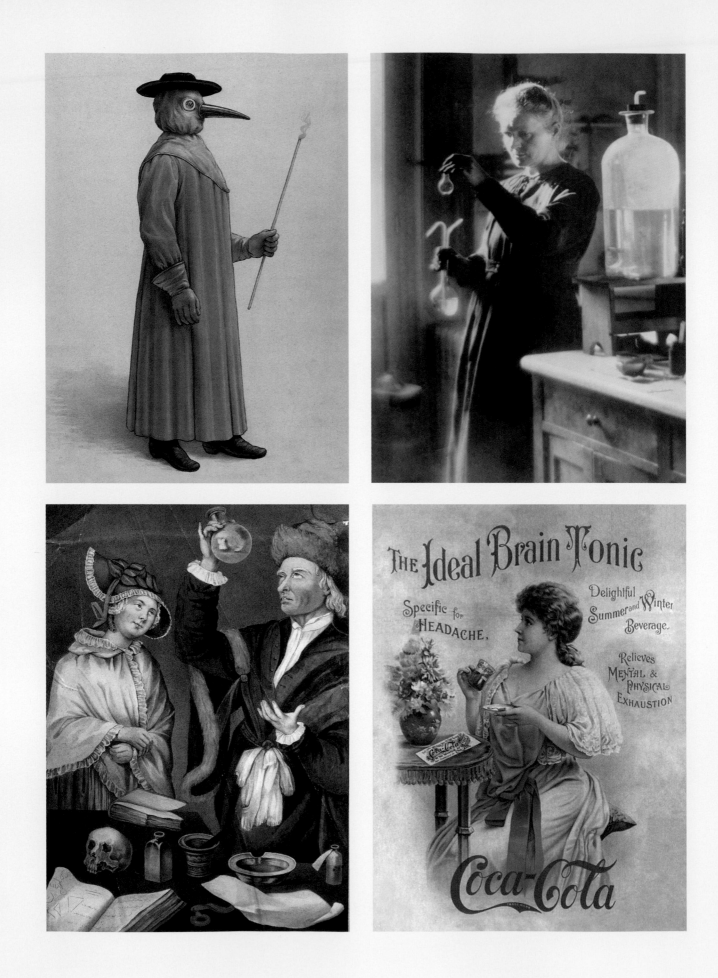

Contents

Preface

Man being subject to as many and more distempers than his famous structure can boast variety of parts, all the faculties of his soul have been continually employed to find out the Remedies for the preservation and restauration of his decaying body.

Robert Talbor (1642–81), English quack doctor who discovered a "secret" remedy for malaria

Medicine is both a science and an art, and has been called "the greatest benefit" to humankind. The challenges to find remedies to alleviate, treat, and cure illness have engaged the minds of doctors, healers, and patients since ancient times. Medicine is also about the art of listening to the patient, diagnosing diseases, and understanding or preventing their causes. Physicians and patients have wrestled to make sense of the plagues and pestilences of the past and, many discoveries later, scientists continue to unravel the mysteries of the body and mind.

The achievements and practices that have transformed medicine are many: Jenner and vaccination; Pasteur and Koch with their "germ theory"; Florence Nightingale and her nursing reforms; Lister and antisepsis; Röntgen and X-rays; Crick and Watson with the DNA double helix. But there are also stories of trauma and tragedy—patients who experienced unimaginable pain under the surgeon's knife in the centuries before anesthesia, and the fear of the poor in the 19th century that after death their bodies would be dug up by body snatchers to end up on the anatomist's dissecting table. There are dramatic episodes such as John Snow's removal of the Broad Street pump handle in 1854 to prevent the spread of cholera in London. There are also endless intriguing questions: for example, why did the ancient practice of bloodletting and use of opium remain so popular over the centuries? And there are momentous occasions such as the vaccination of the first child for smallpox in 1796; the young boy who was given insulin shots for diabetes in 1922; the identical twins who made the dream of organ transplant a reality in 1954; and the patient who received the world's first artificial organ created from his own stem cells in 2011.

This book highlights some of the themes and key milestones in the story of medicine. The first part explores the development of ideas about the causes of disease from the Greco-Roman humoral theory to the discoveries of germs and genes in the modern era. The second part looks at medical practice: at the physicians, nurses, surgeons, dentists, and others who have played a role in treating and caring for the sick at home and in hospitals. The third part describes treatments and therapies including bloodletting, acupuncture, and healing herbs, as well as dangerous narcotics added to quack and patent medicines. The fourth part traces the development of modern drugs and vaccines: from the arrival of antibiotics and early breakthroughs in cancer treatments to the growth of biotechnology encompassing breathtaking advances in ways of modifying and harnessing living organisms to obtain previously undreamed-of products, such as genetically engineered human proteins, vaccines, and monoclonal antibodies.

Life expectancy in many countries is now over seventy or eighty years – double that of the mid-19th century. Lifesaving drugs, vaccines, and surgical interventions, improvements in sanitation, nutrition, standards of living, and wider access to health care have all contributed to this result. We have come a long way from leech farms catering for the popular practice of bloodletting to the establishment of global pharmaceutical companies and the power of "magic bullets" and biotechnology to transform lives. Yet challenges remain. Cardiovascular diseases and cancers are leading causes of death, and, while declining in some high-income countries, they are increasingly prominent in lower- and middle-income countries; ancient infections, such as malaria and tuberculosis, and recently emergent diseases, notably, HIV/AIDS, cause a great many deaths; life expectancy in parts of sub-Saharan Africa is twenty or thirty years less than in the West. Antibiotic resistance is a huge concern to all societies along with fears of new or untreatable infections; Alzheimer's disease and other dementias are a major and rapidly increasing problem for our aging populations. Some of these challenges can and will be met in the future with advances in medical knowledge and technologies, healthier lifestyles and, it is hoped, a reduction in the global inequalities in human health.

Meanwhile, the importance of a good "bedside manner" and the care of a patient, whether by physician, nurse, family, or friends is an important factor both in recovery and in the easing of the last months or hours of a life. As the physician William Osler (1849–1919), who witnessed some of the greatest developments in medicine, aptly advised: "the old art cannot possibly be replaced by, but must be incorporated in, the new science." In the integration of all that is best in the "science" and the "quiet art" of medicine lies the future health of the world.

Mary Dobson,
St John's College, Cambridge

March 2013

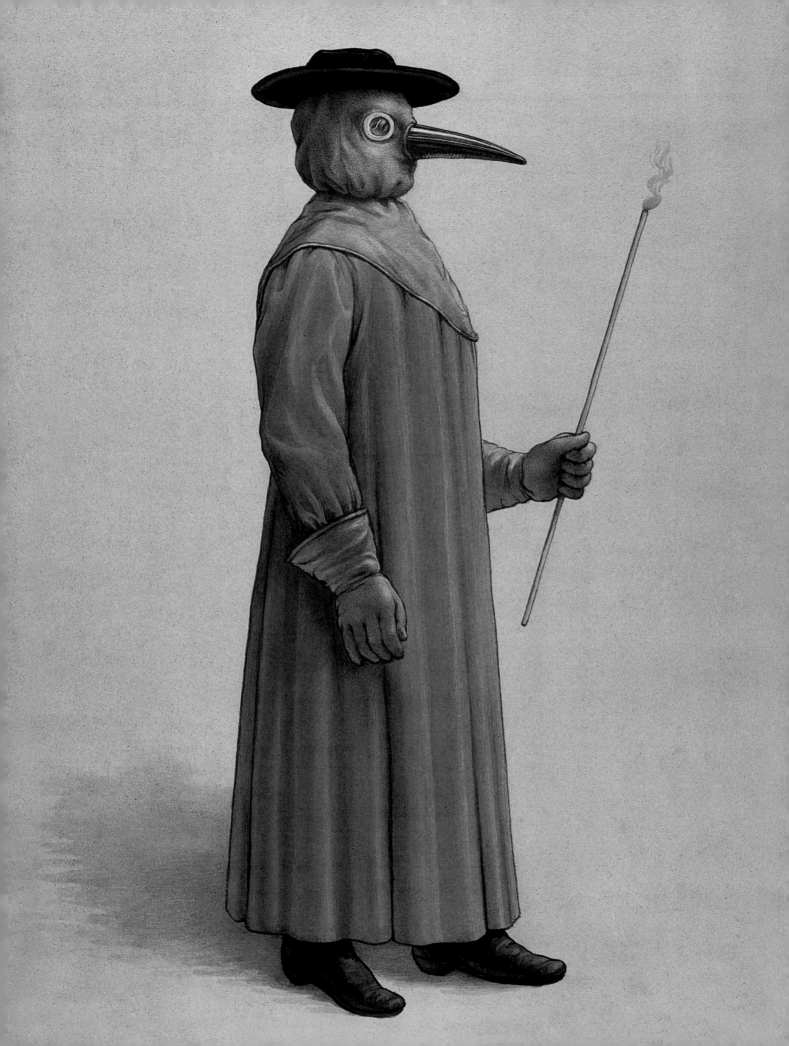

Bad Blood and Bad Airs

He knew the cause of every malady
Were it of hot or cold, of moist or dry,
And where engendered, and of what humour;
He was a very good practitioner.

Chaucer, *The Canterbury Tales*, Prologue "The Physician" (14th century)

From ancient times, plagues, pestilences, and ill-health were attributed to a range of overlapping causes—from demons and supernatural influences to divine retribution and human failure. Greco-Roman humoral theory was one of the most dominant ideas for explaining sickness in an individual, and followers of Hippocrates and Galen emphasized that diseases stemmed from natural, rather than sacred causes. Black bile was the humor considered to cause most serious illnesses—both physical and mental. It was also thought that an excess of "bad blood" could be relieved by bloodletting. Over the centuries, physicians also debated whether diseases like plague and cholera were "contagious," spread from person to person, or were caused by "bad airs" and foul smells. Even before scientists unraveled the causes of many mysterious diseases and found "magic bullets" to treat them, there were some remarkable interventions from smallpox vaccination to improved sanitation.

Concepts of disease: from ancient Egypt to the East

Magic is effective together with medicine; medicine is effective together with magic.

Ebers Papyrus *c.*1500 BC

Medicine has always involved an understanding of the human body—both in sickness and in health. The ancient world saw the birth of several great medical traditions, some of which have largely disappeared, while others, with changes over the centuries, continue to this day.

OPPOSITE A physician wearing a 17th-century plague costume. During plague epidemics, specially appointed "plague doctors" wore protective garments with aromatic herbs in their "beaks" along with fumigating torches.

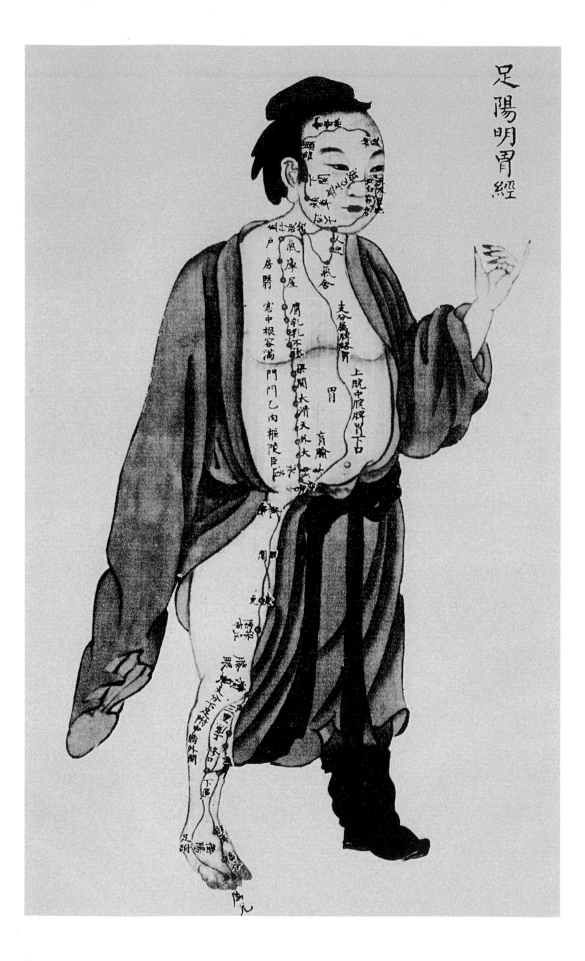

Concepts and theories of disease

Ideas about disease, as well as remedies, have been exchanged across the globe, transmitted between different cultures and adapted to local settings and beliefs.

Egyptian papyri dating back to over three and a half thousand years ago give us a fascinating insight into the medical beliefs, practices, and treatments of the ancient world. Ancient Egyptian medicine, for example, appears to have been a combination of clinical observation intertwined with the rich mysticism and religion of Egypt. The medical papyri, on the one hand, make specific reference to benign and malign influences that entered the body from the outside or, as written in the Ebers Papyrus: "the breath of life enters into the right ear and the breath of death enters into the left ear." The Egyptians also believed in disease "demons" that needed to be appeased by healers or priest-magicians in order to cure the patient, often using a variety of incantations. Pestilence was thought to be an infliction brought by Sekhmet, the Egyptian goddess of plagues and the protection thereof.

On the other hand, the papyri also show that there was an empirical component to medicine alongside its magico-religious bent, describing numerous herbal and other natural remedies that might be prescribed by a physician or "*swnw*." One prescribed remedy, a rejuvenating potion, was based on an oil from bitter almonds:

> *Annoint a man with it. It is something that repels a cold from the head. If the body is wiped with it, what results is rejuvenation of the skin and repelling of wrinkles, any age spots, any sign of old age, and any fever that may be in the body. (Proved) good a million times.*

Good health was associated with clean and correct living, being at peace with the gods, spirits, and the dead. Being "prepared" for the afterlife in every sense—morally, spiritually, and physically (as in mummification)—was also important to the Egyptians.

In early Eastern civilizations, such as those of the Indian subcontinent and China, ideas about supernatural and demonic forces as causes of death came to coexist within a more systematized approach to medicine relating disease to the "balance" of vital forces inside the body. "Blocked flows" along meridians or energy pathways resulted in disease. Bound up with spiritual beliefs as well as rooted in ancient Eastern philosophies, these complex medical systems are holistic and see the body, mind, and spirit as one, governed by flowing and balanced energies.

Two ancient Indian treatises, the *Caraka Samhitā* and *Sushruta Samhita*, were written more than two thousand years ago and Ayurveda (from the Sanskrit words for "life" and "knowledge," *āyus* and *veda*) is one of the oldest surviving continuing medical systems. In China, the *Huangdi Neijing* (or the Yellow Emperor's Inner Canon) was a fundamental source of Chinese medicine for some two millennia and continues to be studied today by practitioners of Traditional Chinese Medicine (TCM). Chinese medicine reached Japan between the 6th and the 9th centuries, mainly via the Korean Peninsula, and was developed in Japan as Kampo ("the way of the Chinese"). Prayer and respect for the gods, as, for example, Dhanvantari, the god of Ayurvedic medicine, remains an important part of Eastern medicine.

OPPOSITE The channels of the body according to Chinese medicine in an illustration from the Kangxi reign (1662–1722) of the Qing dynasty. This incorporated the principle of *yin-yang* balance, the concept of *qi* and the practice of acupuncture —to preserve or restore a healthy balance.

Blood, bile, and the humoral doctrine of "dis-ease"

The humoral theory of disease is, perhaps, one of the best known of the ancient doctrines in the West. It is most closely associated with the Greek physician Hippocrates (c.460 BC–c.375/370 BC), and the later Greco-Roman physician Galen (AD 129–c.210). Hippocrates is often known as the "Father of Western Medicine" and his compendium of sixty to seventy written works—the output of a number of scholars—is known as the Hippocratic Corpus. This contains a wealth of influential information about medical practice and beliefs in ancient Greece. There were various competing interpretations of the causes of disease but through Galen's influence the humoral theory (as well as his ideas on anatomy, see page 28) dominated late antiquity and early medieval thought.

At its simplest, the humoral doctrine of disease was based on the idea that the body was made up of four "humors" or fluids: black bile, yellow bile, phlegm, and blood. If the humors became unbalanced, disease, or "dis-ease" (humoral disequilibrium), resulted. A perfect balance was always under threat from variations in climate, seasons, diet, and lifestyle. Too much or too little of one or more of the humors was not good news.

The physician would look for signs in bodily fluids and features as indicators of imbalanced humors: a flushed face might signal fever; a runny nose a sign of winter colds; discolored or bloody urine or stools were explained in terms of imbalances. The Hippocratics also emphasized that diseases were not influenced by supernatural forces but by natural causes. This can be read at the beginning of a treatise on epilepsy called *On The Sacred Disease* (5th century BC):

> *It is thus with regard to the disease called Sacred: it appears to me to be nowise more divine nor more sacred than other diseases, but has a natural cause from which it originates like other affections.*

Nature, too, thus had a way of redressing balance. One of the Hippocratic aphorisms was: "Natural forces are the healers of disease." Diarrhea, vomiting, urinating, and sweating were natural ways of evacuating and expelling any excess humor.

The best and most "natural" way to achieve health and prevent imbalance of the humors was to follow a moderate regimen. Therapies were aimed at restoring the balance of disease and identifying the specific needs of the individual patient. The Greek concept of *diaita* (or daily way of life) encompassed everything needed to take care of an individual and was concerned with the enhancement of the quality of life as well as disease prevention. However, if nature or a balanced lifestyle did not restore a patient's health, other more drastic interventions might be needed. In the case of blood—too much blood, too little blood, or just bad blood—bloodletting was seen as the most appropriate course of action to get rid of any corrupt humor (see Bloodletting and Purging).

While stressing and observing humoral imbalances and natural causes of disease, the Greeks and Romans, additionally, put their faith in religion—again, an important reflection of the overlapping or intertwining roles of the secular and the divine in healing. Illness, as a result of imbalance, could be restored by being at peace with the gods. The Greeks worshipped Asclepius and his daughters Hygieia (goddess of health, cleanliness, and sanitation); Panacea (universal remedy); Iaso (recuperation from illness); Aceso (healing process); and Aglæa (beauty and splendor). The sick went to temples of Asclepius—at Epidaurus, Cos, and Athens —for a healing ritual or "incubation cures."

Egyptian medical papyri

Ancient Egyptian books were rolls of papyrus made from the pith of the native wild papyrus plant. These were first manufactured in Egypt as far back as the 3rd millennium BC, and twelve principal medical papyri still exist today. They detail disease, diagnosis, and remedies, which include herbal remedies, surgery, and magical spells. The Ebers Papyrus was discovered in a tomb in Thebes in 1862 and purchased at Luxor (Thebes) by German Egyptologist Georg Ebers (1837–98), in 1872/3.

The copy of this text was written in c.1500/1550 BC but is believed to have incorporated content from over 1,000 years earlier. It is currently in the University of Leipzig library, Germany. The Edwin Smith Surgical Papyrus (c.1600 BC and the oldest known surgical treatise on trauma) was purchased

from a merchant in Luxor in 1862 by American Egyptologist Edwin Smith (1822–1906), and is now in the New York Academy of Medicine.

Other medical evidence for disease in ancient Egypt comes from paleopathological studies of mummies, art, and hieroglyphic carvings in tombs. Using noninvasive technology to "look inside" mummies, scientists have found evidence, for example, that schistosomiasis, a parasitic-worm disease, has existed continuously in Egypt for at least 5,000 years.

ABOVE A reproduction of the Ebers Papyrus, one of the oldest extant medical books in the world. Egyptian physicians thought disease arose not only from supernatural causes but also from an imbalance in a physical substance, *wekhdw*, produced by internal body processes—analogous to the Greek notion of humors.

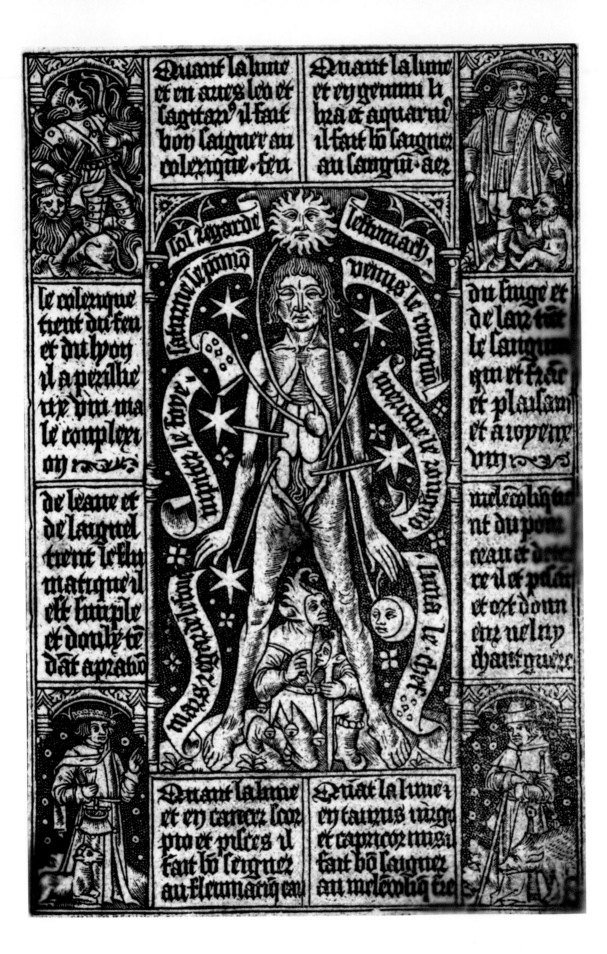

Greek and Roman medicine reaches medieval Islam and Europe

Following the Fall of Rome, few in the West had access to the numerous written works of these ancient authorities. However, many of the ancient Greek and Roman manuscripts found their way to the Byzantine (Eastern Roman) Empire, the capital of which was Constantinople, now Istanbul. More significantly, from the mid-8th century onward they were translated into Arabic.

In a period stretching over five hundred years, Arab and Persian, Muslim, Christian, and Jewish scientists, physicians, and philosophers in the medieval Arabic-speaking regions helped develop a scientific understanding of the world. The expansion of Islam, combined with extensive networks of trade and exchange between the Middle East, the Near East, India, and the Far East, led to spices and silk, ideas and innovations (such as paper from China), texts and traditions being widely disseminated.

Many centers of Arabic science flourished at this time. Baghdad (now the capital of Iraq) became the greatest intellectual center of its time, attracting scholars from all over the Islamic Empire. Between the mid-8th and early 10th centuries, translators of Greek, Persian, and Indian-Sanskrit texts proliferated. The translations of these works into Syriac and Arabic by the physician Hunayn ibn Ishāq (*c.*809–73) in the 9th century were said to be worth their weight in gold. He became known as the "Sheikh of translators." It is the medical work of Galen that is his most important legacy, for not only did it open up the Islamic world to ancient Greek and Roman medicine, but it is through the Arabic translations that much of Galen's work reaches us today.

Adopting and assimilating these translated texts into Islamic medicine, most Arabic-speaking physicians venerated Hippocratic and Galenic ideas, including humoralism. They also wrote their own major works. *The Comprehensive Book of Medicine* by Muhammad ibn Zakariya al-Razi (*c.*865–*c.*925) and *The Canon of Medicine* by Ibn Sina (980–1037) are two of the most comprehensive and best-known Arabic treatises of learned medicine. Razi (known in the West as Rhazes), Ibn Sina (or Avicenna), and others pioneered many areas of medical science. Razi was the first to describe smallpox and measles as distinct diseases. He even challenged the Greek notion of the four humors in his book *Doubts About Galen*. However, this was not followed up and the humoral theory was subsequently brought back into medicine and remained fundamental to Ibn Sina, whose influence on medical teaching and practice lasted for over half a millennium.

By the early 11th century, the Middle-Eastern translations of the Greek Hippocratic-Galenic works and the classic Arabic texts were being translated again, this time into Latin, by medical scholars and schools in Western Europe.

While the Greek texts made their way back to Europe, their Arabic translations were disseminated across South Asia, following the Muslim domination of the Indian subcontinent from the 12th century onward. One of the last surviving legacies of the Hippocratic "humoral" heritage is Unani Tibb (Greek Medicine), still practiced in India, Pakistan, and Bangladesh.

OPPOSITE A 15th-century woodcut illustrating the four humoral temperaments (choleric, sanguine, phlegmatic, and melancholic). In line with the humoral theory, Greek and Roman physicians held that cancer was the result of an excess of black bile. By the medieval period, temperament also became associated with the humors.

Plagues and pestilence

Epidemics of every kind would periodically sweep across wide areas of the world affecting and killing many people, while leaving others unscathed. The Hippocratic works included a book on *Epidemics* but it was hard to fit these widespread and deadly scourges, such as the "Plague of Athens" in 430–427 BC (its cause much debated, but now thought to have been typhoid), into any humoral theory. Why did so many die during these pestilential outbreaks? Why and how did others survive?

A major epidemic of "plague" (possibly the first epidemic of bubonic plague) occurred in AD 541–4 during the reign of the Byzantine Emperor Justinian. Spreading from Egypt to Europe, the "Plague of Justinian" killed, at its peak, up to 5,000 people a day in Constantinople and spread like wildfire through coastal ports and towns. This epidemic, together with further onslaughts throughout the 6th to 8th centuries, was identified by swollen buboes in the groins, armpits, or necks of its victims and may have killed as many as 25 million people overall. Writers of the time, such as the Byzantine historian Procopius of Caesarea (AD *c*.500–565) in his *History of the Wars*, were at a loss to know how to explain this terrible pestilence:

> *It is quite impossible either to express in words or conceive in thought any explanation, except indeed to refer it to God. For it did not come in a part of the world nor upon certain men, nor did it confine itself to any season of the year, so that from such circumstances it might be possible to find subtle explanations of a cause, but it embraced the entire world, and blighted the lives of all men ... For much as men differ with regard to places in which they live, or the law of their daily life, or in natural bent, or in active pursuits, or in whatever else differs from man, in the case of this disease alone naught prevailed.*

Similar sentiments were expressed, again, during the Black Death (as it was later known) of 1347–53, which is estimated to have wiped out between one-quarter and one-half of the population of Europe. It spread via the Silk Road from the Steppes of Central Asia to Europe, the Middle East and the northern shores of Africa. It was as frightening as it was puzzling. The Italian poet Petrarch (1304–74) lost his beloved Laura to the plague in Avignon, France, in 1348, and grieved:

> *Where are our dear friends now? Where are the beloved faces? Where are the affectionate words, the relaxed and enjoyable conversations? What lightning bolt devoured them? What earthquake toppled them? What tempest drowned them? What abyss swallowed them? There was a crowd of us, now we are almost alone.*

Mass graves "stacked high with putrefying corpses in which the layers of corpses were separated with sprinklings of dirt" were grimly likened by one Italian writer to "cheese between layers of lasagna."

Many explanations were put forward for the plague epidemics, including God's reaction to the sins of humanity or some ominous configuration of stars and planets. Giovanni Boccaccio (1313–75), writing in *The Decameron,* described the Black Death as "a deadly pestilence, which, [came] either because of the operations of the heavenly bodies, or because of the just wrath of God mandating punishment for our iniquitous ways." The Saints Cosmas, Damian, Sebastian, and Roch were traditionally invoked in the Christian world for protection from the plague. As plague continued to rage in the centuries following the Black Death, citizens and the clergy even

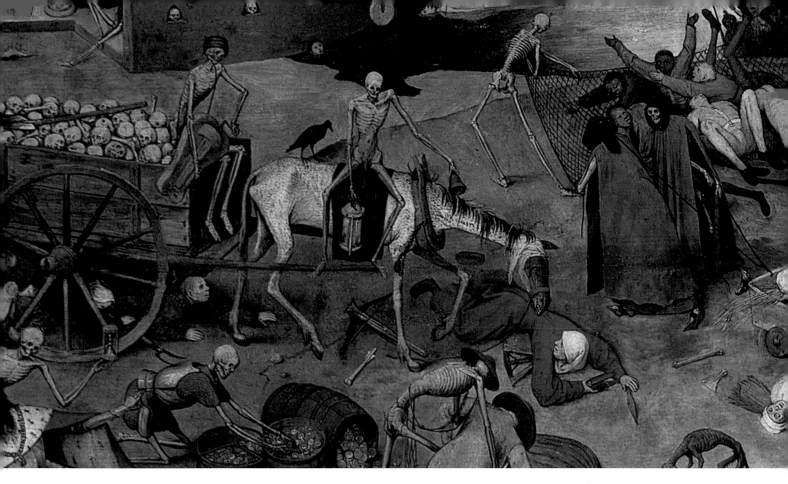

The Triumph of Death (detail) by Pieter Brueghel the Elder, *c.*1562, shows an army of skeletons wreaking havoc across a desolate landscape. It reflects the ever-present threat of death in medieval Europe brought on by the Black Death and subsequent plague epidemics.

built churches in the hope of appeasing the Almighty's wrath. In Venice, the Redentore Church, designed by the architect Andrea Palladio (1508–80), was built as a votive church following the 1575–6 plague, when up to a third of the population of Venice died. The *Festa del Redentore*, on the third Sunday of July each year, still celebrates Venice's deliverance from the plague.

Focusing on sin as the ultimate cause of plague, the London clergyman Thomas White (*c.*1550–1624) claimed that theaters were a corrupting influence and argued that: "the cause of plagues is sin, if you look to it well, and the cause of sin is plays: therefore the cause of plagues are plays." Some people, known as flagellants, took penance to extremes, flogging themselves or one another with knotted strips of leather or iron spikes. Yet more horrific was the mass torture and murder of thousands of Jews and others in Europe accused of poisoning wells and spreading disease.

There were also down-to-earth explanations of the plague: earthquakes, unusual weather and, above all, the rot and decay of garbage accumulating in streets and dungheaps, emitting foul miasmas that poisoned the air. The filthy channel of the Fleet Ditch in London was described as "a nauceious and abominable sink of nastiness" into which the tripe dressers, sausagemakers, and catgut spinners flung their variety meat. In 1580, Nicholas Woodroffe in London ordered that the streets be cleansed and the kennels (street gutters) run "for the avoydinge of the infection of the plague and the loathsome stinkes and savours that are in the severall streets of this cyttie." Overcrowded houses, prisons, pest hospitals—the congested places of the poor, sick, and institutionalized—were often viewed as "places of a thousand stinks."

Precautions against the risk of contagion carried both a religious and secular purpose. The words "Lord have mercy upon us" and red crosses marked the doors of those shut up because of the plague ...

Then there were the people themselves: whether sinful, smelly, or sickly, humans were somehow thought to be bound up with the pestilential corruption of the world, and also capable of spreading sickness by contagious vapors from breath, buboes, or clothes. Attempts were made to prevent and protect oneself from the plague, mirroring the multicausal ideas of what caused the disease. Individuals sought to save themselves by various means including smoking tobacco, sitting under a foul-smelling latrine, or sniffing roses.

During the Great Plague of London of 1665–6, Samuel Pepys (1633–1703), the famous English diarist and Fellow of the newly founded Royal Society of London for Improving Natural Knowledge, was "put into an ill conception of myself and my smell" and felt "forced to buy some roll tobacco to smell and chaw—which took away the apprehension"; tobacco was regarded as a way of preventing infection. Perfumes, along with prayers, wafted through the churches. Daniel Defoe, in his 1722 account of the Great Plague of London, described the churches, filled with the grieving, sick, and penitent, as "like a smelling bottle; in one corner it was all perfumes; in another, aromatics, balsamics, and a variety of drugs and herbs." Viper fat, spider's webs, toad poison, woodlice, and crabs' eyes were just a few of the various antidotes offered for sale.

The wealthy and, even, the elite physicians often fled from plague-infected areas, while those employed as "plague doctors" wore protective garments and carried aromatic herbs in their "beaks" along with fumigating torches, protecting themselves from infection and foul smells. Authorities ordered both the cleaning up of foul-smelling dungheaps and the killing of cats, dogs, hogs, and pigeons—as well as putting into quarantine the infected and those who had had contact with victims. Precautions against the risk of contagion carried both a religious and secular purpose. The words "Lord have mercy upon us" and red crosses marked the doors of those shut up because of the plague in cities like London. The use of quarantine (from the Italian *quaranti giorni*, forty days) to prevent contagious diseases from spreading dates back to the 14th century. The Italian states imposed stringent quarantine regulations during times of plague, and other countries soon followed suit.

A bacterium, *Yersinia pestis*, which spread from infected black rats, via fleas, to humans, was eventually identified in the late 19th and early 20th centuries as the cause of bubonic plague. However, medical historians are still debating whether or not some past plagues, such as the Black Death, were rat-flea-borne.

Contagious poxes and fevers

One of the theories to account for the mysterious plagues of the medieval and early modern world was the idea of contagion (from the Latin *contingere* meaning "to touch closely"). Leprosy (Hansen's disease), prevalent in Europe between the 11th and 14th centuries, was also thought to be contagious, leading to "Leper houses" being set up to isolate and care for sufferers.

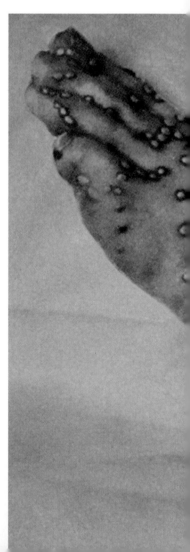

The concept of contagion gained particular momentum when, shortly after the opening up of the "New World," Europeans in the late 15th century were struck by a deadly "pox," later called the Great Pox or syphilis. Whether or not syphilis came from the New World to the Old is still much debated but, whatever its route, it caused terrible symptoms for those who contracted it. One of its sufferers, the German scholar Ulrich von Hutten (1488–1523), wrote:

> The [physician] cared not even to behold it ... for truly when it first begun, it was so horrible to behold. They had boils that stood out like acorns, from whence issued such filthy stinking matter, that whosoever came within the scent, believed himself infected.

It did not take long, however, for a connection to be made between the spread of the disease and sexual encounters. Indeed, syphilis (as well as gonorrhea) became known as venereal diseases (VD)—from Venus, the Roman Goddess of Love. The Italian physician Girolamo Fracastoro (c.1476/8–1553) first named syphilis in 1530 and described it in his 1546 treatise *De contagione et contagiosis morbus et eorum curatione* ("On contagion, contagious diseases and their cure").

Smallpox and measles spread rapidly along trade routes and, as formerly isolated countries and "new worlds" were discovered and opened up to outsiders, they could have devastating consequences. The sparsely populated Japanese archipelago had remained relatively free of

An early stage of smallpox with pustules on the leg and foot (*c.* 1908). Known as the "speckled monster," smallpox appeared to be spread by immediate contact with a sufferer of the disease, killing princes and peasants alike.

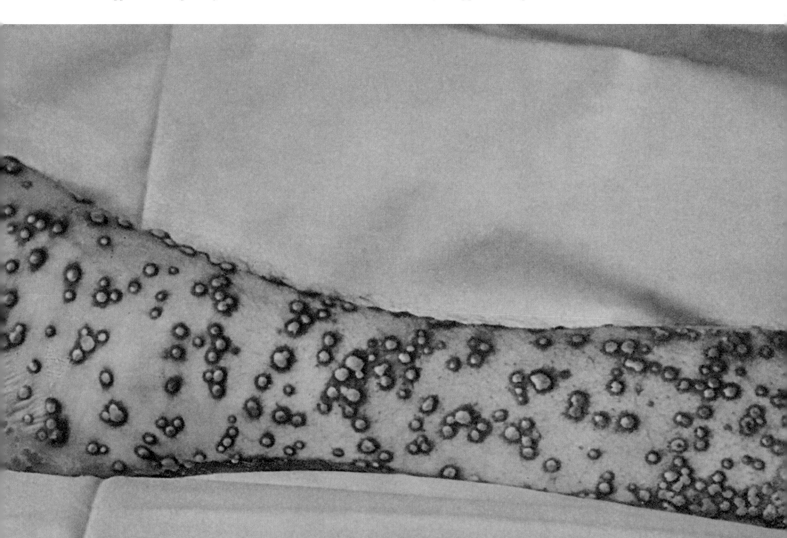

major epidemics in the early centuries. But as cultural and trading links increased from the 6th century AD between China (where smallpox was already established) and Japan, smallpox began to take its toll. A major epidemic devastated Japan's first city, Nara, in the early 8th century. Thereafter, smallpox, as well as measles epidemics, broke out every few years. These two diseases were probably partly responsible for the near annihilation of Native Americans when sailors from Europe discovered the "New World" in the late 15th century and spread these and other infectious diseases to indigenous peoples who had not previously encountered them, and so had no immunity to them.

From the late 18th century, these diseases reached Australia and New Zealand, with deadly consequences for the indigenous populations. A century later, some island communities such as the Faroe Islands, Hawaii, and Fiji suffered devastating epidemics following the introduction of smallpox or measles. These epidemics, like others, were dramatic, and suggested that some contagious agent was responsible.

Astrology—the influence of the stars

Samuel Jeake (1652–99), an English merchant, suffered from fevers and agues, and depression. His *Diary of the Actions and Accidents of my Life* detailed the symptoms and timing of his illnesses. He noted the precise timing of his cold and hot sweats and tried to link them to astrological phenomena, though Jeake recognized that there was no single explanation for his illnesses.

The idea of the stars, or heavenly bodies, influencing disease led to the naming of influenza (from the Italian word and its Latin equivalent, *influentia coeli*, meaning "heavenly influence"). Thomas Willis, describing an epidemic in 1658, said it was as if "it was sent by some blast of the stars, which laid hold on very many together, that in some towns, in the space of a week above a thousand people fell sick of it."

These widespread and spasmodic episodes of influenza were immensely puzzling. Today, we see influenza pandemics resulting from global travel or infectious migrant birds, as in the avian "bird" flu pandemic of 1997 and onward.

Astrological influences, specifically the pull of the moon, were thought to play a part in mental illness, hence the root of the old words "lunacy" and "lunatic" from the Latin *luna* or moon.

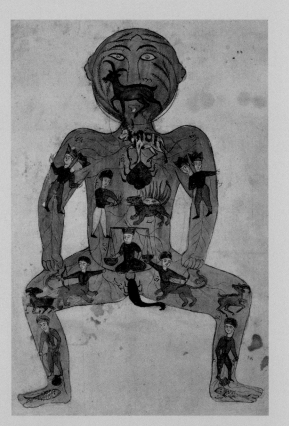

This 19th-century figure made after a Persian source shows a "Zodiac" or "Astrological" man. In medieval times the signs of the zodiac were seen to control specific groups of the body parts and functions. Aries, for example, was associated with the head and eyes, while Scorpio was linked to the rectum, bladder, pelvis, and reproductive organs.

An interesting reflection of the early ideas about the infectious nature of smallpox led to the empirically based preventive practice of smallpox inoculation and in the late 18th century Edward Jenner's cowpox vaccination (see Vaccination and Preventive Medicine). Long before there was any scientific understanding of the causes of smallpox, it was recognized that by deliberately giving a healthy patient a mild dose of smallpox or cowpox, they would be less likely to catch the full-blown disease from an infected patient.

Yellow fever was another terrifying disease that spread along trading routes, especially via slave ships from the mid-17th century. From Africa, it was carried to the Caribbean and the Americas and, occasionally, to Europe. It proved a lasting threat to the eastern seaboard of North America and some towns, such as Charleston and Philadelphia, lost many lives to the disease. Quarantine measures were frequently imposed. Affected ships were obliged to carry a "Yellow Jack" flag and to wait for 40 days before anyone was allowed to disembark. The flag became such a distinctive emblem that it was often used as a nickname for the disease itself.

Swamp fevers: miasmas and mal'aria

As usual, the atmosphere has proved a complete malaria to me. How, indeed should it be otherwise, when it is a compound of fen-fog, chimney-smoke, smuts, and pulverized horse dung! The little leisure I have is employed in blowing my nose, with interludes of coughing.

Robert Southey (1774–1843), *Letter from England*, 1808

Airs, Waters, and Places, a 5th-century BC Hippocratic work, warned about the dangers of living in swampy places—and they were indeed dangerous. As physicians in later centuries began to ask why, they became increasingly convinced that noxious, odorous smells and stenches —or "miasmas" (from the Greek *miainein*, meaning "to pollute")—emanating from marshy areas were the direct cause of deadly fevers. These were variously known as swamp fevers, Roman fevers, agues, or the shakes. The Italian Pontine marshes near Rome were notoriously unhealthy, as were the English marshes. The writer Daniel Defoe (*c.*1659/61–1731) in his tour through "the whole island of Great Britain" was very glad when he got out of the East Anglian Fen country for "tis a horrid air for a stranger to breathe in." In England, even the clergy pleaded with their bishops to be excused from living in marsh or Fenland parishes, as summed up by one 18th-century vicar:

> *The Thames having a very foul shore in this parish which is inclosed within land by many salt marshes I soon found myself attacked by so many repeated agues that my physician ... told me I must not ... reside there.*

As European explorers and others began to travel to tropical regions, notably the west coast, rivers, and interior of Africa, many were struck down by fevers in these torrid zones, reinforcing the role of environmental and atmospheric causation. The west coast of Africa became known as "White Man's Grave."

The word "mal'aria" (from the Italian *mala aria*, meaning "bad air") was adapted into the English language in 1740 by Horace Walpole (1717–97). While traveling in Italy, he wrote home: "there is a horrid thing called the mal'aria, that comes to Rome every summer and kills one." In 1827 John MacCulloch (1773–1835) wrote an influential book, *Malaria: An essay on the production and propagation of this poison and on the nature and localities of the places by which it is produced*. He set out to show that any number of diseases, in all sorts of poisonous localities —from swamps to slaughterhouses, prisons, sewers, ships' bilges—were caused by "malaria." He noted: "this is the unseen, and still unknown, poison to which Italy applied the term that I have borrowed, Malaria. This is the cause of fevers, both ordinary and intermitting."

The puzzle of malaria was still being debated at the outset of the American Civil War in 1861 when the newly founded journal *Scientific American* highlighted its threat to soldiers but added: "What malaria is nobody knows ... there is no doubt, however, that malaria is some mysterious poison in the atmosphere, and that it is confined strictly to certain localities."

Over the centuries, some astute observers made a tenuous connection between mosquitoes, swamps, and fevers but it was not until the later 19th century that the pieces of the puzzle were finally solved and the disease, which we now call malaria, was shown to be transmitted by the bite of a female mosquito (see page 178).

Evil airs and tuberculosis

Another ancient disease, pulmonary tuberculosis, was known by a number of names including "phthisis" (meaning "dwindling" or "wasting away") and consumption. The Greeks and Romans put it down to "evil airs," while, centuries later, the English preacher John Bunyan (1628–88) reminds us of its seriousness in his book *The Life and Death of Mr Badman* (1680):

> He was dropsical, he was consumptive, he was surfeited, was gouty, and, as some say, he had a tang of the pox in his bowels. Yet the captain of all these men of death that came against him to take him away, was the consumption, for it was that that brought him down to the grave.

As towns and cities grew rapidly over the course of the 18th and 19th centuries, many generated squalid slums, and tuberculosis (TB) soon became one of the most painful chronic illnesses of all time. Its victims (often depicted in art, literature, and opera) seemed to be literally "consumed" by the disease, becoming pale and emaciated. Its cause was much debated, with one explanation being that the individual's constitution affected the severity and final outcome of the disease. Even the "sorrowful passions of young lovers" was mooted as a cause. Increasingly, TB became associated with squalor and poverty, as it seemed to be most prevalent among those who lived and worked in overcrowded, damp, or dusty conditions.

For those who could afford the time or money, a change of air was recommended by physicians. When the English poet John Keats (1795–1821) coughed up blood he wrote "that drop of blood is my death warrant. I must die." He duly left his home in London and sought refuge in Rome. But for Keats, it was already too late: he died from TB in Rome in 1821, aged 25. His apartment, which can still be visited at the foot of the Spanish Steps, was fumigated and his furniture burned in the hope that this would destroy whatever it was that caused this mysterious, deadly infection. When, in the 1880s, pulmonary tuberculosis (one of several forms of TB) was found to be caused by an airborne bacterial infection, institutionalized sanatoria (see Hospitals and Nursing Care) proliferated, isolating patients with diseased lungs in healthy airs.

> The cause of tuberculosis was much debated ... Even the "sorrowful passions of young lovers" was mooted as a cause.

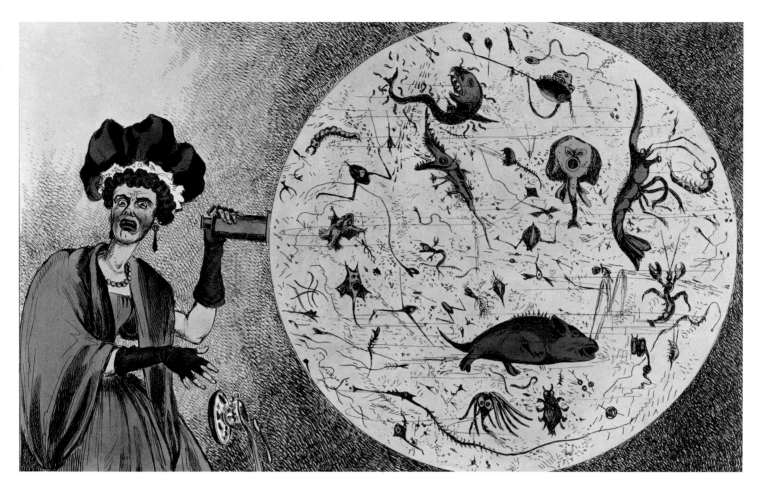

The impurity of London water was renowned throughout the 18th and 19th centuries. In this 1828 colored etching by W Heath, entitled *Monster Soup Commonly Called Thames Water*, a lady drops her teacup in horror upon discovering the monstrous contents of a magnified drop of Thames drinking water.

Epidemics of cholera—the "contagionists" versus the "miasmatists"

One of the greatest epidemiological shocks to the West in the 19th century was the arrival of cholera (Greek *cholē*, meaning "bile" and *rhein*, "to flow"). The first Asiatic cholera pandemic to reach Europe from its heartland in the Ganges Delta in the Indian subcontinent was in 1831–2. The disease was characterized by appalling symptoms—violent vomiting and uncontrollable diarrhea with the presence of profuse "rice water" stools—invariably followed quickly by rapid dehydration and death. In the 1830s the disease struck Moscow, Hamburg, Sunderland, London, Paris, Quebec, and New York City—putting Asiatic cholera well and truly on the world map.

Carrying a mortality rate of at least 50 percent, and conveyed unwittingly over land and sea by travelers, from soldiers and pilgrims to traders and refugees, each pandemic (lasting from five to thirty years) followed different trajectories. Cholera affected young and old, rich and poor, but its striking epidemiological characteristic was its devastating impact on centers of pilgrimage such as the Ganges and Mecca, and on the stinking slums of the rapidly expanding industrial towns of Europe and America.

Opposing views as to the likely cause led to varying approaches of prevention. "Miasmatists" (also known as anticontagionists) thought cholera should belong to a group of "filth diseases," which included typhoid and typhus. Their answer was to clean up the insanitary mess of the industrialized towns, cities, and slums. Quarantine was proposed by the "contagionists," who feared it was transmitted by a poison passed from person to person, but quarantine was seen as posing a threat to the commercial activities of the industrializing nations, and sanitary conferences were set up to debate the question.

Edwin Chadwick (1800–90), an English lawyer by training, was one of the most vocal of all the miasmatists and became a leading figure in the public health movement. He was the author of a key text, *Report of an Inquiry on the Sanitary Conditions of the Labouring Population of Great Britain* (1842) and captured succinctly the miasmatists' viewpoint that "all smell is disease!":

> *All smell is, if it be intense, immediate acute disease; and eventually we may say that, by depressing the system and rendering it susceptible to the action of other causes, all smell is disease.*

William Farr (1807–83), the English medical statistician, said that lethal miasmas were like a mad dog prowling forth from the city's cesspools. Chadwick, Farr, and others in Europe and the USA, including Bostonian Lemuel Shattuck (1793–1859), amplified their arguments with "sanitary" or "effluvia" maps and vital statistics that showed a direct correlation between the filthiest, most overcrowded or poorest parts of the cities and the highest mortality rates. Awareness of these links was high as an appeal reported in *The Times* of London in 1849, indicates:

> *Sur …We live in filth and muck. We aint got no priviz, no dust bins, no drains, no water-splies, and no drain or suer in the hole place. The Suer Company, in Greek Street, Soho Square, all great, rich powerfool men take no notice watsomdever of our complaints. The Stenche of a Gulley-hole is disgustin. We all of us suffer, and numbers are ill, and if the Cholera comes Lord help us.*

The contagionists, the miasmatists, those on the fence, and those who "blamed" the poor, continued to debate their cause against a background of increasingly worrying times. In 1853, as the third great cholera pandemic was making its way across Europe toward Britain, the editor of the medical journal *The Lancet* expressed bewilderment as to the nature of the disease:

> *What is cholera? Is it a fungus, an insect, a miasma, an electrical disturbance, a deficiency of ozone, a morbid off-scouring of the intestinal canal? We know nothing; we are at sea in a whirlpool of conjecture … Every analogy leads to the conclusion that the essential cause of cholera consists in a morbid poison, which under certain congenial conditions becomes developed into activity, and ferments in the blood.*

As the debate rumbled on, a London doctor, John Snow (1813–58), came up with an answer that challenged the various confusing viewpoints. Following what can only be described as brilliant medical detective work, by 1854 Snow became convinced that it was something in the water that caused cholera.

Snow's "ghost map"

The story of John Snow and the disabling of the Broad Street pump to prevent further outbreaks of cholera is legendary. During an oppressively hot August in 1854, the baby daughter of Thomas and Sarah Lewis of No. 40, Broad Street, Soho—in the Golden Square area of London—fell ill with vomiting and green watery stools that emitted "a pungent smell". Sarah, desperately trying to cope with her baby's soiled diapers, washed them in a bucket and threw some of the water into a cesspool in the basement at the front of their house. The next day their upstairs neighbors fell ill, and a few days later whole families in the surrounding area began to sicken—often dying together in their dark, squalid rooms. Within ten days, 500 locals were dead—10 percent of the area's population.

John Snow, then a local practitioner, had already been convinced that cholera might be caused by swallowing "some as-yet-unidentified" infective particle in sewage-contaminated water and had published the first account of his waterborne theory in 1849. As the 1854 epidemic raged in

> Within ten days, 500 local residents were dead—10 percent of the area's population.

the Soho district, Snow inspected with meticulous detail the drinking habits of the victims of the outbreak. He noted that most of those who caught cholera were drawing their drinking water from the Broad Street pump—which was right outside No. 40 Broad Street. In a nearby workhouse and brewery, both of which had their own private water supplies, there were almost no casualties. On September 7 1854, two weeks after the local outbreak began, Snow persuaded the authorities to remove the handle of the Broad Street pump. Cholera abated. In the fall of 1854 Snow produced a "ghost map" of cholera deaths and the location of water pumps in the Golden Square area of London. This correlation of water sources and disease was not immediately appreciated, and by the time the pump had been disabled, the worst had passed.

Snow died before his hunch could be proven. In 1858, the year of his death, London experienced a long hot summer, but also the so-called "Great Stink." During that summer the stench of untreated sewage floating in the River Thames was so horrendous that it became almost impossible for members of the House of Commons to conduct their business. The windows were draped with drapes soaked in chloride of lime. But even that was not enough. Politicians choked and retched and threatened to leave London. It was, moreover, generally believed that the very smell itself was the cause of the deadly fevers that frequently plagued the city. The Great Stink would, it was feared, lead to further outbreaks of pestilence. One writer at the time remarked: "stench so foul, we may well believe, has never before ascended to pollute this lower air. Never before, at least, had a stink risen to the height of an historic event." Ironically, when the British physician William Budd (1811–80), having been intrigued by dire predictions that the overpowering stench would lead to a huge rise in mortality, later examined the reports for sickness and death in the years 1858–9, he noted:

> Strange to relate, the results showed, not only a death-rate below the average, but ... a remarkable diminution in the prevalence of fever, diarrhoea, and the other forms of disease commonly ascribed to putrid exhalations.

Snow's waterborne theory was later proved to be correct by Robert Koch (1843–1910), who, in 1883–4, identified the "cholera bacillus" (a bacterial infection) in drinking water, and in stools and intestines of infected patients. By this stage, huge efforts were already underway to build new underground sewer systems and improve public health. The Victorian engineer Joseph Bazalgette (1819–91), who was instrumental in revolutionizing London's sewerage system from the 1860–70s following the Great Stink, has been credited with saving more lives than any other 19th-century public official. Like Jenner with his smallpox vaccine, such extraordinary feats showed what could be done to prevent disease even before scientists had unraveled their mysterious causes.

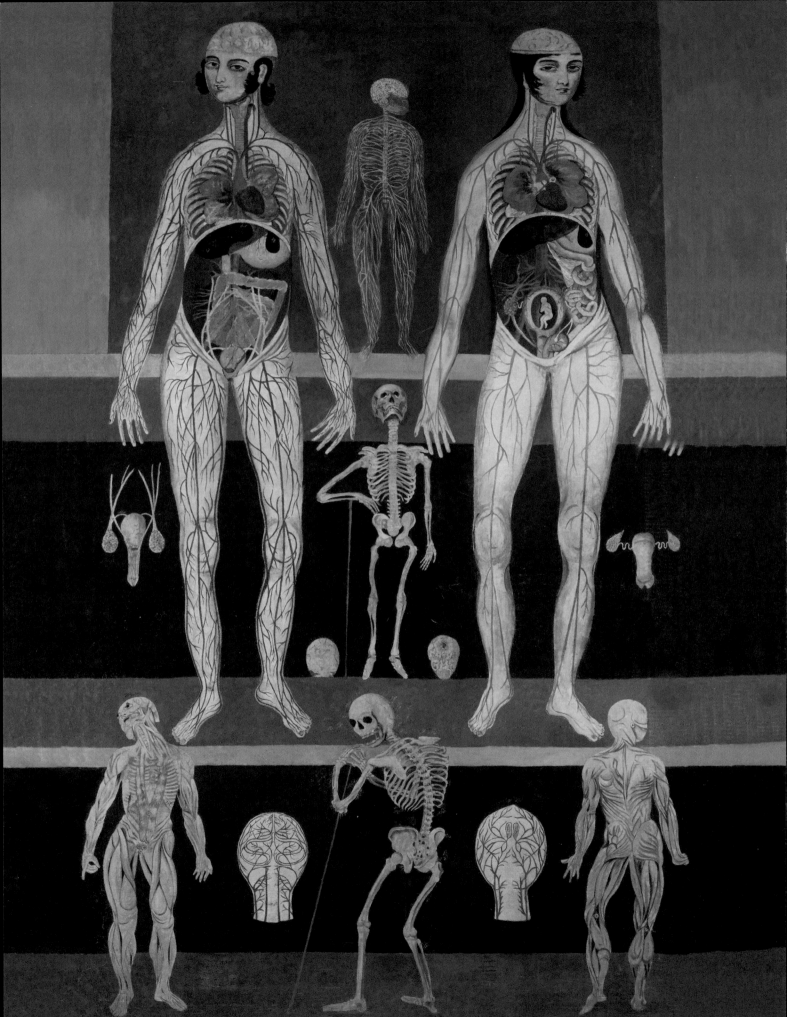

Bones and Bodies

The inner parts … are for the most part unknown; at least, those of man are, and hence we have to refer to those of other animals, the natural structure of whose parts those of man resemble, and examine them.

Aristotle (384–322 BC)

While physicians and scientists debated the role of mysterious disease-causing humors and miasmas, they also began to investigate the inner structures of the body. Galen based most of his anatomical investigations on animals but it was Andreas Vesalius who in the 16th century transformed our understanding of the human body through his dissections of executed criminals. This practice expanded over the centuries, leading to many scientific and medical discoveries, including William Harvey's discovery of the circulation of the blood. From the 18th century, important insights about pathological changes in the human body were also made through postmortem examinations. Surgery benefited hugely from anatomical studies, but stories of the notorious "body snatchers" in the 18th and early 19th centuries are chilling reminders of the more gruesome side of some of these endeavors. Knowledge of the role and function of both abnormal and normal organs, tissues, and cells was developed in the 19th century, especially by Rudolf Virchow—often known as "Hippocrates with a microscope."

Opening up the body: the first dissections

The ancient Greeks and Romans forbade human dissection on religious grounds. This was largely out of respect for the dead and the, then popular, belief that dead human bodies still had some "awareness" and therefore retained an absolute right to be buried intact. The word "dissection" is from the Latin *dissecare*, "to cut apart," while "anatomy" is an almost direct borrowing of the Greek *anatomē,* a compound of *ana-*, "up or through" and *tomē,* "a cutting." There was one brief period in Hellenic Alexandria, Egypt, in the 4th to 3rd centuries BC, when

OPPOSITE A 19th-century Persian anatomical study. Medical illustration remained important to the study of anatomy through the 19th century, and many books, including Henry Gray's *Anatomy of the Human Body,* contained large numbers of detailed drawings.

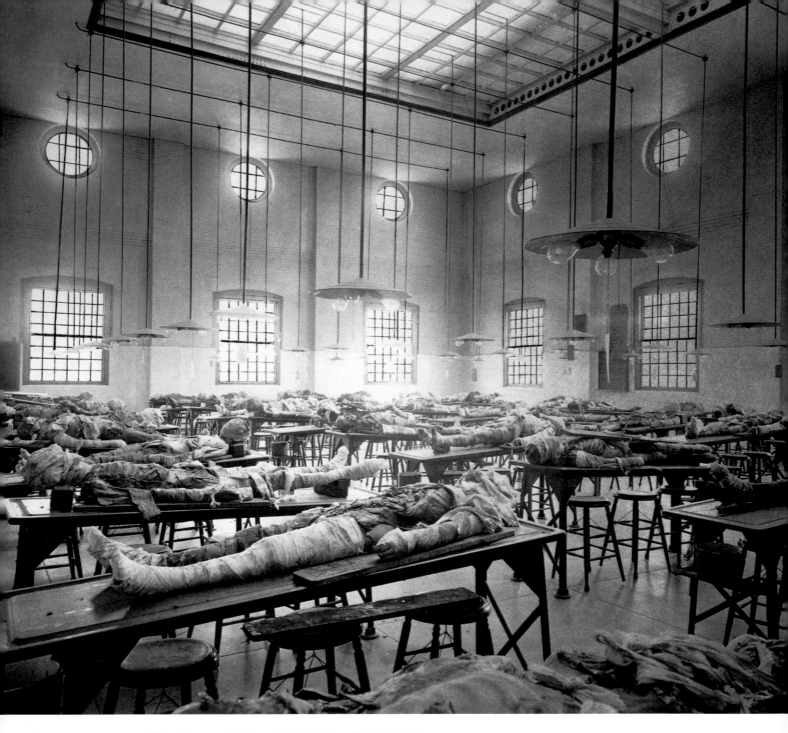

A dissecting room in Jefferson Medical College, Philadelphia, in 1902.

human dissections were permitted in the ancient world and Herophilus of Chalcedon and Erasistratus of Cos investigated the internal body and dissected criminals.

Later, in the 2nd century AD, Galen had to base his ideas of the anatomy of the human body on his dissections of dead (or even live) animals. Pigs, goats, and barbary apes, and on one famous occasion, the emperor's pet elephant, enabled him to study the nervous system, brain functions, the heart, and various other organs. He advised his students to cut "without pity or compassion"—even into a living animal (vivisection). It was said that his favorite public stunt was to sever the nerves of a live piglet's spine until, with a final slice at the neck, it stopped squealing. Galen did, no doubt, acquire knowledge of the human body in his capacity as physician to the Roman gladiators and was able to examine the digestive system from the exposed guts of a defeated gladiator wounded in the stomach. However, his descriptions of anatomical structures were mostly extrapolated from animals to humans and his major writings went unchallenged for centuries.

In Christian Europe, the first recorded public dissection of a human body took place in Bologna, Italy, in 1315/16. The Roman Catholic Church gradually became more accepting of human dissection as a teaching aid in medicine—although the numbers of cadavers permitted each year were limited to a few executed criminals who would then receive a reverent Christian burial. It was generally left to assistants to do the dissections, while the "great" professors read out the words of the revered Galen.

The gory gallows and Vesalius's images of bones and bodies

Father of patient
Your reasoning is most eloquent, of course. There is but one thing which surprised me: that's the positions of the liver and the heart. It seems to me that you got them the wrong way about; that the heart should be on the left side, and the liver on the right.

Pretend Doctor
Yes, it used to be so; but we have changed all that. Everything's quite different in medicine nowadays.

Molière (1622–73), *Le Médicin malgré lui*

On a dark night in the year 1536, or so the story goes, the young Flemish anatomist Andreas Vesalius (1514–64) was walking home when the cadaver of an executed criminal hanging from a gibbet outside the city walls of Louvain caught his eye. With the help of his friend, the mathematician-physician Gemma Phrysius, he smuggled the body into the city. Far from being overcome by the stench of rotting flesh, he carefully boiled all the bones and then put the skeleton back together—replacing missing parts from other cadavers. Now he had a complete example of the structure of the human body. Over the next few years, Vesalius dissected many bodies—mostly of executed criminals or stolen from cemeteries.

Vesalius was one of the few who dared to challenge Galen, correcting many of his anatomical errors, such as the erroneous missing or "Adam's rib," clarifying that men have twelve on each side just as in the female. Vesalius produced precise descriptions and illustrations of the skeleton,

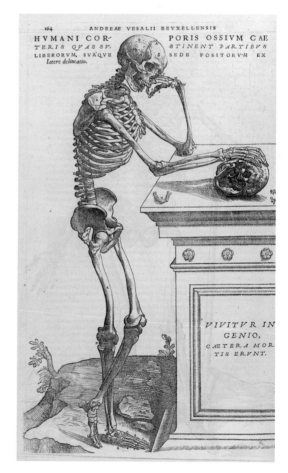

The publication in 1543 of his remarkable illustrated work, *De humani corporis fabrica* ("On the structure of the human body"), marked Vesalius out as one of the most influential anatomists of all time. In this engraving, the skeleton's naturalistic pose enables the viewer to understand how it is articulated as if it were a living being. Contemplating the skull, the image acts as both an anatomical representation and a reminder of the temporal nature of life.

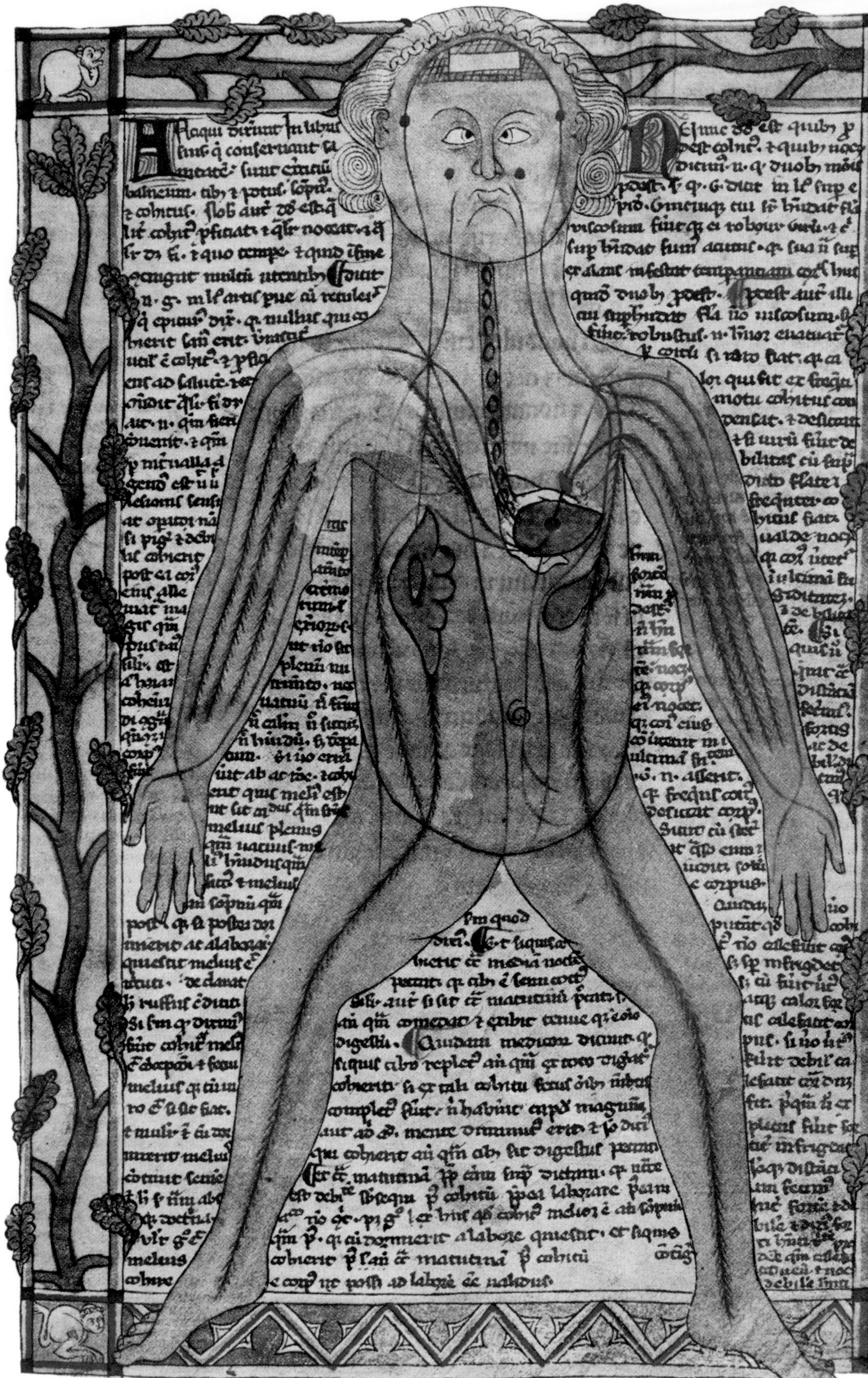

muscles, blood vessels, the nervous system, and the soft internal organs of the body, especially those contained within the abdominal and thoracic cavities. For a while, many learned physicians stuck to the long-cherished teachings of Galen, despite evidence to the contrary —some tried to argue that the human body must have changed in the intervening centuries.

Dissections in the 16th century became a public spectacle, and anatomy "theaters" were built in the great centers of medical and surgical learning, especially in Italy. Perfectly preserved or reconstructed anatomy theaters include those in Padua, Edinburgh, Uppsala, Barcelona, and Leiden. In 1543, Vesalius conducted a public dissection of the body of Jakob Karrer von Gebweiler, a notorious felon from the city of Basel in Switzerland. He assembled the bones and donated the skeleton to the University of Basel, where it can still be seen today: the world's oldest anatomical preparation.

William Harvey and the circulation of the blood

In 1628, the English physician William Harvey (1578–1657) published his now-celebrated text, *Exercitatio anatomica de motu cordis et sanguinis in animalibus* ("An anatomical exercise on the motion of the heart and blood in living beings"). Best known for his discovery of the circulation of the blood, Harvey studied at Cambridge University before traveling to the University of Padua, Italy. Padua, the foremost scientific university in Europe, was where Galileo (1564–1642) was professor of mathematics and where Vesalius in the 1540s had performed public dissections in the magnificent purpose-built anatomy theater, accompanied by lute music.

On his return to England, Harvey rapidly gained prominence as a practitioner, a royal physician, and a keen experimentalist. He carried out animal dissections and vivisections, and based his theories on "experiments and observation." Harvey was able to give an accurate description of the pulmonary circulation of the blood. The heart, Harvey recognized, acts as a pump, keeping the blood circulating. It was, he said, the "foundation of all life, and author of all." He proved conclusively that blood "moves around in a circle," constantly circulating through the veins and arteries, continuously returning to the heart. Dark venous blood flows toward the right ventricle of the heart and bright red arterial blood flows away from the left ventricle of the heart. The blood passes through the lungs (rather than "invisible pores" in the septum as Galen had speculated) in its passage between the right and left ventricle of the heart.

Harvey attributed his achievements to his Padua days: "I profess to have learnt and teach anatomy, not from books but from dissections; not from the positions of philosophers but from the fabric of nature." He was also influenced by the findings of other scientists, including his medical teacher at Padua, Hieronymus Fabricius of Acquapendente (1537–1619), who had described the valves of veins. One intriguing question is whether Harvey and others knew of the 13th-century description by Syrian Ibn al-Nafis (1210/13–88), of the "lesser circulation of the blood." Nafis had "speculated" that blood is carried from the right side of the heart to the left via the lungs, contradicting Galen's idea of two separate systems of arteries and veins moving blood through the body.

OPPOSITE Historical artwork of a human figure showing internal organs and blood vessels. William Harvey, in 1628, showed that blood circulated around the body, rather than simply flowing outward from the heart and liver to the extremities, to be consumed and somehow "regenerated," as Galen had claimed earlier.

Exploring and naming the human interior

Although Harvey's concept of the blood circulation was not universally accepted for several years, his impact on science has been profound. Many other experiments were carried out in the 17th century, enabling scientists to begin to describe more precisely the role of the heart, blood, lungs, arteries, veins, capillaries, glands, the lymphatic, and nervous systems and, later, to understand digestion, respiration, reproduction, and muscle functions.

New parts of the human body were discovered and named on a regular basis. Across Europe, anatomists vied with each other to identify previously uncharted parts of the human

These 17th-century anatomical figures give a basic, if simplistic, layout of the main organs. By the 19th century, medical understanding of the structural components of the human body was starting to take shape.

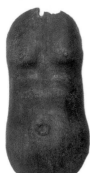
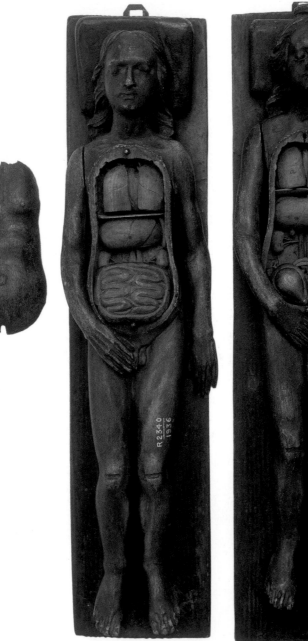
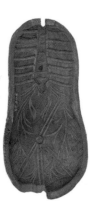

body, staking their claim to a "new" piece of the human interior. The Fallopian tubes, the Eustachian tube, the "Circle of Willis," the aqueduct of Sylvius, the Malpighian layer, and Scarpa's ganglion and triangle are just a few of the "body parts" with which surgeons today will be familiar and are named after their "discoverers." The works of the English physician-anatomist Thomas Willis (1621–75), after whom, the "circle of Willis" (the arterial circle at the base of the brain) is named, contain descriptions of the brain, the spinal cord, and the nervous system. When he dissected his own patients, he tried to relate the symptoms of different diseases, including "mania," "melancholia," and "hysteria," to brain pathology. The brain is still seen as one of the most complex organs of the human body.

Some anatomists also left their own body parts for their successors to study. The Italian anatomist and surgeon Antonio Scarpa (1752–1832) was one such donor and his pickled, dismembered head, kidneys, and four of his fingers can still be seen in the University History Museum in Pavia, Italy.

Microscopes—but not, yet, microbes ...

If anatomy shew us neither the causes nor cures of most diseases I think it not very likely to bring any great advantages for removeing the pains and maladys of mankind.

John Locke, c.1668

The invention of the microscope in the late 16th century was also of great importance for scientists. English natural philosopher Robert Hooke (1635–1703) coined the term "cell" from his observations of a sliver of cork viewed through the new microscopic lens. Meanwhile, Dutch draper Antonie van Leeuwenhoek (1632–1723) looked through the microscope to discover *animalcules* or "little animals" in specimens such as saliva and sputum. At the time, these *animalcules* were not understood as "living germs" or microbes capable of transmitting disease—that part of the puzzle would be solved in the 19th century by Louis Pasteur and Robert Koch (see pages 42 and 43).

Indeed, as exciting and revolutionary as these experiments were—and they initiated the beginnings of modern scientific medicine—there abounded a whole range of diverse concepts of disease causation for physical, as well as mental, ill-health. Pepys witnessed many of the experiments being carried out in the late 17th century, including the first attempts at blood transfusion. He described Robert Hooke's 1665 book, *Micrographia*—which reproduced his sightings through the lens, including a magnified flea—as "the most ingenious book that I have ever read in my life." Yet, when it came to trying to understand his own frequent episodes of ill-health, he attributed them to a range of factors and sought various opinions and solutions.

He, invariably, stressed "cold" and therefore the role of phlegm, and on over a hundred occasions in his diary, kept from 1660–9, he recorded "taking cold." This was dangerous because it "clogged the pores" and thus prevented the healthy expulsion of "corrupt humors." He generally blamed it on the weather, which also gave rise to other complaints such as pimples, itching, tickling, and pissing pains. Sometimes he confessed it was his own folly: forgetting to wear his wig, standing in drafts, wearing unaired clothes. On November 2 1662, he scribbled: "and so home and to bed, with some pain in making water, having taken cold this morning in sitting too long bare-legged to pare my cornes."

From bedside to the morgue: the "seats of disease"

From the 18th century, physicians extended their methods of understanding disease by following up the clinical examinations of hospitalized patients who had died with autopsies to correlate symptoms with pathological changes. The Italian anatomist Giovanni Morgagni (1682–1771) conceived the bold project of a work "of diagnoses based on the anatomies of morbid cadavers." In 1761 he published hundreds of reports in his book *De sedibus et causis morborum per anatomen indagatis* ("On the seats and causes of disease investigated by anatomy"). This newly developing field of clinicopathology or pathological anatomy became especially associated with the large municipal hospitals of Paris, built following the French Revolution of 1789–99.

"Open up a few corpses: you will dissipate at once the darkness that observation alone could not dissipate" wrote the Parisian anatomist Marie-François-Xavier Bichat (1771–1802). It is said that he sometimes slept in the morgue of the Hôtel-Dieu in Paris to maximize his dissecting opportunities. Paris became known as "the capital of the cadaver," attracting students from all over Europe and America. Nowhere was this development more helpful than in the study and understanding of fevers.

Fevers had always been a complex area for physicians. They were variously described by their appearance or disease symptoms: scarlet, yellow, spotted, bilious, inflammatory, or hysteric; by the periodicity or severity of the feverish symptoms: intermittent, malignant, putrid, or pestilential; by the seasonality or locality: autumnal, ship, famine, or gaol fever.

By observing the feverish symptoms on the ward and examining the internal "seats" of disease at postmortems, physicians began to distinguish between diseases with new precision. Different fevers left their hallmark or lesions in certain organs and tissues. Typhus and enteric (typhoid) fever were, by the mid-19th century, differentiated by their pathological signs rather than their feverish symptoms. Typhoid victims showed inflamed lesions in their small intestines at autopsy; these were absent from typhus victims. But this was only part of the puzzle. It would be a few more decades before the underlying causes of these infectious diseases were tracked down and a distinction drawn conclusively on scientific grounds. In the 1880s typhoid was found to be transmitted through contaminated water; and in 1909–10 typhus was shown to be transmitted by the body louse. Both were associated with filth, poverty, and poor sanitation.

Tuberculosis—also known as consumption or "phthisis"—was one of the leading causes of death in the 19th century and was poorly understood. It was not until the early 19th century, that the tubercle (a small swelling) in the lungs, gut, liver, or brain was identified—by French physician René Laënnec (1781–1826), famous for his discovery of the stethoscope—suggesting that the disease might have a single cause. In 1882, Koch discovered the bacterium that caused tuberculosis (the abbreviation TB originally stood for *tubercle bacillus*). Laënnec himself died of TB aged 45 after having also coined the terms "cirrhosis"(the growth of small tissues that cause liver degeneration) and "melanoma" (a darkened area indicative of skin cancer).

The importance of anatomy for surgery

Dissecting the dead soon became seen as the key to saving the living in the form of surgery. Anatomy and surgery became closely intertwined and it was increasingly recognized by the medical profession that it was vital for surgeons to be trained and to have a thorough knowledge of the human body before inflicting their saws or knives on the patient. As the

London surgeon John Abernethy (1764–1830/1) informed his students at St Bartholomew's Hospital: "there is but one way to obtain knowledge ... we must be companions with the dead." The stories of the surgeon-anatomists' quest for this vital knowledge are some of the most fascinating, if gruesome, accounts in the history of medicine.

A number of influential doctors set up their own private medical schools to dissect, and to teach students surgery and anatomy. The Scottish-born surgeon-anatomist and obstetrician William Hunter (1718–83) had one of the most famous schools in London. His brother, John Hunter (1728–93), was also a keen dissector. When the young Philadelphian Philip Syng Physick (1768–1837) visited John Hunter with his father in 1789, Physick's father demanded to know how he was planning on teaching his son surgery. "These are the books your son will learn under my direction ... the others [printed books] are fit for very little," Hunter replied, gesturing at his dissection room and several open cadavers. Physick later imported the Hunterian model to America. London surgeon Astley Paston Cooper (1768–1841) noted:

> Without dissection there can be no anatomy ... I would not remain in a room with a man who attempted to perform an operation in surgery who was unacquainted with anatomy ... he must mangle the living if he has not operated on the dead.

The "sack-'em up men"

There was soon a desperate need for more bodies for dissection or autopsy. In 16th-century Britain, for example, the Barber-Surgeon's Company was allowed the annual right to dissect the bodies of four hanged criminals; increased to six a century later. By the mid-18th century, judges could sentence murderers to death followed by dissection. Still, the supply of "legal" corpses was far from adequate for the growing numbers of anatomists. So what was the alternative?

Robbing freshly buried corpses from their graves appeared to be an option. Gangs of men, often including medical students, would dig up graves in the dead of night. They would prize off the coffin lid with a crowbar and carefully lift out the corpse, ensuring that no clothing or other items were removed. The latter would have been regarded as "theft," whereas the corpses were not considered "property" (even if the practice of grave-robbing, itself, was illegal). Often known by the public as the "sack-'em up men" or, by the anatomists, as the "resurrection men," the gangs would put the bodies in a sack and quickly whisk them to a back door of one of the anatomy schools. Here a porter would negotiate prices and pay for the bodies. Adults were known as "larges," while children's bodies or "smalls" were sold by the inch. The duties of one porter, David Paterson, at the private anatomy school of the surgeon-anatomist Robert Knox included:

> Keeping the door, cleaning and sweeping out the rooms, putting on and mending the fires, scrubbing the tables, and carrying away and burying the offals of the dissecting rooms; washing and cleaning subjects preparatory to their being brought into the class-room; attending on the students, and doing little jobs for them – such as cleaning and scraping bones, getting their dissecting clothes washed [done by Paterson's mother and sister] ... and be ready at all times to receive packages [i.e. the bodies] and go for them.

On the dissecting table—spilling the blood and guts

The surgeon-anatomists and their students had to work deftly to open up the corpse on the dissecting table. Wearing aprons (but no gloves), the process of dissection followed a logical sequence according to the rate of decomposition of the various body parts. First, the abdomen was opened up to remove the guts, the lengthy meters of intestines, the spleen, gall bladder, and pancreas; next came the lungs—removed by sawing open the rib cage with a hacksaw. This would be followed by removal of the heart, recognized by the later 17th century as the center of the physiological system—plus the remaining key organs: the brain, liver, bladder, kidneys, and reproductive parts. Finally, the muscles, which decayed slowest, were removed, leaving the bones, which could then be wired together as articulated skeletons.

The organs were usually dried and pickled, and often preserved in alcohol (superseded by the use of formaldehyde from the late 19th century). Colored resins and waxes were injected into organs, blood vessels, and soft tissues. Medical students were encouraged to touch and examine each of the organs and even to taste the bodily juices, such as the gastric juices and the mucus from the urethra. For some, the stench and horrors of the dissecting table were too much to bear, but for others, the acquisition of knowledge and an intimate understanding of the human body promised to deliver lifesaving techniques. As one highly critical newspaper journalist wrote: "scarcely a day passes but reports are circulated of the supposed sacrifice of fresh victims to the 'interests of science.'"

Many people were petrified at the prospect of being dissected after death, especially those with the belief that the body needed to be whole to rise on the Day of Judgment. Cages of iron, called "mortsafes" were invented to protect wealthy corpses from body snatchers. John Hunter managed to "acquire" the cadaver of Charles Byrne (1761–83). Known as the "Irish Giant" at nearly 96in (8 feet) tall, Byrne had earned his living as "the tallest man in the world." According to one version of his story, he persuaded his friends that when he died they were to bury his body at sea in a leaden coffin rather than let it be "anatomized." Despite his plans, a few years after his death his skeleton appeared in a splendid new glass case in the museum of John Hunter. Almost certainly Hunter had bribed Byrne's friends, paying well to secure the body. Rather than dissecting the cadaver, Hunter probably boiled it down to be prepared as a skeleton. The skeleton of the "Irish Giant"—now thought to have suffered from a pituitary tumor, a rare genetic mutation that caused his gigantism—can be seen in the Hunterian Museum in London.

Burking mania

Burke's the Butcher, Hare's the Thief,
Knox, the man who buys the Beef.
(Unknown)

The notorious reputation of body snatchers finally came to a head in 1828. William Burke and William Hare, residing in a cheap lodging house in Edinburgh, Scotland, had discovered that there was serious money to be made handing over corpses to the local surgeon-anatomist, Robert Knox. The first body to be delivered to Knox's porter, Patterson, was an old man who had died of natural causes. The next bodies handed over were all poor vagrants or prostitutes who had not had natural deaths. Burke and Hare had dosed their victims with alcohol and, once they were unconscious from its effects, had smothered them to death.

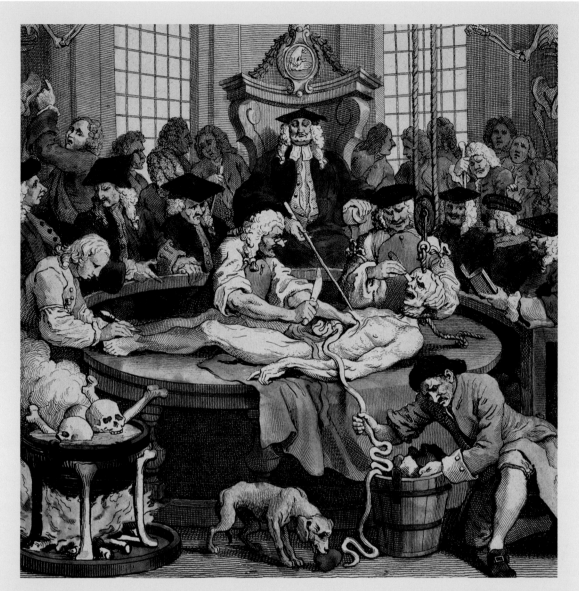

The gory reality of dissection

The 18-year-old future composer Hector Berlioz (1803–69) followed his father's wishes to enter medical school in Paris, only to give it up a few years later. As he recalled in his *Memoirs*:
When I entered that fearful human charnel-house, littered with fragments of limbs, and saw the ghastly faces and cloven heads, the bloody cesspools in which we stood, with its reeking atmosphere, the swarms of sparrows fighting for scrapings, and the rats in the corners gnawing bleeding vertebrae, such a feeling of horror possessed me that I leapt out of the window, and fled home ... firmly resolved to die rather than enter the career which had been forced upon me.

He revealed the stark reality of a medical training: filthy hospitals, dreadful medical students, hideous corpses, the shrieks of patients, the groans and death-rattles of the dying. It seemed to be "the utter reversal of the natural conditions of my life—horrible and impossible."

ABOVE William Hogarth's engraving, *The Reward of Cruelty* (1751), depicts the horrors of a public dissection of a criminal.

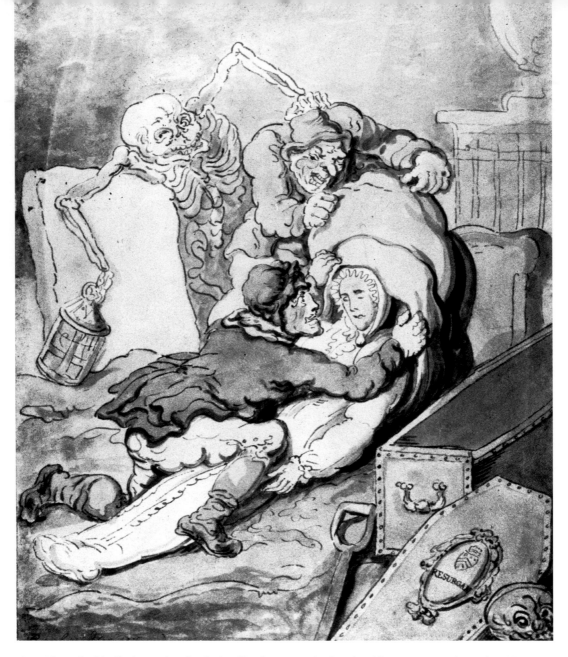

The grisly work of the "body snatchers," as depicted by Thomas Rowlandson (1775), became more and more lucrative during the 18th and 19th centuries on both sides of the Atlantic, as well as "down under" in Australia.

They were, finally, caught with their 16th victim, an elderly Irish woman Mary Docherty, whom they murdered on October 31 1828. Before delivering her to Knox's anatomy school, Burke and Hare held a Hallowe'en party and, in jest, told their guests not to go near Burke's bed. Intrigued, the guests did precisely that. There they discovered Mary Docherty's dead body hidden under a bale of straw. Burke and Hare hastened her off to Patterson, but it was too late: the police were on the case. They were arrested: Hare turned King's evidence and Burke was hanged, after which his body was dissected. His death mask and a pocket-book bound with his skin are on display at the Surgeon's Hall Museum of the Royal College of Surgeons of Edinburgh —as the magistrate at the time put it: "so that posterity may remember your repulsive crimes." Hare disappeared and Knox got off scot free.

Still, the body snatching trade continued in parts of the Western world. In Britain an Anatomy Act was passed in 1832 that made it legal for the anatomists to be supplied with the corpses of the "unclaimed poor" for "anatomical examination." This meant, in principle, that anyone who had died in a hospital, workhouse, prison, or other charitable institution and who had not left specific instructions saying they did not want to be dissected or who were not claimed by relatives within 48 hours, could legally become the "property" of the anatomists.

The famous medical textbook *Gray's Anatomy* (1858), illustrated by Henry Vandyke Carter (1831–97), which is still in print today, may well have been based on these "legally sanctioned" bodies. Henry Gray (1827–61), of St George's Hospital, London, intended the work "to furnish the Student and Practitioner with an accurate view of the anatomy of the Human Body, and more especially the application of this science to Practical Surgery."

Laboratory science and the cell

By the 19th century, the laboratory, as well as the hospital morgue and the dissecting table, was of increasing importance in enabling scientists and physicians to experiment and develop new specialist fields. Experimental physiology was one such area. The famous French physiologist Claude Bernard (1813–78) developed the concept of the "intérieur milieu" (homeostasis), which helped explain how organisms function by keeping, within a narrow range, many physiological parameters such as temperature and blood sugar. He conducted important work on the function of the pancreas gland and the liver, and, based on animal experiments, argued that the laboratory was the true sanctuary of medical science.

Another leading scientist of the time was Rudolf Virchow (1821–1902), the German "father of pathology" or "Hippocrates with a microscope." He placed slivers of flesh and smears of blood under his microscope and noticed that a mass of flesh that looked undifferentiated to the eye was, in fact, made up of millions of microscopic cells. He realized that cells were fundamental to life, recorded his ideas in his *Die Cellularpathologie* (1858), and is best known for the aphorism: "all cells come from cells." Virchow also recognized the condition he named leukemia (from the Greek *leukos*, "white," and *haima*, "blood"), which was characterized by a proliferation of abnormal white blood cells. Disease, he argued, arose from abnormal changes within cells, and these could multiply out of control through division and spread to the rest of the body; so began the modern study of oncology (cancer).

Diseases were, by the mid-19th century, increasingly recognized in Western medicine as being "situated" in organs, tissues, and cells rather than in the "humors." But there was still the question of finding what caused many fatal and debilitating diseases in the first place and how to solve the debates of the sanitarians and contagionists.

The "walking stomach"

Some ... will have it that the stomach is a mill, others that it is a fermenting vat, others again that it is a stew pan.
(William Hunter)

The question of how digestion works was asked by the ancient Greeks and rumbled on in scientific circles down the centuries. One bizarre incident on the Canadian border in 1822 enlightened US army surgeon William Beaumont. While treating a large bullet wound to a young fur trader's stomach, Beaumont had to add a stopper, secured by a bandage, to stop the contents of his stomach from leaking out of a gaping hole. This hole, however, gave Beaumont an incredible insight into digestion processes and he was able to show based on a number of experiments that gastric juices dissolved food in the stomach and played a key role in digestion.

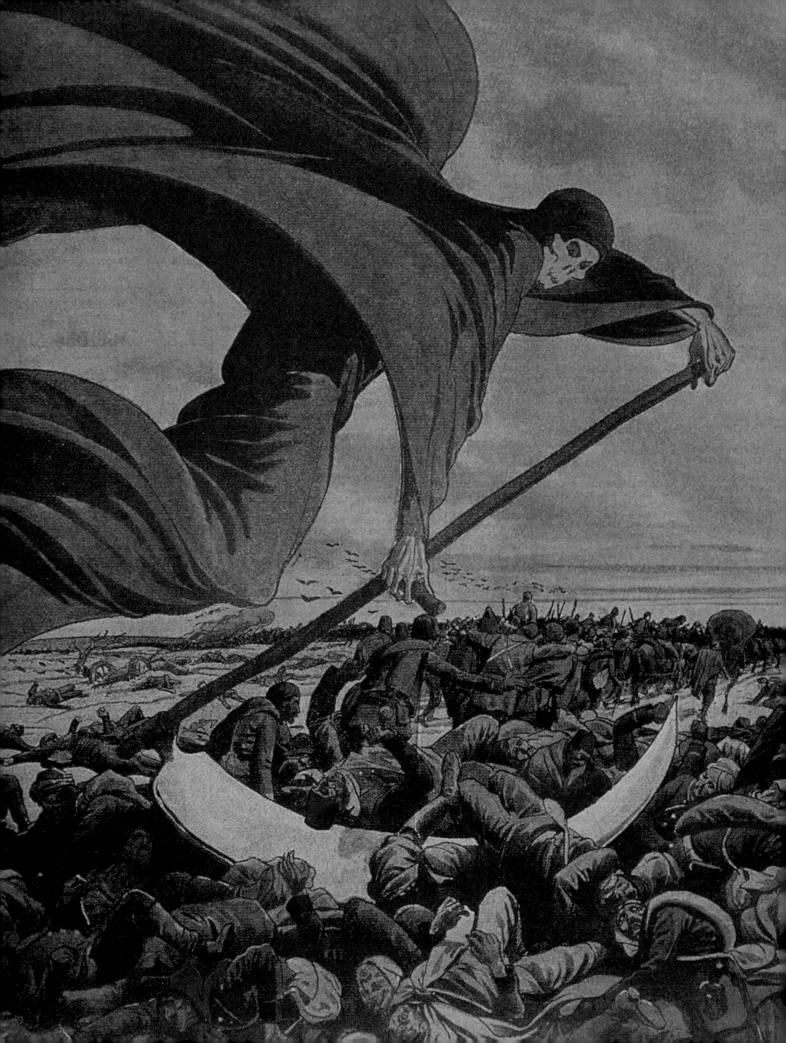

Germs and Genes

The microbe is so very small
You cannot make him out at all,
But many sanguine people hope
To see him through a microscope.

Hilaire Belloc (1870–1953), 'The Microbe' from *More Beasts for Worse Children* (1897)

A remarkable discovery made in the 1860s by French chemist Louis Pasteur showed that 'microbes' did not develop through 'spontaneous generation', as some believed, but were present in the air. Pasteur's studies led to an understanding of 'germ theory', one of the greatest medical milestones of all time. Robert Koch, a German physician, also made major contributions to this area and in the 1880s identified the bacteria responsible for some of the most frightening killers of the day, tuberculosis and cholera. Other causes of infectious diseases were discovered, such as the transmission of the malaria parasite by mosquitoes. By the 1930s, viruses including those causing influenza and polio were identified. New insights have also been made into the make-up of the human body, adding biochemical, physiological, immunological and genetic factors, as well as 'lifestyle' risk factors, as determinants of whether we stay healthy or get sick. The discovery of the molecular structure of DNA in 1953 and the launch of the Human Genome Project in 1990 have given an added dimension to our modern understanding of the causes of both infectious and non-infectious diseases.

Early ideas of a 'germ theory' of disease

Louis Pasteur (1822–95) became professor at the universities of Strasbourg and Lille and held various academic posts in Paris. His studies of fermentation solved practical problems for wine-makers and brewers. He found that by heating wine to 50°C he could kill the yeast responsible for its deterioration, and that heat treatment applied to milk stopped it souring. These experiments, moreover, showed that the widely held belief in 'spontaneous generation' of microbes (the idea that living organisms can emerge from inanimate matter) was incorrect. Pasteur then went on to solve the problem of an infectious disease of silkworms that was threatening the French silk industry. He established that the disease was caused by living organisms and began in the 1870s to talk about a 'germ theory' of human disease.

OPPOSITE Death striking down troops with cholera during the Balkan Wars (1912–13). Cholera is a frightening disease and the identification in 1883-4 by Robert Koch of its causative agent, a bacterium called *Vibrio cholerae*, transmitted through drinking water contaminated with human faeces, was one of the major advances in the history of medicine.

Louis Pasteur challenges old medical theories

I am afraid that the experiments you quote, M. Pasteur, will turn against you.
The world into which you wish to take us is really too fantastic.

La Presse, 1860

Pasteur's demonstration of an animal anthrax vaccine in 1881 was perhaps his most daring public experiment. His great rival, Robert Koch, had already investigated the 'germ' responsible for anthrax (see page 43). Pasteur's experiment would be as much a proof of the role of germs in causing disease as of the value of the vaccine. Anthrax is a potentially fatal disease that can kill both animals and humans. He developed an anthrax vaccine by reducing the virulence of the anthrax bacterium, by exposing it to air. At the time, there was still strong opposition to the 'germ theory' and no one was more sceptical than the esteemed veterinarian Hippolyte Rossignol, editor of *La presse veterinaire*. Rossignol challenged Pasteur to test his vaccine on his own farm, south-east of Paris, fully expecting to humiliate this 'upstart' scientist.

A group of sheep, goats and cows were vaccinated with Pasteur's vaccine and another group of farm animals were left 'unprotected'. A month later, all the animals were injected with three times the lethal dose of anthrax. Two days later, on 2 June 1881, Pasteur and his colleagues Charles Chamberland (1851–1908) and Émile Roux (1853–1933) entered the farmyard in full view of the waiting press. They were greeted by the vaccinated animals – all in good health. Meanwhile, against a backdrop of unvaccinated animals stiff with rigor mortis, two of the surviving unvaccinated sheep staggered out and died in front of the assembled company. The Paris correspondent from the *London Times*, Henri de Blowitz, wired 'the experiment at Pouilly-le-Fort is a perfect success' immediately to London; the newspaper declared Pasteur as 'one of the great scientific glories of France'.

The 'Institut Pasteur', founded in 1888, was funded largely by public subscription, and Pasteur remained its director until his death in 1895. His name lives on in our everyday lives whenever we drink pasteurized milk or eat pasteurized cheese.

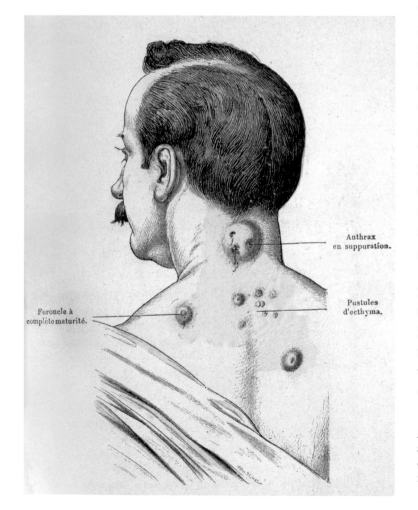

Anthrax is a dangerous disease that affects both animals and humans and can prove fatal. This print details the symptoms. Pasteur developed a vaccine for anthrax, as well as one for rabies.

Robert Koch and the development of the germ theory

Does disease follow bacteria, or do bacteria follow disease? We still don't know the answer ...
My heart says 'yes' to bacteria, but my reasons say 'wait, wait'.

Karl Thiersch, c.1875

The same age as Pasteur, the German surgeon Karl Thiersch (1822–95) was one of many to raise questions about the role of bacteria in disease. While it was Pasteur who had set the stage for the proof of the 'germ theory', it was his rival, Robert Koch (1843–1910), who was able to identify *specific* microbes that caused *specific* diseases and provide answers to numerous tantalizing questions. Koch, like Pasteur, became intrigued by the possibility that microbes might be responsible for many of the infectious diseases that had plagued humans over millennia. His mentor, Jacob Henle, had published a paper in 1840 on the subject of miasma and contagion, suggesting the role of invisible living organisms in causing infection and concluding that their importance was potentially very significant. Koch must have taken note of this idea as he became increasingly determined to prove the case.

His first success in bacteriology was his work on anthrax in 1876. Starting from the research of the French physician Casimir Davaine (1812–82), who had proposed in 1863 that the disease was caused by small rod-like structures in the blood, Koch succeeded in describing the full life cycle of what became known as *Bacillus anthracis*, and to reproduce the disease in animal experiments. He confirmed that the bacteria could be transmitted from animal to animal, and later made the important discovery that the bacteria can form 'resting spores' that lie dormant in the soil for many years. This would account for the apparently spontaneous outbreaks of anthrax in animal herds. A leading botanist and bacteriologist, Ferdinand Cohn, recognized the significance of Koch's work and strongly supported him.

Working in Breslau and then Berlin, Koch developed many innovative new techniques for observing, staining and growing bacteria. He used dyes – such as methylene blue added to caustic potash – to stain bacteria preparations and found a solid medium with which to culture bacteria; this gave better results than the usual liquid medium. His first choice was a potato, then a colleague's wife suggested trying agar, an extract of seaweed, as this could be used to make perfect jelly. His assistant, Julius Richard Petri (1852–1921), designed a glass dish to incubate and grow bacterial colonies for study. The Petri dish is still used by medical scientists. Spreading agar onto Petri dishes, Koch and his team had found a way of cultivating virtually any bacteria, minimizing the usual problem of contamination. He also described a number of conditions necessary to 'prove' that a disease was caused by a 'germ'. These became widely known as Koch's postulates.

Koch's major triumph was the identification in 1882 of the bacterium *Mycobacterium tuberculosis* as the cause of TB, which killed one person in four in Europe and the United States. He presented his new findings to a stunned audience in Berlin on 24 March 1882, complete with paraphernalia from his lab: test tubes with cultures, glass slides with stained bacteria, dyes, and glass jars with tissue samples. The young Paul Ehrlich (1854–1915) was in the audience and later described it as 'the most important experience of my scientific life'. Koch was awarded the Nobel Prize in Physiology or Medicine in 1905 for his 'investigations and discoveries in relation to tuberculosis'.

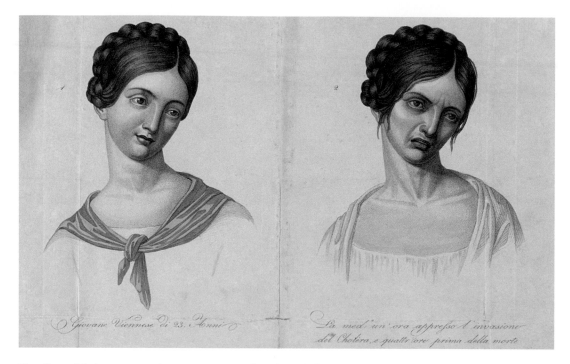

The effects of cholera: a young Viennese woman, aged 23, shown before and after contracting the disease (c.1831). Cholera wiped out vast swathes of people in areas affected, so there was a real sense of urgency – and professional rivalry – to discover the cause and then a possible preventive or cure.

The race to find the cause of cholera

Following the outbreaks of cholera in mid-19th-century London, the physician John Snow had become convinced that cholera was transmitted by drinking contaminated water (see pages 24–5). In Italy, the physician and microscopist Filippo Pacini (1812–83) had in 1854 observed the microbes that cause cholera in the excreta and intestinal contents of victims in Florence – but his valuable work was overlooked.

In 1883, two rival teams – one French, one German – were dispatched to Alexandria in Egypt where cholera was raging, in a race to find its cause. The expedition of the French 'Pasteurians' was marred by failure and tragedy, and they returned to France when one of their team succumbed to the disease. The German team, headed by Koch, had more success investigating twelve patients with cholera. They performed autopsies on ten of the victims, identifying a specific bacterium in their intestinal mucosa. Koch was convinced that these bacteria 'stand in some way to the cholera process'.

The following year, in the teeming, cholera-infested suburbs of Calcutta (now Kolkata), India, Koch found the same 'comma'-shaped cholera bacterium (*Vibrio cholerae*) in both the local drinking water and the 'rice water stools' of victims. He was confident that he could 'prove that we have found the pathogen responsible for cholera'.

John Snow and Filippo Pacini had the right idea: cholera was a waterborne disease, communicated mainly by polluted water and transmitted through the faecal-oral route. Some remained unconvinced, however, and one of Koch's sceptical colleagues, the German hygienist Max Joseph von Pettenkofer (1818–1901), had his own complex theory based partly on the older view that cholera was caused by 'miasmas' or particles emanating from rotten material polluting the air and infecting people who inhaled them. In an extreme form of public testing, von Pettenkofer, having secured from Koch a flask containing a culture infected with cholera 'germs', proceeded to swallow it in 1892. For unexplained reasons – although unusually high levels of stomach acid might be the answer – this merely resulted in a mild bout of diarrhoea. Von Pettenkofer failed to acknowledge the importance of filtering and boiling drinking water as a preventive measure, and when a major outbreak of cholera hit Hamburg in 1892, which killed upwards of 8,000 people, it eventually tarnished von Pettenkofer's reputation and led to his suicide in 1901. The implementation of a sand-filtering water plant helped free Hamburg from recurring epidemics of cholera, as well as typhoid – another bacterial waterborne disease. Indeed, such public health measures, designed to separate sewage-contaminated water from drinking water, played a major role in helping to control the spread of the 'filth' diseases in many parts of the Western world. Cholera remains a problem in countries with poor sanitation, however, and in 2010 a serious outbreak followed an earthquake in Haiti.

The dawn of the bacteriological age

Sir Patrick: *Suppose there's no germ ...*

Sir Ralph: *Impossible ... there must be a germ: else how could the patient be ill?*

G B Shaw, *The Doctor's Dilemma*, 1906

By the early 20th century, the majority of scientists and physicians, at least in the Western world, were eventually coming round to a Pasteurian way of thinking. Constant discoveries were being made into disease-causing bacteria and by 1906, germ theory had become so popular that it was mocked by the playwright George Bernard Shaw. Laboratory science blossomed, with technicians and physicians eagerly peering down microscopes of increasing sophistication, magnification and discrimination. Hospital laboratories enabled urine, faeces, sputum, pus, blood and tissue biopsies to be analyzed on site. The new generations of medical practitioners could put the ancient texts and humoral theories of Hippocrates, Galen and others of the past behind them. They were qualifying in one of the most exciting eras in the history of medicine and witnessing some of the most rapid and fundamental changes in the concepts and theories of disease for over 1,500 years.

The triumph of germ theory as an explanation of disease ratified the search for vaccines and drugs to prevent and kill the invading organisms. Serum therapy (an anti-toxin) was introduced for diphtheria in the 1890s after it was discovered that some bacteria produce harmful toxins (poisons) that cause the illness. It was subsequently replaced by a vaccine for diphtheria, but its contribution to saving lives, especially those of children, provided positive publicity for bacteriology. A number of new vaccines for

The HeLa cells – the oldest human cell line

In 1951, George Otto Gey (1899–1970), of Johns Hopkins Hospital, Baltimore, received a sample of cells from a young patient, Henrietta Lacks (1920–51), with cervical cancer. Usually such samples died but her cells could be cultured and kept alive. Gey propagated these into an immortalized human (HeLa) cell line. They have been used worldwide ever since, helping develop new treatments: polio vaccine; biomedical research into cancer; gene mapping; and *in-vitro* fertilization. Although at the time Henrietta's family was unaware of the use of her cells, they later discovered her 'immortality' and the unique contribution she had made to medical science.

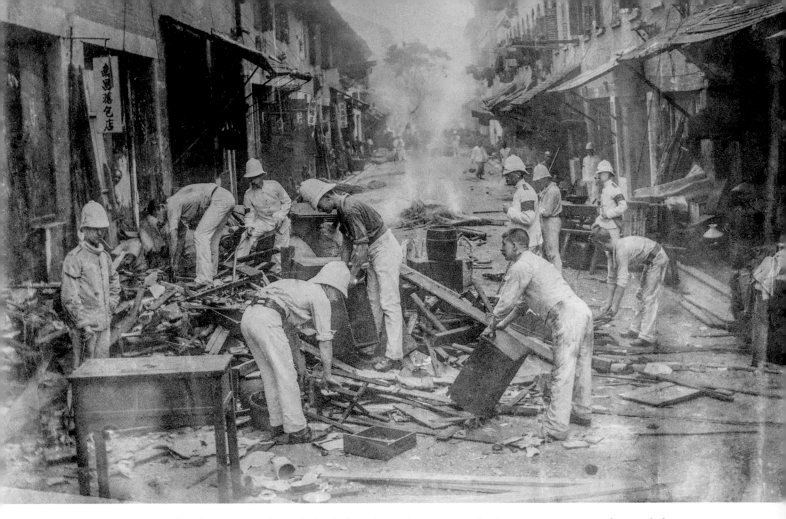

The Staffordshire Regiment clearing bubonic plague houses in Hong Kong, 1894, in an attempt to prevent the spread of the disease. Bacteriologist Alexandre Yersin (1863–1943), also there at the time, discovered the bacterium that causes the plague. The discovery in 1898 of rat-to-human transmission via flea bites led to major public health campaigns.

infectious diseases were developed, and disease prevention through immunization became a success story of the early bacteriological age (see Vaccination and Preventive Medicine).

The first 'magic bullet' in 1910 was Salversan for syphilis (see pages 185–6). It took some time for therapies, such as antibiotics, to be found to match the evolving bacteriological knowledge, and also for scientists to recognize that some diseases, such as rickets, beri-beri and pellagra, were caused not by the *presence* of germs but by the *absence* of an essential nutritional factor. But the germ theory did give credence to the benefits of public health measures, such as sanitation and isolation of infectious patients, that could now be fitted into a bacteriological model of disease causation. It also led to important improvements, for example the adoption of antiseptic and aseptic principles in hospitals and surgery.

The idea of germs, albeit invisible, also began to capture the public imagination. Cleanliness in the home and the workplace began to take on a new meaning, with messages promoting ways to prevent diseases from spreading. The main selling point of the new linoleum floor covering was that it was easy to clean 'after a TB sufferer had finished coughing around the house'. Domestic kitchens, toilets and washbasins were viewed as dangerous havens for bacteria. 'No Spitting' and 'Swat the Fly' signs were put up in public places and the danger of sneezing and coughing in other people's faces was advertised. It even had an effect on fashion: women's skirts were shortened to avoid bringing germ-laden dirt from the streets into the home.

The tropical disease detectives

The ancients were quite right – the disease [malaria] is caused by the emanation of the marsh.
That emanation, however, is not a gas, nor even a contagium vivum, *but an insect.*

Ronald Ross, 1910

The hazards of the tropics, whether trading, fighting or exploring, had exposed Westerners to a range of deadly 'tropical' diseases: elephantiasis, malaria, schistosomiasis (bilharzia), trypanosomiasis (or African sleeping sickness), leishmaniasis (kala azar), onchocerciasis (river blindness), hookworm, dracunculiasis (Guinea worm) and Chagas disease (or American trypanosomiasis).

Patrick Manson (1844–1922), a Scottish physician, made the first significant discovery in tropical medicine in 1877, and became known as 'Mosquito Manson'. Working in Amoy (now Xiamen), China, he followed up earlier ideas that microscopic 'thread-like' worms (larval microfilariae) might be the cause of elephantiasis, or lymphatic filariasis – a terrible disease that leads to gross swellings, especially in the legs and male genitals, as well as internal damage to the kidneys and lymphatic system. He then speculated that mosquitoes might be involved in the transmission of the microfilariae.

Manson experimented on his gardener and was the first to demonstrate conclusively the insect-borne transmission of any disease. Manson's ideas were followed up by others and by the early 20th century the role of the infective mosquito bite and the complex life cycle of

Patrick Manson conducting an experiment on his gardener, Hinlo, *c.* 1876–77, in a painting by Ernest Board. Manson suspected that mosquitoes might be responsible for transmitting microfilariae (larval worms) as a cause of lymphatic filariasis (elephantiasis). He kept Hinlo, in whose blood he found microfilariae, in a 'mosquito house'. When he subsequently dissected the mosquitoes that had fed on Hinlo's blood, he found larval stages of the filarial worm. The experiment was the first to show without a doubt that a disease could be transmitted by insects.

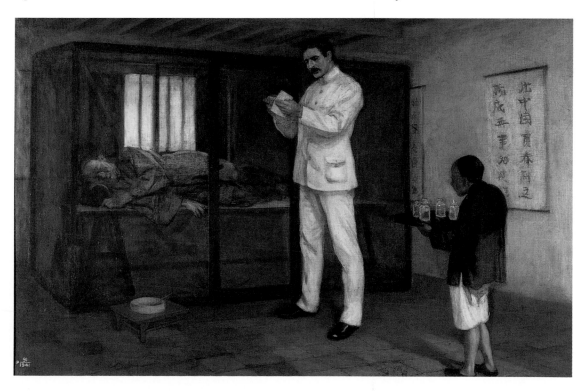

lymphatic filariasis had been established. The term 'parasite' (Greek, *para-*, 'alongside or near', and *sitos*, 'food') gradually entered into medical terminology as a disease-causing agent that lives in two hosts.

Manson's protégé, Ronald Ross (1857–1932), a British army surgeon in the Indian Medical Service, is credited with doing the first key experiments in 1897 and 1898 to identify malaria parasites in mosquitoes that had fed on the blood of an infected patient. He also unravelled the malaria cycle in birds. Italian scientists, including Giovanni Battista Grassi (1854–1925), in 1898 worked out the next crucial step by establishing the role of mosquitoes (of the genus *Anopheles*) in transmitting human malaria. In 1900 Manson's pathologist son, Patrick, tested the mosquito hypothesis by exposing himself to the bites of infective *Anopheles* mosquitoes. On developing malaria he was able to identify the parasite in blood films and used quinine to treat himself.

In spite of the use of mosquito nets, environmental measures to eliminate the vector and antimalarial drugs, tragically this deadly disease still kills a child in Africa every minute.

Another disease found to be transmitted by mosquitoes, yellow fever, is characterized by jaundice, haemorrhaging and its appalling symptom of black vomit often followed by coma and death. Like malaria, yellow fever had for centuries affected both tropical and temperate

Members of the British Roman Campagna Malaria Commission on their way to an area of Italy where the disease was prevalent *c.*1900. They tested the mosquito-malaria theory by sleeping in a mosquito-proof hut. Unlike everyone around them, they did not catch the disease.

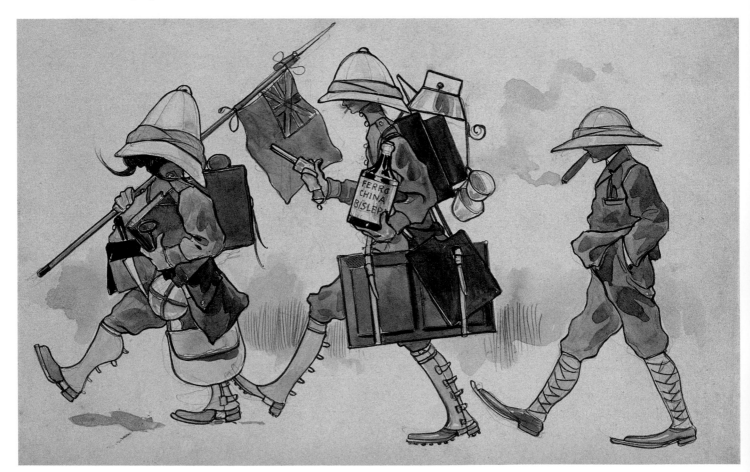

CONCEPTS AND THEORIES OF DISEASE

areas. The 1793 American yellow fever epidemic killed around 5,000 people in Philadelphia, Pennsylvania, roughly 10 per cent of the town's population. Medical student Stubbins Ffirth went to extraordinary lengths to prove that it was impossible to 'catch' this mystery disease in 1804. He smeared 'fresh black vomit' from yellow fever patients into cuts on his arms, drank it, and, when still uninfected, repeated his experiments using patients' blood, saliva and urine. In the 1880s Cuban doctor Carlos Finlay (1833–1915) suggested a link with mosquitoes. This was confirmed in a 1900 experiment by Walter Reed (1851–1902) of the US Army in Cuba, proving that it was not filth or contaminated clothing and bedding but the bite of an infective mosquito that caused the disease (later identified as a virus transmitted by the mosquito species *Aedes aegypti*, which also transmits dengue fever).

Many other important discoveries of the role of insect vectors (as well as the part played by intermediate and animal hosts) in transmitting disease followed. Various species of mosquitoes, tsetse flies, blackflies, the South American 'assassin bug', lice, fleas, sandflies, leeches, mites, houseflies and ticks have all now been implicated in the seemingly bizarre biting, feeding and defecating habits of creatures that can cause human disease, while parasitic worms play a role in the complex life cycles of a number of diseases. Major public health initiatives have looked for sustainable ways to fight diseases such as malaria, yellow fever and hookworm, and in 1913 the Rockefeller Foundation was established as a philanthropic organization 'to promote the well-being of mankind throughout the world'.

Today, the World Health Organization (a 1948 agency of the United Nations), as well as charitable organizations, such as the Bill & Melinda Gates Foundation, support global programmes in health and disease. These help raise awareness and provide funding for 'Neglected Tropical Diseases' or 'diseases of poverty'.

The virus hunters

The first clues that a large number of diseases from smallpox to the common cold were caused not by bacteria but by 'viruses' (smaller than bacteria, these replicate only inside the living cells of organisms) came from a study by Dutch scientist Martinus Beijerinck (1851–1931) of the 'invisible' causal agent of tobacco mosaic disease in 1898.

Early evidence for the existence of viruses (Latin: 'poison') was obtained from experiments with filters that had pores too small for bacteria to pass through. The fluid that passed through the filters, such as sap from diseased tobacco leaves, was shown to transmit disease to healthy tobacco plants, so proving that disease agents ('soluble living germs') existed that remained invisible to existing technology – until the introduction of the electron microscope in the 1930s. The examples of polio and influenza illustrate how the emerging field of virology enabled scientists to transform our understanding of these viral diseases.

The summers of 1916 and 1917 saw one of the first major polio epidemics in history – in the USA – leading to widespread panic and suspicion as to the cause. People feared that flies and filth of all kinds, stray cats and dogs, contaminated milk bottles or even bananas infected by tarantula spiders might be the cause. Over 6,000 people, mostly children, died and many others were left paralyzed, with New York City especially badly affected. By the late 1940s, scientists at the Boston Children's Hospital in Massachusetts succeeded in growing the polio virus in non-neurological human tissue in the laboratory, paving the way for the development of a vaccine – thanks to which the disease is now close to being eradicated (see page 225).

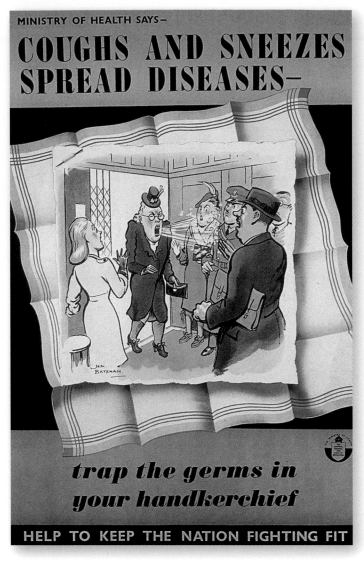

MINISTRY OF HEALTH SAYS—

COUGHS AND SNEEZES
SPREAD DISEASES—

*trap the germs in
your handkerchief*

HELP TO KEEP THE NATION FIGHTING FIT

A British Ministry of Health poster from the 1940s promoting awareness of the spread of germs. After millions of deaths from influenza, in the 1930s it was identified as a viral disease spread from person to person in airborne droplets generated by coughing, sneezing and unwashed hands.

In 1918–19, at the end of the First World War, an influenza or 'Spanish flu' pandemic circled the entire globe killing at least 50 million people in just a few years. This was the highest death toll of any single pandemic in the annals of human history. Public health initiatives promoted disinfecting streets and homes, sterilizing water fountains, banning spitting and shaking hands, quarantining ships, and enforcing the wearing of gauze masks. It did not help that scientists mistakenly identified a bacterial cause and created misconceived vaccines. Finally, in the 1930s, influenza was identified as a viral disease spread from person-to-person in airborne droplets generated by coughing, sneezing and unwashed hands. Based on victims buried in permafrost, Spanish Flu has been identified, retrospectively, as influenza type A, subtype H1N1. Complications caused by secondary bacterial pneumonia may have accounted for the fatal impact of the pandemic.

By the second half of the 20th century, scientists were generally confident that they knew the causes and routes of transmission of most infectious diseases. With effective treatments and vaccines in place, the disease pattern shifted from infectious diseases to 'non-communicable' diseases, such as cancer, heart disease and stroke, associated with ageing populations, genetic and lifestyle risk factors.

So it was a shock, when an entirely new – and devastating – human infectious disease, AIDS (acquired immune deficiency syndrome), came to medical and public attention in the early to mid-1980s, just after the global eradication of smallpox had been announced a few years earlier (see page 218). The cause of AIDS, one of the most destructive pandemics in recorded history, was shown in 1983–4 by two teams of scientists in the USA and France to be a retrovirus, ultimately named human immunodeficiency virus (HIV), which is transmitted mainly through sexual contact and by exposure to infected blood products or contaminated needles. Although there are now anti-retroviral drugs that control the symptoms of HIV/AIDS, the search for a vaccine to prevent or stop its transmission continues to be a major goal of virologists and immunologists today. TB has also re-emerged, especially in developing nations, where it is closely associated with HIV/AIDS, and is proving difficult to treat especially with the development of widespread antibiotic drug-resistance.

Other alarming new viral and bacterial diseases had also been identified from the late 1960s onwards: Ebola virus (1976), Lyme disease (1975) and SARS (severe acute respiratory syndrome) in 2003. Some of these diseases, including HIV/AIDS, have jumped the species barrier from an animal host to humans, becoming increasingly virulent along the way. These belong to a large group of diseases known as 'zoonoses'. The recent outbreaks of H5N1 avian (bird) flu beginning in 1996/7 and the H1N1 'swine' flu pandemic from 2009 onwards have caused widespread panic and tragic loss of life. They have also revealed critical insights into the role of infected birds and animals in the influenza story. Today, there are antiviral drugs to treat the primary cause of influenza, antibiotics to treat secondary bacterial infections, and vaccines to protect people from catching flu – but it is still seen as a potentially major threat to humans.

Discovering the 'secret of life': DNA and the Human Genome Project

When we saw the answer we had to pinch ourselves.

James Watson

On a wintery day, 28 February 1953, two Cambridge scientists, Francis Crick (1916–2004) and James Watson (b.1928), walked into a 17th-century Cambridge pub, *The Eagle*, to celebrate the fact that they had unravelled the structure of DNA (deoxyribonucleic acid), saying (according to a BBC news report): 'We have discovered the secret of life!' That morning they had worked out the double helix structure of DNA – the molecule that carries genetic information from one generation to another. The understanding of life had moved from organs to tissues, cells and molecules.

This was an achievement that promised countless advances in medicine and solved a mystery that had long puzzled scientists. On 25 April 1953, Watson and Crick published their, now famous, paper in the journal *Nature*, which began: 'We wish to suggest a structure for the salt of deoxyribose nucleic acid (DNA). This structure has novel features which are of considerable biological interest.' Nine years later, in 1962, Crick and Watson shared the Nobel Prize in Physiology or Medicine with Maurice Wilkins (1916–2004) of King's College, London, 'for solving one of the most important of all biological riddles'. Sadly, another scientist, Rosalind Franklin (1920–58), who had done much of the key experimental work in Wilkins' laboratory, had died of cancer in 1958.

Genetics is the branch of biology dealing with the transmission of certain physical and biochemical traits of organisms from one generation to the next. It dates back to the work in the 1850s and 60s of the Austrian monk Gregor Mendel (1822–84), who studied the inheritance of easily identifiable traits in pea plants. His work on inheritance was overlooked until 1905, when the word 'genetics' was coined by the English scientist William Bateson (1861–1926), a champion of Charles Darwin's theory of evolution. Although advances followed, it was the discovery of the double helical structure of DNA that laid the foundations for 'cracking the genetic code'. This enabled scientists to sequence and determine the exact order of DNA's four chemical bases – commonly abbreviated to A, T, C and G – which, ultimately, led to the establishment of the Human Genome Project (HGP) in 1990 to map the whole of the human genome. Sponsored and funded primarily by the US government through the Department of Energy and the National Institutes of Health, and the Wellcome Trust in the UK, along with other groups from around the world, the results have been made freely available on the internet for all researchers.

Just ten years later, a working draft of the genome was complete. Bill Clinton, then President of the United States, was able to announce from the White House:

With this profound new knowledge, humankind is on the verge of gaining immense, new power to heal. Genome science will have a real impact on all our lives – and even more, on the lives of our children. It will revolutionize the diagnosis, prevention and treatment of most, if not all, human diseases.

The Human Genome Project soon revealed that humans have fewer genes than was previously thought – around 20,000–25,000 protein-coding genes instead of the expected 100,000 plus – not so very different from those of the fruitfly genome! It appeared that only a tiny proportion of our DNA codes for proteins – just 1.2 per cent. The results of another multi-national project, ENCODE (the ENCyclopedia Of DNA Elements), which began in 2003, are revealing even more intriguing secrets of human DNA. What had been dismissed by some as 'junk DNA' (the bulk of DNA that does not constitute a gene and which does not directly

James Watson (left) and Francis Crick (right) with their model of part of a DNA molecule. One interpretation of DNA is that it is 'the book of life'.

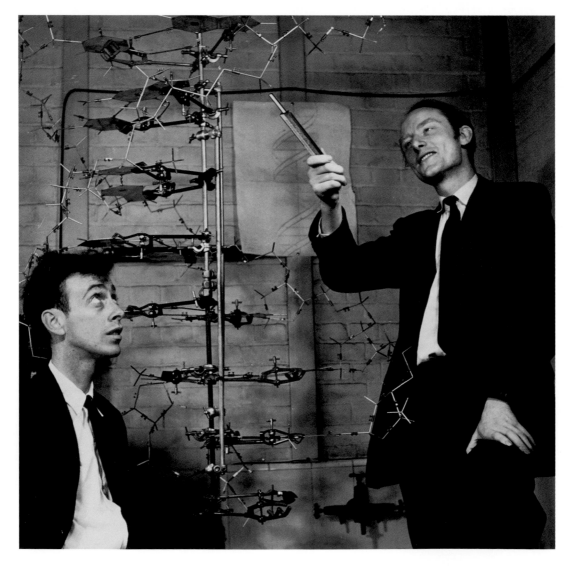

Concepts and theories of disease

code for the creation of a particular protein) now appears to be vital for the functioning of our cells, perhaps by turning certain genes on and off.

The first decades of the 21st century have seen a phenomenal acceleration in genome science, which is especially important for the field of oncology and the discovery of cancer-causing genes. Increasingly sophisticated genetic tests, including pre-natal tests and embryo screening, are being developed by biotechnological companies to detect faulty genes in people (or unborn babies) suspected of having particular diseases or of being at risk of developing them. The diagnostic, preventive and therapeutic implications of this project, as Clinton foretold, are exciting medical applications of DNA science with predictions that personalized (or stratified) medicine, based on the newly developing field of pharmacogenomics, will offer hope that appropriate or 'custom' drugs can be tailored to a patient's genetic profile and targeted to specific sites in the body. The Human Genome Project, however, also recognizes the ethical, legal and social issues – a huge field of enquiry, legislation and debate – that these prospects entail.

Today, developments in science and medicine move at ever-increasing speeds and the fields of 'translational' research and medicine continue to promise that basic findings in laboratories will eventually be translated into cures for the future, though the challenges and huge costs involved are not to be underestimated. As Eric Lander, Director of the Whitehead Institute Center for Genome Research in the USA, reminds us:

> We are standing at an extraordinary moment in scientific history. It's as though we have climbed to the top of the Himalayas. We can for the first time see the breathtaking vista of the human genome. For many years to come, we will be exploring the intricate details of the terrain ahead. We've got a long way to go before we will ultimately understand all the secrets that the genome has to tell us.

Many diseases, including cancers, are, moreover, extraordinarily complex, with genetic susceptibility being only one of many factors involved. Multiple sclerosis, a highly debilitating inflammatory disorder of the brain and spinal cord, for example, appears to be triggered by environmental factors, or even viral infections, in individuals with complex genetic-risk profiles relating to their immune system. Viruses and bacterial infections have now also been implicated in a number of cancers, notably cervical cancer, liver cancer, Burkitt's lymphoma, Kaposi's sarcoma and stomach cancer. Research carried out in the 1980–90s by Australian scientists Robin Warren and Barry Marshall proved that a bacterium, *Helicobacter pylori,* causes peptic ulcers – and won them a Nobel Prize. A course of antibiotics together with omeprazole (which reduces gastric acidity) is now a standard treatment for peptic ulcers.

Medical mysteries: prions to protein-misfolding diseases

A century after Pasteur and Koch developed their germ theory, the scientific world woke up, in 1982, to read in the prestigious journal *Science* about a completely new kind of infectious agent called a 'prion' (proteinaceous infectious particle). The publication of US physician-research scientist Stanley Prusiner's paper 'set off a firestorm'.

About 35 million people are living with some form of dementia, with predictions that this number will rise to over 100 million people by 2050.

Prusiner was intrigued by a number of mysterious, horrific diseases of animals and humans such as Kuru, linked to pre-1950s human brain-eating rituals in Papua New Guinea, and Creutzfeldt-Jakob disease (CJD), a rare degenerative brain disorder, resulting in sponge-like holes in the brain. Drawing on experimental work on hamsters, he produced evidence to show 'a new biological principle of infection' and that the cause of these diseases was not the 'unconventional slow virus' (favoured by US Nobel laureate Carleton Gajdusek, 1923–2008, and colleagues since the 1960s) but an aberrant form of protein he called a prion. Although able to self-replicate, prions – unlike other conventional infectious agents such as bacteria, viruses, parasites and fungi – seem devoid of nucleic acids.

Some scientists were initially sceptical, but the alarming outbreak of bovine spongiform encephalopathy (BSE) or 'mad cow disease' in cattle in the mid-1980s, followed by human cases ('variant' CJD or vCJD), linked to eating contaminated beef products, convinced most people that Prusiner was right. BSE and vCJD are prion-related diseases. Prions multiply in an incredible way by converting normal protein molecules into dangerous ones simply by inducing the benign molecules to change their shape. In 1997, Prusiner was awarded the Nobel Prize for his discovery.

Other fascinating scientific work is also transforming our understanding of a whole range of neurodegenerative and indeed other types of disease. Over the past ten years or so, as a result of the work of, among others, Christopher Dobson and colleagues at the University of Cambridge, it is increasingly apparent that prion diseases are infectious forms of a much larger group of medical disorders including: Alzheimer's (named after Alois Alzheimer, 1864–1915), Parkinson's (after James Parkinson, 1755–1824) and Huntington's (after George Huntington, 1850–1916) diseases, as well as type 2 diabetes, and also rare conditions such as 'fatal familial insomnia'. This class of diseases is associated with a phenomenon in which proteins can 'misfold' and clump together to form toxic deposits in various types of tissue in the form of amyloid fibrils or plaques. In the case of neurodegenerative conditions such as Alzheimer's disease, these damaging forms of proteins accumulate in the brain, leading to cognitive impairment, while in the case of type 2 diabetes they form in the pancreas.

The reasons for the aberrant deposition of misfolded proteins is currently being explored and include factors such as genetic mutations (in familial diseases like Huntington's and early-onset Alzheimer's), and lifestyle risk factors including obesity (linked to type 2 diabetes), while most forms of dementia (including Alzheimer's and Parkinson's disease) are associated with increasing longevity. Understanding these currently incurable diseases is of enormous importance given the effects of an ageing population on society and health care. About 35 million people are living with some form of dementia, with predictions that this number will rise to over 100 million people by 2050.

With medical sciences constantly pushing forward the frontiers of our fundamental knowledge of the human body and an ever-increasing understanding of the aetiologies (causes) of disease, who knows what other agents of disease or novel pathways are awaiting discovery in the coming decades of the 21st century.

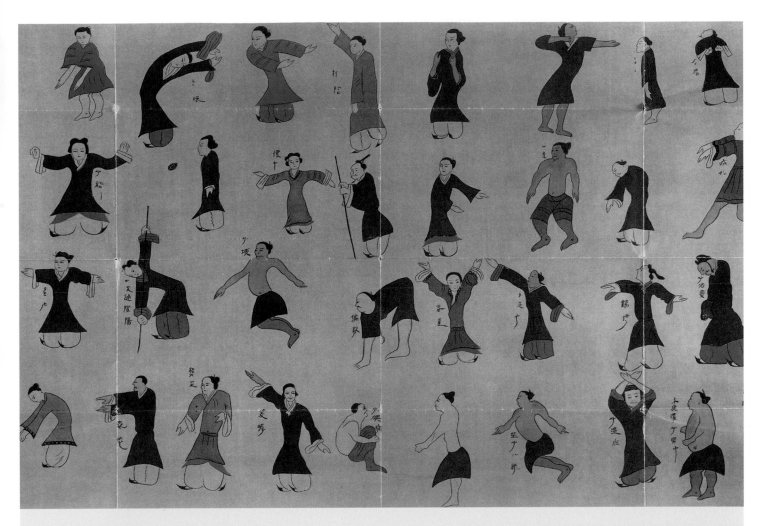

Lifestyle risk factors

From ancient times, certain 'lifestyle' patterns have been recognized as factors that can lead to ill-health, disability and premature death: eating too much, drinking too much alcohol, not exercising enough; and occupational hazards – in mines, mills, manufacturing industries or sedentary occupations.

In recent decades, studies based on population surveys have confirmed the link between smoking and lung cancer, as well as chronic obstructive pulmonary disease (COPD) and cardiovascular diseases (CVDs). CVDs (disorders of the heart and blood vessels) are the number one cause of death globally: an estimated 17.3 million people die from CVDs annually, with lower-income countries disproportionately affected.

It is estimated that behavioural risk factors, from physical inactivity to alcohol abuse, are responsible for about 80 per cent of CVDs and over 30 per cent of all cancers. Obesity is a major factor explaining the recent rise in type 2 diabetes. 'Prevention is better than cure' is an important message in reducing the toll of many of the non-communicable diseases.

This 20th-century Chinese exercise chart (*Daoyin tu*) contains animal postures such as the bear walk. It is based on a 'Guiding and Pulling Chart' found in a 168 BC tomb in the former kingdom of Changsha.

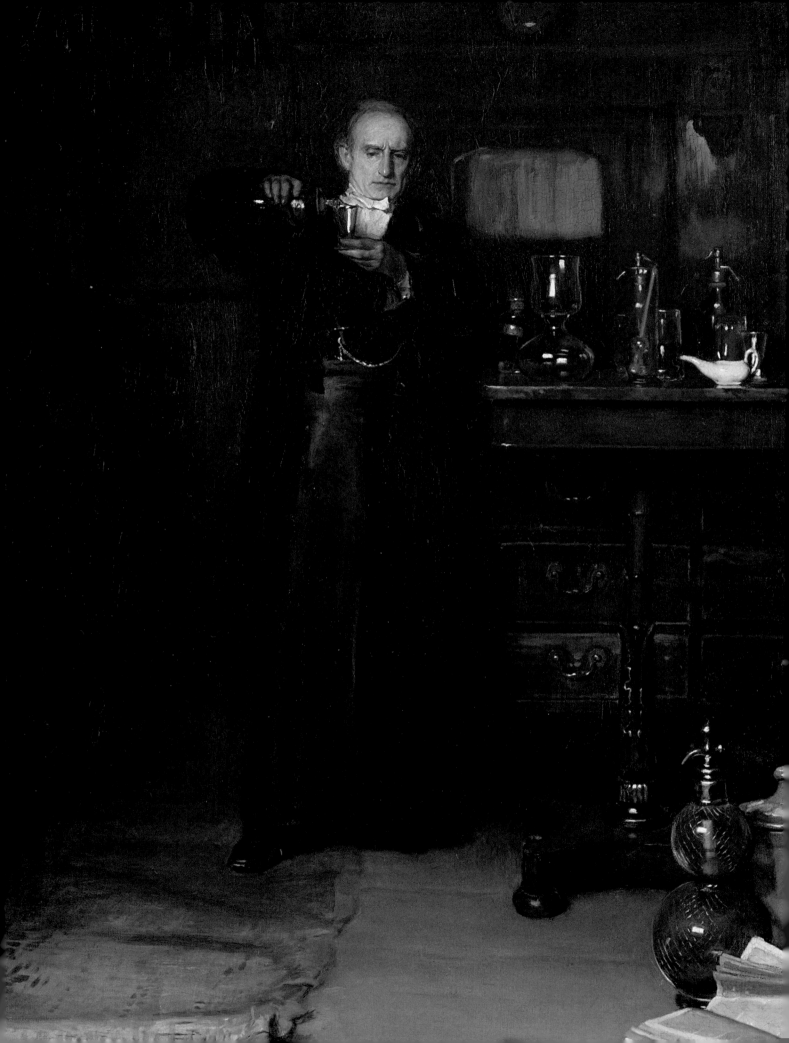

Physicians and Healers

We doctors have always been a simple, trusting folk!
Did we not believe Galen implicitly for fifteen hundred
years and Hippocrates for more than two thousand years?

William Osler, 1909

Over the centuries, countless men and women have devoted their lives to tending, healing, and curing the sick. Some physicians have achieved fame and even fortune; some have been infamous. Many early physicians received their training by following their mentors and learning "on the job." There were also several important medical schools in antiquity and in the medieval Islamic world, while formal medical education in the Christian West began in the Middle Ages with the School of Salerno in Italy. Within the medical marketplace of the medieval and early modern period, there were many types of healers and medical practitioners: quack doctors, alchemists, plague doctors, barber-surgeons, apothecaries, herbalists, spiritual healers, priests, midwives, and nurses who offered their services (often for a fee) to the sick and dying. In the modern era, there are still various different groups of healers, from doctors and nurses trained in Western medicine, to practitioners of traditional, alternative, or complementary medicine.

Doctors in the ancient world

The art has three factors, the disease, the patient, the physician. The physician is the servant of the art.

Hippocrates, *Epidemics I*

It is difficult to gauge how far back in time human societies selected key members to act as healers, the equivalent of the medicine man or shaman still found in traditional cultures today. Cave paintings found in various localities, including France (*c.*17,000 years old), depicting men masked in animal heads, performing ritual dances, are possibly the oldest surviving images of medicine men.

OPPOSITE *Doubtful Hope* by Frank Holl (1875) shows a doctor preparing medicine for a sick child. The title and physician's expression are poignant reminders that while a doctor might care for his patients he was not always able find a cure. One in six babies died in their first year at this time and life expectancy was 43 years, compared to around 80 in Britain today.

Egyptian practitioners used a range of methods and treatments, including surgery, pharmacy as well as magic spells, rituals, and prayers.

Looking at the early civilizations in Mesopotamia (largely corresponding to modern Iraq), we get some fascinating glimpses of a range of healers as well as our first insight into medical negligence. There are about a thousand extant clay tablets with cuneiform writing, from the 1st millennium BC, bearing the professional writings of ancient healers. These are chiefly "medical omens" and therapeutic prescriptions, incantations, and rituals. In the *Diagnostic-Prognostic Handbook*, sometimes on the basis of certain symptoms, named diseases are diagnosed, such as eye disorders, distended bellies, and even a "stinking disease," but more often the only "diagnosis" was to attribute the malady to a particular deity.

The Code of Hammurabi, named after the Babylonian King and dating from around the 18th century BC, provided for malpractice and liability for negligent medical care. Babylonian healers—diviners (*Bōrû*) and priests-exorcists (*Āshipu*)—could not be held responsible for illness caused by the gods or evil spirits, but a physician (*Asû*) using a "bronze lancet" to treat a patient was accountable for direct human error. Penalties were varied, and one rule states: "if a physician makes a major incision on a man with the operating knife, and kills the man, or opens a man's temple with the operating knife, and blinds the man's eye, his hand shall be cut off."

In ancient Egypt, there is evidence of a variety of physicians, including royal and court physicians, temple and priest-physicians, magicians, as well as specialist *swnw*, as for example, a "herdsman of the anus." According to the 5th-century BC Greek historian Herodotus:

> The art of medicine is so divided among them that each physician applies himself to one disease, and not more. All places abound in physicians; some physicians are for the eyes, others for the head, others for the teeth or the belly, and some for hidden maladies (internal disorders).

Egyptian practitioners used a range of methods and treatments, including surgery and pharmacy, as well as magic spells, rituals, and prayers. In diagnosing disease, as described in the medical papyri, the doctor asked the patient about symptoms and examined outward signs of disease—studying the sputum, urine, feces, and other bodily emanations—including in one case smelling a skull wound that was likened to "the urine of sheep." They then checked the pulse for "it is there that the heart speaks … it is there that every physician and every priest of Sekhmet places his fingers." They might also palpate the "belly" and feel for swellings.

One of the most fascinating reflections on early Chinese medicine was written by the Chinese polymath Shen Guo in the 12th century AD:

> The ancients treated patients, they became familiar with the cycles of yin and yang and of time, and with the exhalations of qi from mountain, forest, river and marsh. They discerned the patient's age, body, weight, social status, style of life, disposition, likes, feelings, and vigour. In accord with what was appropriate to these characteristics, and avoiding what was not, they chose among drugs, moxa, acupuncture, lancing with the stone needle, decoctions and extracts. They straightened out old habits and manipulated patterns of emotions … and would go on to regulate the patient's dress, rationalize his diet, change his living habits.

This ancient "holistic" approach to healing is still a characteristic of contemporary Traditional Chinese Medicine, Ayurveda, and other Eastern medical traditions. It also bears similarities to the ancient Greek and Roman approach to healing. Hippocrates was one of the most famous and influential of all ancient physicians. Born on the island of Cos, in the Aegean, around 460 BC, it is believed that he spent much time traveling around Greece and Asia Minor. While the Hippocratic approach to medicine was objective and rational, he also reminds us that medicine is an "art" and a "long" one! One of his many aphorisms: "art is long, life is short, opportunity fleeting, experience dangerous, judgment difficult," reads in Latin:

ars longa, vita brevis, occasio praeceps, experimentum periculosum, iudicium difficile.

In Hippocratic medicine, diagnosis relied on asking the patient a series of questions and effective treatment was achieved by considering the individual patient as a whole. Diet, sleep, work, and exercise were all seen as important ways of restoring health following an imbalance in humors that was believed to result in illness. Prognosis (foreseeing and foretelling the outcome of the disease) was a favorite topic of the Hippocratic healers. The well-known ancient code of medical practice, the Hippocratic Oath, was introduced in ancient Greece (probably by one of Hippocrates's followers)—an ethical framework to be recited by those entering the medical profession.

One of the most famous formal Greek medical schools of antiquity, at Alexandria in Hellenic Egypt, flourished from the early 4th century BC to the late 3rd century AD. The Greek physicians Herophilus and his contemporary Erasistratus taught there, carrying out what may have been the first human anatomical dissections (see page 28). The Greco-Roman physician Galen received some of his early training and experience at Alexandria in the 2nd century AD. Later in Rome he was a physician for leading senators, dignitaries and, from AD 169, the households of emperors, including Marcus Aurelius (while also treating ordinary people). He was renowned for practising on patients with a crowd of spectators around him— also spectacular were his public dissections of animals.

Like Hippocrates, Galen's influence on medical theory over the following 1,700 years cannot be underestimated. As a practitioner in the "art" of medicine, Galen prided himself on being a "fine physician," though as one doctor writing in the 1780s noted, "he shewed the greatest impudence and temerity towards all regular practitioners; and ... went so far as to assert that he himself was the only [physician] who deserved that title."

As in other epochs, there was a wide range of other spiritual healers in ancient Greece and Rome—priests, diviners, and exorcists. Empirics, guided by practical experience, were all too eager to offer their services. Self-help was universal and families were very much involved with the healing process.

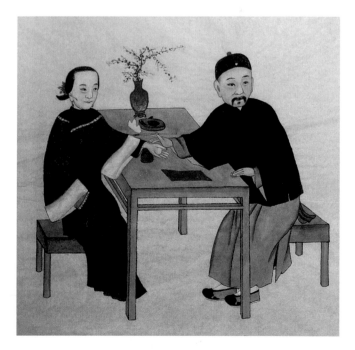

A Chinese doctor taking the pulse of a patient, *c.* 1890. In traditional Chinese medicine, different diseases are associated with particular qualities of the patient's pulse.

Medical education from medieval Islam to Renaissance Europe

In the medieval Islamic world there were impressive hospitals (*bimaristans*) for treating patients and teaching aspiring physicians. The polymath and physician Razi (AD *c.*865–*c.*925), practiced medicine at a number of these hospitals, including Baghdad, an unrivaled center for the study of medicine, science, and the humanities, until its destruction during the Mongol invasion of Baghdad in AD 1258. The advice given by one 10th-century Arabic physician, Haly Abbas, in his *Complete Book of the Medical Art* to medical students is as timely today as it was then:

> *One of the requirements for the student of this art is that he should be in attendance at the hospitals and the places of the sick; that he consult extensively with the most skilled teachers among the physicians about their patients' situations and circumstances; and that he examine frequently the conditions of the patients and the symptoms apparent in them, calling to mind what he has read about these conditions and what they indicate of good and ill.*

Razi, however, recognized that even highly skilled physicians did not have all the answers and wrote the aptly titled text *On the Fact that Even the Most Skilful of Physicians Cannot Heal All Diseases.*

In the 10th century, a confluence of Christian, Arabic, Greek, and Jewish medical thought from around the Mediterranean basin came together at the first medical school in Christian Europe in Salerno, southern Italy. Roger of Salerno expressed the formality of its medical

Kill or cure!! This quack promises cures for social situations and professions, including "Scandal Drops for Olde Maids" and "Sublime Elixir for Poets" in this satirical print, *c.* 1802.

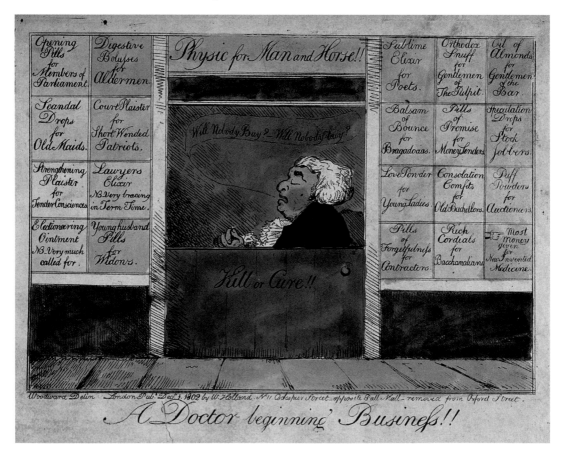

education: "who, from now on, wishes to practice medicine, has to present himself before our officials and examiners, in order to pass their judgment." The Salerno course took five years, preceded by three years' study of logic. The famous, lengthy 13th-century poem or "home health manual" "Regimen Sanitatis Salernitanum" ("Salernitan Regime of Health") was also a product of this school. It is well remembered for its couplet [in a 1608 translation]:

> Use three Physicians still; first Doctor Quiet,
> Next Doctor Merry-man, and Doctor Dyet.

By the Renaissance, medical teaching was flourishing in European universities: Bologna, Padua, Naples, and Pavia in Italy; Paris and Montpelier in France; and Oxford and Cambridge in England. Latin was, originally, the language of medicine and much was taught by reading and learning the ancient texts. There is only one recorded case of a qualified woman doctor, Dr Laura Bassi (1711–78), who was appointed Professor of Anatomy at the University of Bologna, Italy, in 1732.

There were tensions at this time, especially in northern Europe, between medical practitioners. Physicians were those qualified or licenced to practice medicine using drugs, while surgeons or barber-surgeons practiced a "handi-craft"—sometimes combining cutting hair, cutting corns, extracting teeth with bloodletting, and amputating limbs. A curious hangover from the old days is that male surgeons today in parts of the English-speaking world—however eminent—are still referred to as "Mr" (a variant of Master) rather than "Dr" (the word "doctor" is from the Latin, *docere*, "to teach").

Quacks in early modern Europe

Quacks are the greatest liars in the world except their patients.

Benjamin Franklin (1706-90)

So-called "quack" doctors in early modern Europe, as in earlier centuries, offered their services alongside the elite and professionally trained physicians, leading to considerable rivalry. In England, a small group of physicians led by the scholar Thomas Linacre (*c.*1460–1524) petitioned King Henry VIII (1491–1547) to establish the College of Physicians in London in 1518 (the Royal College of Physicians from 1674), similar to those founded in several other European countries. They wanted the power to grant licenses to men qualified to practice medicine and to punish unqualified practitioners and anyone engaged in malpractice.

The first mention of quacks in English literature appeared in *Schoole of Abuse*, printed in 1579, which referred to "a quacksalver's budget of filthy receites." Its derivation may be from the Dutch *kwaksalver*, meaning hawker of salves, or the German *quacksalber* for quicksilver or mercury, a treatment for syphilis—one of the specialties of the quack doctor.

Quacks such as the "horse mountebanks" were often itinerant salesmen—proclaiming from the saddle and selling their wares with much fanfare, quickly moving on before their dubious pills, powders, and cordials were discovered to be useless. An advertisement in the Bristol press in 1783 by a Mr Farland claimed he could cure:

> Broken bodies ... in six weeks without trusses; Cancers ... without incision ... all Diseases of the
> eye even when blind; ... Hare-lip in eight days; venereal disease of ever so long standing.

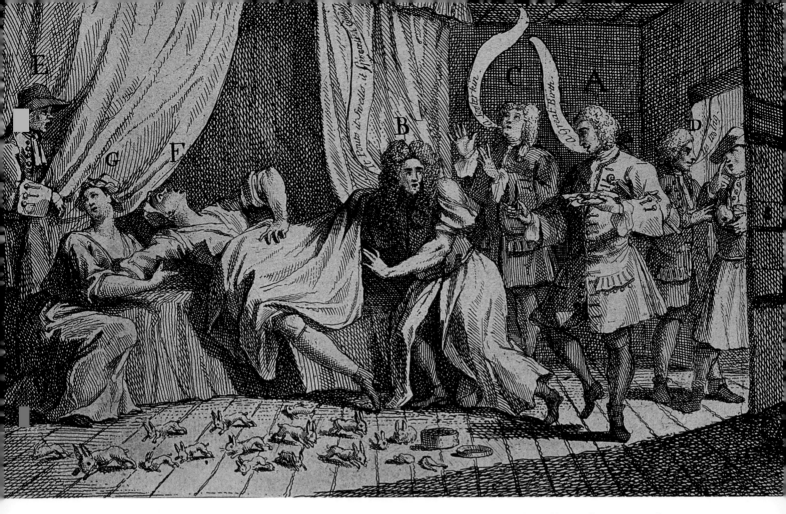

Medical hoaxes made for sensational headlines. In 1726 Mary Tofts reportedly gave birth to rabbits. In fact, an accomplice had inserted into her vagina parts of a cat and dead baby rabbits. Bridewell Gaol was her reward.

Some empiric quack healers might claim a specific skill, such as bonesetting or urine casting ("piss-prophets'). There were even "ass-doctors" who believed that all diseases must be expelled *per anus*. Female quacks were known as "petticoat quacks."

The early modern period was a high peak of quackery. Individuals such as Mrs Sally Mapp, or Crazy Sal the "bonesetter" (d. 1737), and James Graham (1745–94), who set up his extraordinary Temple of Hymen in Pall Mall, London, designed to help couples with their sexual problems, became famous.

Alchemists, astrologers, and the Royal Touch

Alchemists were another group of interesting and diverse practitioners found in many parts of the world, including Egypt, China, India, the Middle East, and Europe. Alchemists taught that earthly substances were controlled by supernatural powers, and attempted to create new metallic and natural compounds by mixing existing elements together. They wanted to make valuable gold and silver, but some also searched for the "philosopher's stone" and the "elixir of life." Some form of alchemy was practiced by Jabir ibn Hayyan and Razi in medieval Islam. In Britain, well-known followers of alchemy included Roger Bacon (1214–94), George Ripley (c. 1415–90) and John Dee (1527–1608), trusted advisor to Queen Elizabeth I. Alchemical scrolls, known as Ripley scrolls, with symbolic drawings and secrets, can be seen in a number of museums and libraries.

Alchemy in medicine was promoted by the Swiss healer Theophrastus Philippus Aureolus Bombastus von Hohenheim (c.1493–1541), who called himself Paracelsus. He traveled widely and gained considerable knowledge: "I have not been ashamed," he wrote, "to learn from tramps, butchers, and barbers." These influences led him to reject much of Galenic and university-taught medicine. He was also dismissive of the traditional view of the four humors. He argued that the body was a chemical system that had to be balanced both internally and in harmony with the environment. On the basis of this idea, Paracelsus introduced new chemical substances into medicine, including the use of the metal mercury for the treatment of syphilis. In 1527 he was appointed to the University of Basel, Switzerland, where he overthrew convention by publicly burning the books of Galen and Ibn Sina, and was expelled from Basel a year later.

Some physicians, including Paracelsus, combined their medical or alchemical skills with the ancient practice of astrology. Simon Forman (1552–1611) was one of London's best-known physicians and self-proclaimed master of the occult during the Elizabethan era. When a patient visited him with a question, such as "what is my disease?," "am I pregnant?," "will I die?," Forman would "cast a figure," an astrological computation of the stars. Thousands of celestial configurations were possible and the chart would result in a verdict. He was highly popular in London among a large clientele and was consulted by more than 2,000 patients a year. The medical establishment, by contrast, branded him the worst of the "unlearned and unlawful practitioners, lurking in many corners of the city." Forman and his pupil, the clergyman-astrologer-physician Reverend Richard Napier (1559–1634), kept over 50,000 case notes—which are currently being digitized by Cambridge historian Lauren Kassell. Among the cases of "deep depression," over fifty were attributed to grief following children's deaths.

Somewhat bizarrely, royalty in France and England for centuries fancied themselves as Godly medical healers of one specific disease—scrofula or the "King's Evil" (a glandular form of tuberculosis). They laid their hands on sufferers in a ceremony known as the Royal Touch, occurring on special days. In England the practice dates from the early 11th century. Samuel Pepys (1633–1703) and John Evelyn (1620–1706) gave graphic descriptions of overcrowded ceremonies during Stuart times: some people were crushed to death. Charles X of France (r. 1824–30) gave the last performance in 1825. The term "scrofula" is the diminutive of the Latin *scrofa*, meaning "a breeding sow"—the puffy appearance of someone with swollen lymph glands in the neck apparently resembled "a little pig."

Bedside medicine: observing and listening to the patient

Thomas Sydenham (1624–89) is often called the "English Hippocrates." While many of his bookish contemporaries were sniffing and peering at urine (uroscopy) without even visiting their patients, dissecting the dead in the cause of "science," or gaining fame or fortune from their quackish enterprises, Sydenham valued observation and experience. In his clinical descriptions of disease observed at the bedside, he left many graphic accounts of gout, hysteria, smallpox, and other illnesses. He began to classify diseases (nosology) and recognized that the same disease produced the same symptoms in different people. He treated many poor people using trial and error to work out the best cures and advised students: "as for anatomy, my butcher can dissect a joint full and well; no young man ... you must go to the bedside, it is there alone that you can learn disease."

Hermann Boerhaave (1668–1738), of the University of Leiden in the Netherlands, closely studied his patients at a hospital designed specifically for teaching; he attracted many students from all over Europe. His case report of a man who died from a ruptured esophagus inaugurated the sequence of clinical history, examination and autopsy findings. Boerhaave's introduction of a medical curriculum of natural science, anatomy, physiology, and pathology was to influence the new schools of 18th-century medicine in Edinburgh, Vienna, Göttingen, and Philadelphia.

With the appointment, in 1726, of Leiden-trained Alexander Monro, *primus* (1697–1767) to the Edinburgh school, a special twelve-bedded ward was set aside to teach students—including many Americans who received medical degrees from Edinburgh. The Edinburgh-educated US physician Benjamin Rush (1745–1813), a student of the influential physician William Cullen (1710–90), the "Scottish Hippocrates," learned to place great emphasis on the medical history of the patient by interrogation: "endeavour to get the history of the disease from the patient himself," he advised:

> *How long has he been sick? When attacked and in what manner? What are the probable causes, former habits and dress; likewise the diet, etc., for a week before especially in acute diseases … in chronic diseases enquire their complaints far back and the habits of life.*

The real transformation in "bedside" medicine occurred in the late 18th and early 19th centuries, especially in post-Revolution France, where large new municipal hospitals enabled students from Europe and the USA to learn on the wards rather than from ancient Greek and Latin texts. Prodding and probing the patient, as far as decorum permitted, was encouraged. One simple but revolutionary innovation was the stethoscope invention of 1816 by the French physician René Laënnec. While working at the Neckar Hospital in Paris, he had wanted to listen to the heart of a young, somewhat plump, female patient, but felt it inappropriate to do anything as intimate as putting his head so close to her bosom. So he rolled up his notebook and put one end on the young lady's chest and the other to his ear. He could clearly hear not only the sounds of her heart but also her breathing. Soon a hollow wooden stethoscope was being used, later developing into a flexible version. As Roy Porter wrote:

> *By giving access to body noises – the sounds of breathing, the blood gurgling around the heart – the stethoscope changed approaches to internal disease and hence doctor-patient relations. At last, the living body was no longer a closed book: pathology could now be done on the living.*

There were no great breakthroughs in treatment and therapy over the course of the medieval and early modern period, and physicians came in for a good deal of mockery as Matthew Prior quipped in 1714: "cur'd yesterday of my Disease, I died last night of my Physician." On the other hand, there was much imagined illness—most of us know a hypochondriac! In anatomical terms the *hypochondrium* is the region of the abdomen just below the ribs, and the organs beneath this area were believed by the ancient Greeks to be the source of disordered emotions. The term describes a fear of illness or a preoccupation with bodily symptoms. Charles Darwin, troubled by numerous puzzling ailments, wrote: "many of my friends, I believe, think me a hypochondriac."

OPPOSITE This 19th-century doctor is looking at (and probably smelling or even tasting) a patient's urine sample. This practice of uroscopy for diagnosing disease dated back to ancient times.

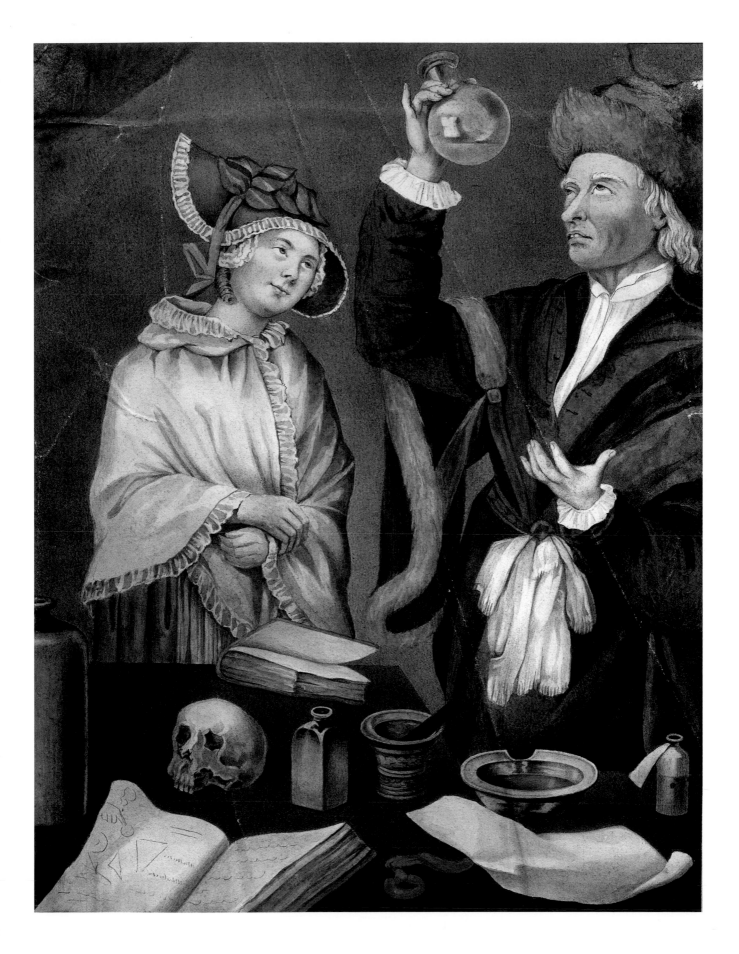

The "Elephant Man"

Joseph Merrick (1862–90) was known as the "Elephant Man" after a childhood condition of disfiguring tumors (now thought to be Proteus syndrome) worsened. He and the owner of a local music hall developed a successful act for the public. On arriving in London, Merrick attracted the attention of doctors, including the surgeon Frederick Treves (1853–1923), who took him to the London Hospital to both examine and care for him. Merrick died unexpectedly in 1890. His skeleton is housed in The London School of Medicine and Surgery, and is now being examined using new scanning techniques.

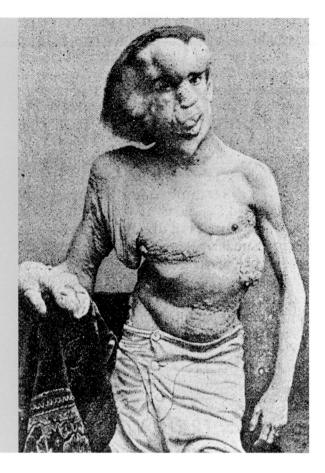

The "Elephant Man" from a photograph taken in 1889 showing the extent of Merrick's deformities.

"Typhoid Mary"

"Typhoid Mary" aka Mary Mallon (c.1869–1938) was described by one magazine in 1910 as "the most harmless and yet most dangerous woman in America." She was a cook for wealthy New Yorkers, and wherever Mary worked, people came down with the dreaded typhoid fever. An investigation followed and it was discovered that her stools contained high concentrations of the typhoid bacilli—she was a typhoid carrier but remained asymptomatic. Mary was quarantined at Riverside Hospital in North Brother Island, New York, and released on condition that she would no longer work as a cook. However, when typhoid broke out in the Sloane Maternity Hospital, she was discovered working there as "Mrs Brown." She spent the rest of her life in an isolation hospital.

Women qualify in medicine

For centuries, it was difficult, if not impossible, for women to enter medicine, although they had always played a role in nursing and midwifery. The Edinburgh-trained army surgeon James Barry, who died in 1865, was revealed as a woman: Margaret Ann Bulkley. Meanwhile in the USA, British-born Elizabeth Blackwell (1821–1910) was the first woman to graduate openly from Geneva Medical College in upstate New York in 1849. In Britain, Elizabeth Garrett Anderson (1836–1917) was awarded a license to practice medicine from the Society of Apothecaries in 1865, and five years later gained a medical degree in Paris.

These doctors were enormously influential in encouraging other women to enter medicine and in establishing some of the first medical training schools and hospitals for women. But it took much longer for young women to establish their role as physicians alongside male colleagues. Today, female applicants to medical school outnumber males in some countries, but women are underrepresented at the professorial and consultant level.

Science and the "quiet art" of medicine

Doctors, together with nurses, played an increasing role in administering to the sick poor in hospitals over the course of the 19th century. Some physicians combined charitable work with lucrative private practices for the wealthy. In London, Harley Street emerged in the late 19th century as the fashionable quarter for eminent—and well-paid—consultants; a knowledge of science and bacteriology added to their air of respectability. Other doctors began to specialize in a particular field of medicine or concentrated on medical research and teaching. There were also a number of physicians who pioneered "alternative" fields of medicine: Franz Mesmer, mesmerism; Samuel Hahnemann, homeopathy; Daniel Palmer, chiropractic; and Andrew Still, osteopathy (see Complementary and Alternative Medicine).

One of the greatest all-round clinical physicians was the Canadian William Osler (1849–1919), who entered medicine just as the understanding of germs as a cause of infection was finally being given scientific verification. Among his widely read works was *The Principles and Practice of Medicine: Designed For the Use of Practitioners and Students of Medicine,* which combined the science and art of medicine. This "father of modern medicine" urged students to learn the scientific principles of medicine and to "observe, record, tabulate, communicate. Use your five senses. It is much more important to know what sort of a patient has a disease than what sort of disease a patient has."

Some practitioners continued to work from private surgeries (often in their own homes). In Britain, from the early 19th century, general practitioners emerged from earlier groups such as the surgeon-apothecaries, broadening their roles from drugmakers and dispensers to general doctors who diagnosed and treated the sick. As Roy Porter noted: "there were thousands of anonymous, unsung, overworked practitioners, haunted by bad debts and dying patients." The nostalgic image of the old-style family doctor was captured by the American physician Carl Binger (1889–1976):

> *Time was ... when the family doctor delivered babies and supervised their nursing, their weaning and their teething, when he vaccinated them and saw them through their measles and chicken pox and whooping cough. He told the boy about the facts of life and treated the girl for her menstrual cramps. He advised about diet and rest, gave spring tonic, clipped tonsils, set a broken arm, reassured father who couldn't sleep because of business worries, pulled mother through a case of typhoid or double pneumonia, reprimanded the cook, who was found on her day out to have a dozen empty whisky bottles in her clothes closet, gave advice about the young man's choice of college and profession, comforted grandma, who was losing her memory and becoming more irritable, and closed grandpa's eyes in his final sleep.*

Despite there still being little in the way of real cures in the early 20th century, that "quiet art" of healing was essential. Arthur Hertzler in his 1938 autobiography, *The Horse and Buggy Doctor,* wrote: "regardless of what the old doctor was able to accomplish in a therapeutic way, the sense of security inspired by the doctor's arrival affected the patients and family favourably."

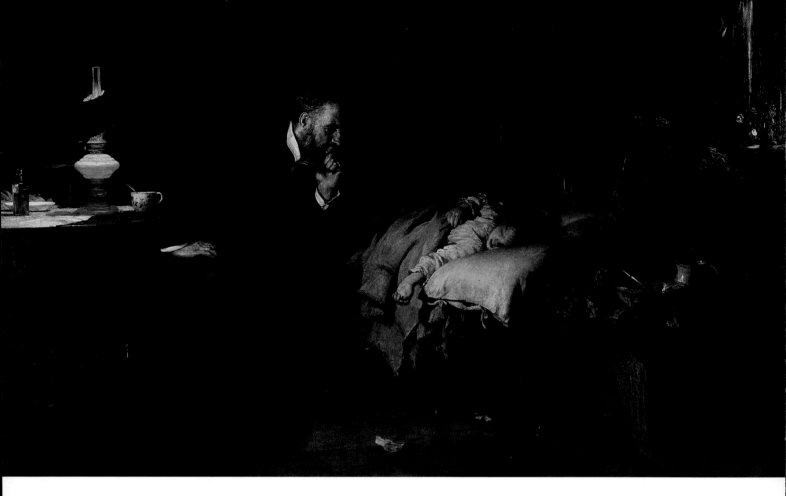

Sir Luke Fildes, *The Doctor* (1891). A family physician on a home visit watches carefully over a sick child, reflecting the "quiet art" of medicine.

Transforming the practice of medicine in the modern age

Infectious diseases like diphtheria, scarlet fever, measles, meningitis, and whooping cough remained frightening killers especially of children well into the 20th century. Medical practice was transformed by the discovery and availability of new therapeutic treatments, especially penicillin from the late 1940s, followed by other "wonder drugs" and vaccines (such as the polio vaccine from the 1950s), as well as improvements in medical education and public health. Primary health-care doctors (general practitioners or GPs in Britain and family physicians in the USA) could now prescribe effective ways of treating patients, or refer serious and surgical cases to hospital specialists.

Reforms to make health care available "for all" have also made a difference in some parts of the world. Otto von Bismarck (1815–98), first Chancellor of Germany, introduced an early "national" health insurance scheme based on shared contributions from employers and employees in 1883. In 1948 the National Health Service (NHS) was introduced to Britain providing free primary and hospital health care "at the point of delivery" and paying the salaries of NHS employees. Japan was the first non-Western country to provide universal health insurance when, in 1961, it introduced *kaihoken*. There is still huge variation in who pays for the ever-escalating costs of medical care and treatments and, with longer life expectancies, the need to care for an increasingly elderly population is one of the major challenges for modern societies.

Global variations in the burden of disease and disability are also compounded by wide disparities in the provision of medical personnel. Data for 2010 show that there is one doctor for every 200–500 or so inhabitants in parts of the world such as North America, Britain, Australia, and Japan. But in some sub-Saharan African countries that ratio can be as little as one doctor for every 30,000–50,000 inhabitants.

Advances in technology are enabling physicians to screen and diagnose diseases more quickly and accurately than previously. Telemedicine enables a physician to "see" a patient remotely. Smartphones and medical apps can be used by patients to monitor, for example, blood sugar levels; blood pressure; heartbeat; suspicious moles; cholesterol; hearing, vision and memory loss; behavioral changes, etc., with the added prospect that results can also be beamed wirelessly to the doctor. In the US scientists are developing a high-tech breath monitor that aims to examine exhaled air for signs of disease—an interesting reflection on the centuries-old medical practice of sniffing and tasting a patient's urine.

As medicine moves into this high-tech age we have much to learn from ancient Hippocratic traditions of "bedside medicine" and also from Traditional Chinese Medicine, Kampo, and Ayurveda, systems that retain the "holistic" and personalized approach to healing. The future for the health of the world lies in the integration of all that is best in the "science" and the "quiet art" of medicine.

X-rays to CT, PET, and MRI scans

The discovery of X-rays in 1895 by Wilhelm Conrad Röntgen (1845–1923), professor of physics at the University of Würzburg, in Bavaria, was a remarkable breakthrough. This image is an early X-ray of his wife's hand, showing a ring she was wearing.

Later diagnostic imaging techniques, include: computerized axial tomography (CAT scans), positron emission tomography (PET scans), and magnetic resonance imaging (MRI). These new tools, developed in the 1960s and 1970s, transformed the way radiologists and clinicians in hospitals could "see" and detect abnormalities in the patient. Ultrasound scanners can be used to provide vivid images of the fetus in the womb.

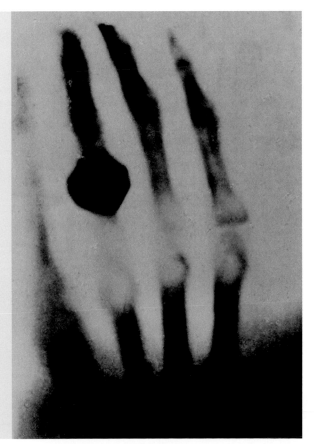

Have you answered the Red Cross
Christmas Roll Call?

Hospitals and Nursing Care

"Six of the patients have died, sir,"
said the hospital nurse to the physician,
as he went on his rounds.

"Why, I wrote medicine for seven,"
mused the doctor, passing to another ward.
"Yes, but one of them wouldn't take his,"
was the naïve reply.

Anon, c.1850

The ancient Greeks had "temples of healing," while the Romans set up *valetudinaria* or military hospitals. In the medieval and early modern period, there were a range of hospitals and "hospices" from the impressive *bimaristans* of the Islamic world to those run by charitable and religious orders offering "shelter" to nurse the sick and poor. By the 18th century, some of the large urban hospitals in Europe were described as overcrowded, smelly, and dirty. Florence Nightingale in the later 19th century was instrumental in promoting reforms in hospitals and nursing care. In the modern era, physicians, surgeons, nurses, and midwives (and ancillary staff) now share the role of offering treatments, care, and comfort to both in- and outpatients, while some hospitals have also become leading centers of medical teaching and research.

Early temples of healing

In ancient Greece healing shrines acted as places where the sick could pray for recovery from a great variety of illnesses from headaches, indigestion, and worms, to infertility and blindness. These were known as *Asclepieia*, after the Greek god of medicine and healing, Asclepius. The surroundings encouraged self-therapy through exercise, mental stimulus, and relaxation; some had a gymnasium, library, and theater.

A distinctive feature was the practice of *incubatio* or "temple sleep" involving ritual purification and a sacrifice to the god, followed by sleep in a special dormitory, where it was hoped Asclepius would interpret their dreams, and either perform a cure, or pass on directions of how to achieve a cure. Sometimes the patient was cured by Asclepius's daughters, Panacea and Hygieia, who were assisted by nonvenomous snakes; the serpent-entwined rod of Asclepius has long been a symbol associated with medicine.

OPPOSITE This American poster calling for volunteers during the First World War highlights the role of nurses as an emblem of medical care. The International Red Cross movement was inspired by Swiss businessman Henry Dunant (1828–1910) in 1863, after he witnessed the appalling suffering of injured soldiers at the Battle of Solferino in 1859.

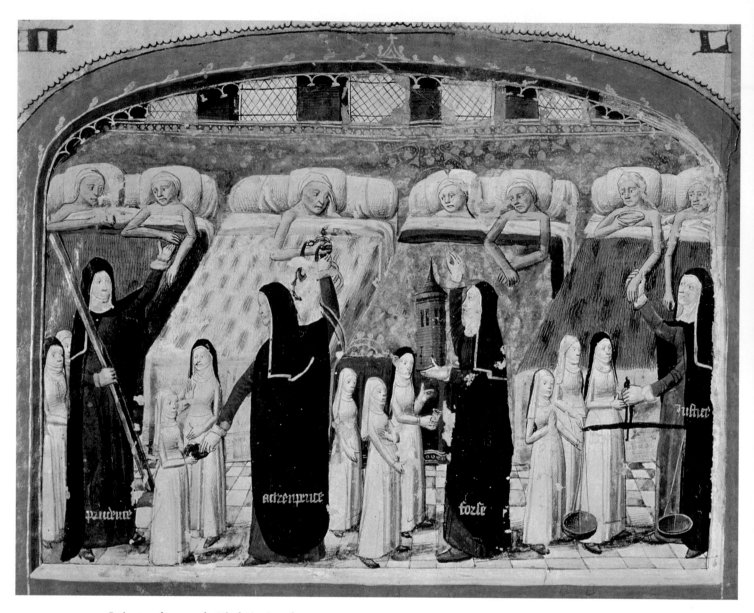

Patients and nuns at the Hôtel Dieu in 15th-century Paris. Early European hospitals provided care, comfort, and spiritual healing for the sick poor. They ranged from small religious houses to cathedral-like buildings, such as the 12th-century Pantokrator in Constantinople.

Numerous inscriptions and votive offerings in the form of clay models of the healed body parts have been left by grateful patients at the sites of these temples. In *c.* 500–400 BC, a patient sought help for a paralyzed hand by visiting Asclepius's shrine at Epidaurus—the most celebrated healing center of the classical world. An inscription of his experience notes: "when he fell asleep he saw a vision ... the god straightened out the fingers one by one ... and asked whether he still doubted the inscriptions. He said: No ... And when the day broke he went out cured."

The Roman *valetudinaria* (Latin, *valetudo*: "a state of health") were some of the first civic hospitals to offer medical and nursing care, especially to soldiers and slaves. As the Roman Empire expanded, field hospitals were set up to treat sick and wounded soldiers—a fighting-fit army was crucial to Rome's expansion plans. Some were permanent constructions at the main forts, others were simple structures, erected near the front lines.

Islamic *bimaristans*

Medieval Islamic *bimaristans* (from the Persian words, *bimar-*, meaning "ill person," and *-stan*, meaning "house") flourished from the 10th to the 12th centuries AD. When Razi was asked to choose a healthy location for a new hospital in Baghdad he selected the place after putting a few pieces of fresh meat in different locations to check which was the least spoilt, giving an indication of the freshest air.

All treatment and recovery in the *bimaristans* was free based on a clear obligation in Islamic belief to treat the sick regardless of their ability to pay. Moreover, they were willing to care for mentally ill and elderly people. Men and women were nursed in separate wards, but both male and female nurses cared for patients. These were secular rather than religious places and often employed Christian and Jewish, as well as Muslim, doctors.

The Nuri Bimaristan in Damascus, Syria, was one of the greatest hospitals in the Islamic world. One visitor commented in the 12th century AD, "doctors come early every day and check up on the patients. They order suitable drugs and foods for each patient." Music therapy and storytelling were used to relieve distress. Patients were given clothes and money on discharge to cover their expenses during convalescence.

Care, compassion, and charity in medieval and early modern Europe

For the majority of patients, hospital-based medical or nursing care was generally the exception rather than the norm and most people relied on home remedies or treatment from a local nurse, midwife, physician, or healer. In medieval and early modern Europe, "hospices" or "hospitals" provided nursing care, food, and shelter for the sick and the poor. Many of these were Christian religious foundations (dating back to the early Byzantine hospitals in the 4th century AD) and were established in the major towns or set up along routes of pilgrimage. Nursing was generally carried out by the "sisters" and "brothers" in religious orders. Benefactors took comfort in the fact that they would be saved from purgatory by the prayers of the grateful poor. Medicine and morality were inextricably linked and saving souls as well as lives was of utmost importance.

The origin of St Bartholomew's, a major London hospital today popularly known as Barts, is a fascinating story. In the early 12th century AD a young courtier and jester, Rahere, decided to go on a pilgrimage to Rome after witnessing one too many royal deaths. As he made his way through the unhealthy Pontine Marshes, near Rome, he contracted a serious fever (probably malaria). He was cared for by monks in a small hospital attached to a church dedicated to St Bartholomew, the apostle, on an island in the River Tiber. Rahere vowed that if God granted him health and a return to England, he would found his own hospital for the sick poor.

Recovered and back in London, Rahere gained the support of King Henry I (r. 1100–35) and the Bishop of London to build both St Bartholomew's Hospital, and a priory church, St Bartholomew the Great, at Smithfield in London, "to give help to ... every kind of sick person and homeless wanderer." In 1552, the hospital claimed to have cured 800 sick poor during the previous five years "of the pox, fistulas, filthy blanes, and sores." William Harvey, of blood circulation fame and physician to Charles I (r. 1625–49), was appointed hospital physician there from 1609–43.

The extent to which hospital patients received medical, rather than just nursing, care varied widely—in many cases, a physician made only occasional visits. Italy led the way in developing in-house medical services and their large hospitals were the envy of other early modern European countries. In 1500, the "splendid" Ospedale di Santa Maria Nuova in Florence focused on medical treatment by physicians, apothecaries, surgeons, and a large nursing staff. The sick were described as "dirty, smelly, and disagreeable," but the nurses, "running to and fro among the sick as they call," were said to be exemplary:

> To some they bring hot water, to others an infusion of barley water, to others a julep or sweet drink. They must hold some up, carry others, dress others, restrain others, and to others bring bedpans. Some of the sick cry out, others shiver, others are delirious. But the nurses bear it all and serve with piety and patience.

King Henry VII (r. 1485–1509) based his 1505 Savoy Hospital in London on this model. Many of the Italian hospitals trained young doctors and by the late 16th century had set up schools of anatomy. An idealistic vision of hospitals was captured by Thomas More (1478–1535) in his fictional work *Utopia* (1516):

> Every city [in Utopia] has four hospitals, slightly outside the walls and spacious enough to appear like little towns. The hospitals are large ... so that the sick ... will not be packed closely and uncomfortably together, and also so that those who have a contagious disease, such as might pass from one to the other, may be isolated. The hospitals are ... supplied with everything needed to cure the patients, who are nursed with tender and watchful care. Highly skilled physicians are in constant attendance ... Hardly anyone in the city ... would not rather be treated ... at hospital than at home.

Isolating the infectious

Although caring for the "sick and infirm with all kindness and mercy" was the aim of most religious and civic hospitals, some patients such as "lepers, the contagious, the insane, and pregnant women"—were often excluded.

For those suffering from the disfiguring disease leprosy (now known as Hansen's disease), separate institutions known as "leprosaria"—as many as 19,000—were set up during the 13th century in Europe. Medical historian Carole Rawcliffe, in *Leprosy in Medieval England* (2006), quotes a 14th-century English sermon, highlighting the role of the priest in providing a spiritual and physical regimen for "lepers":

> He gives us relief from our pain through contrition, and through confession we receive a purgative; he recommends a healthful diet through keeping of fasts; he orders therapeutic baths through our outpouring of tears; he prescribes bloodletting through our recollection of Christ's passion.

Following the spread of syphilis—the "Great Pox"—from the late 15th century, pox-houses were built, first in southwest Germany. In Italy some hospitals accepted incurables (*incurabili*) including syphilis victims. Patients were nursed by priests and nuns while the larger hospitals for such patients usually employed a physician and surgeon for daily visits. In Venice, the Ospedale degli Incurabili was built in 1522 in response to the spread of syphilis. There is a head with a sweetly sad expression over the door for those who did not recover, and a smiling head over a second door for the few who did.

Some of the medieval leper hospitals had been known as "Lock hospitals," referring to

Pest houses and bubonic plague

As leprosy retreated from medieval Europe (for reasons which are still not fully understood), the far more infectious and deadly disease of bubonic plague took center stage. Pest houses for plague were set up, often taking over the old medieval leper hospitals. Temporary shacks were also erected in areas downwind of the "pestilential vapors."

We can only imagine the horrors of these pest houses where the dangerously ill and "contagious" were crammed four or five in one bed. A cardinal in 1630 described the alarming conditions of the pest houses of Bologna, Italy, where he saw people "strip themselves to the skin, others die, others become black and deformed, others lose their minds," adding, "here you are overwhelmed by intolerable smells. Here you cannot walk but among corpses. Here you feel naught but the constant horror of death. This is a replica of hell."

This miniature, from the Swiss manuscript of the Toggenburg Bible, 1411, depicts a couple suffering from the buboes of the deadly Black Death that swept through Europe in the 14th century.

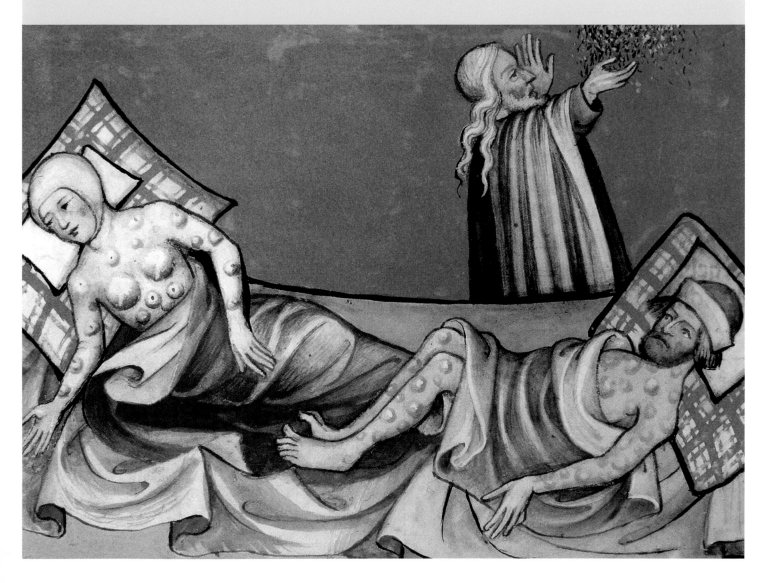

the bandages or "locks" that covered patient's sores. The name lived on in hospitals for the treatment of venereal diseases such as the famous London Lock Hospital, founded in 1746. It had a separate female ward that offered care for "females suffering from disorders contracted by a vicious course of life"—many of whom when admitted arrived "almost naked, penniless, and starving."

Smallpox was one of the most dreaded pestilences of the early modern world. With the disappearance of plague from Western Europe by the early 18th century, some of the old pest houses were adapted to isolate smallpox victims.

Hospitals for the "abandoned"

The Islamic hospitals with wards dedicated to the mentally ill may have been unique in the medieval world. In Catholic countries, religious institutions traditionally cared for those deemed "insane" or "mad," otherwise care rested with the community or families. The notorious "madhouse" of London's Bethlem Royal Hospital (known as "Bedlam") had been founded by Christians in 1247 to care for the homeless. By the 14th century it was admitting patients "deprived of their reason" and gained a grim reputation for its inhumane treatment of inmates.

Another specialist institution was the foundling hospital that took in abandoned babies, and many of these were established worldwide. These facilities often had a receiving cradle attached to a revolving door. The depositor rang a bell to announce the arrival of the "little stranger." The door would turn, accepting the infant into the hospital and protecting the depositor's anonymity. The London Foundling Hospital (1741) was started by Thomas Coram (c.1668–1751), a retired sea captain, who was appalled at seeing "young Children exposed, sometimes alive, sometimes dying" or their corpses heaped on dunghills or in the gutters. He gained the support of rich philanthropists, including William Hogarth (1697–1764) and George Frideric Handel (1685–1759). Tokens, left by mothers along with their babies, can still be seen today at the Foundling Hospital Museum. One poignant heart-shaped metal pendant simply declares: "You have my Heart, Tho' we must Part."

Hospitals in the 18th and 19th centuries: gateways to death?

The Hôtel Dieu (Hostel of God) in Paris was described by the encyclopaedist Denis Diderot (1713–84) as:

> The biggest, roomiest, richest and most terrifying of all our hospitals ... Imagine every kind of patient, sometimes packed three, four, or six into a bed, the living alongside the dead and dying, the air polluted by this mass of sick bodies, passing the pestilential germs of their affections from one to the other, and the spectacle of suffering and agony on every hand.

Founded around AD 651, by the 18th century this medieval hospital housed 3,500 patients crowded into 1,200 beds. The ventilation was so bad that staff would enter it holding a sponge dipped in vinegar to their faces.

As population numbers in the 18th and early 19th centuries soared, especially in the burgeoning urban and industrial areas, some, but not all, hospitals gained a dire reputation for their verminous, filthy conditions and high mortality rates. Physician John Aiken described the worst as "gateways to death," while philanthropist-reformer John Howard (1726–90) found much to criticize during his tour of European hospitals in the 1770–80s. He noted that

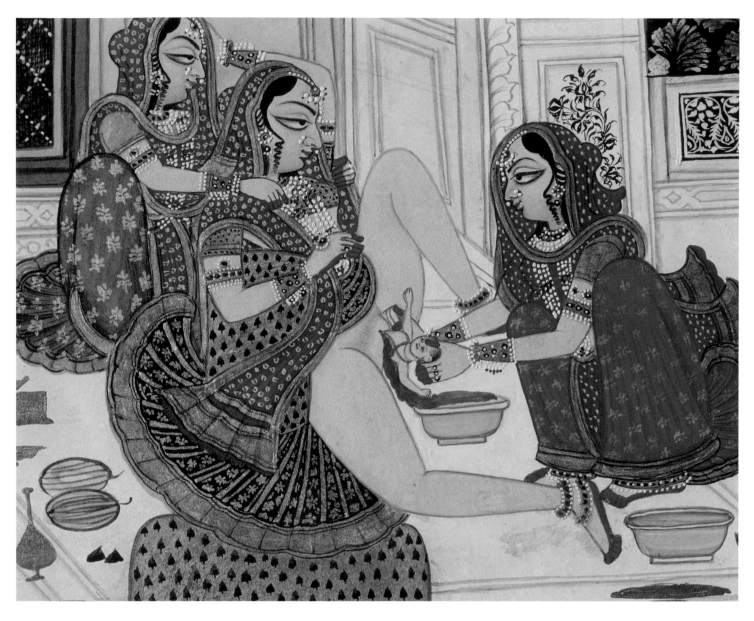

Indian midwives delivering a baby shown in a painting from 1825. Midwifery, like nursing, evolved over the centuries before becoming an established profession in the 20th century with formal training in schools of midwifery.

the old wards at Guy's Hospital, London (established in 1726), had bedbug infested wooden beds—a bug-catcher was on the permanent staff, apparently at a salary equal to the doctors'.

The wealthy continued to give birth and be treated or operated on at home or sometimes in the physician's private consulting rooms. Hospital patients tended to be poor. Medical students were increasingly taught on the wards of larger hospitals and distinctive roles emerged for physicians, nurses, and midwives as hospitals became more medicalized. Although reforms were underway regarding hospital architecture, with the provision of light, ventilation, and space, and, as historians are discovering, not all hospitals were "death trap," there were still occasions when doctors, often unwittingly, did more harm than good. The story of Ignaz Semmelweis and Viennese maternity wards poignantly illustrates the potential horrors of some teaching hospitals in the first half of the 19th century.

Giving birth: hand-washing saves lives

I make my confession that God only knows the number of women whom I have consigned prematurely to the grave.

Ignaz Semmelweis (1818–65)

The 18th century witnessed the beginnings of lying-in (maternity) hospitals offering poor women or unmarried mothers a comfortable place to give birth, providing them with free food, warmth, and shelter. They also served as teaching hospitals for medical students who wished to pursue the new profession of "man-midwifery" (later called obstetrics). However, in some of these hospitals the mortality rate of mothers dying in childbirth from an infection known as puerperal fever was unacceptably high and they soon gained the reputation as "slaughterhouses" or "necropolises." Doctors grappled with the question as to why so many mothers were dying under their care.

Oliver Wendell Holmes (1809–94) in Boston cited one distinguished doctor who removed the pelvic organs at the postmortem of a patient who had died of puerperal fever. He then put them in his coat pocket before going on to deliver a number of women—all of whom subsequently died.

It is, however, the Hungarian physician Ignaz Semmelweis who is now best known for making the connection between corpses and confinements. In 1846 Semmelweis was an assistant in Vienna's famous teaching hospital, the Allgemeines Krankenhaus. There were two obstetrical clinics in the hospital, and expectant mothers were randomly allocated to either one. The one where Semmelweis worked was used for teaching male medical students

Florence Nightingale with a group of nurses at the home of Sir Harry Verney at Claydon House, 1886. These new generations of "Nightingale Nurses" were dedicated to the "calling" and "art" of nursing.

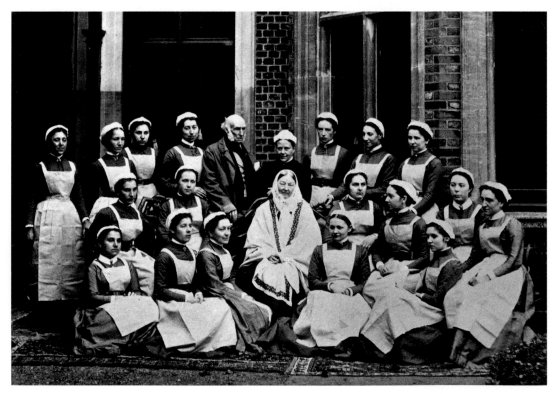

and had a mortality rate of 25 percent, mostly from puerperal fever. The other was for training female midwives, and had a 3 percent mortality rate. When a friend, who was professor of forensic medicine, died, Semmelweis read the autopsy report. His friend had been nicked by a knife while conducting an autopsy, and the report suggested that he had died from the same disease as women who died in childbirth. Semmelweis scrutinized the practices of doctors in his clinic and observed that they would go straight from assisting with autopsies to carrying out vaginal examinations of women in labor—without washing their hands. There had to be a connection.

Semmelweis put forward his "cadaveric theory" and insisted that the students and physicians washed their hands and scrubbed their nails in a bowl of chloride of lime placed at the entrance to the ward, so that "not the faintest trace of cadaver aroma" would be left. Cases of puerperal fever dropped dramatically. But this effective method was not taken up more widely and mortality from puerperal fever (which we now know is caused by the *Streptococcus pyogenes* bacterium) rose in many countries in subsequent years. Decades after Semmelweis's death the significance of his findings was finally realized, and he was hailed a hero.

Today, midwives—either in maternity hospitals or in the home and community—play a major role in childbirth, while district nurses, health visitors, and social workers provide a continuum of care for mothers and babies. In the developing world, however, 65 percent of births among the rural poor take place without a skilled birth attendant. Improving maternal health and reducing child mortality are important goals for global health.

The "Nightingale Nurses"

It may seem a strange principle to enunciate as the very first requirement in a Hospital that it should do the sick no harm.

Florence Nightingale (1820–1910), *Notes on Hospitals*, 1863

Florence Nightingale became famous after nursing the wounded, sick, and dying during the 1854–6 Crimean War. She had offered her services after reading rumors of inadequate medical treatment by *The Times* correspondent William Russell: "Not only are there not sufficient surgeons ... Not only are there no dressers and nurses ... There is not even linen to make bandages." Nightingale and her team of 38 nurses faced filthy conditions:

> *The men lying in their uniforms, stiff with gore and covered in filth to a degree and of a kind no one could write about; their persons covered with vermin ... [underneath the hospital barracks] there were cesspools ... through which the wind blew sewer air up the pipes of numerous open privies into the corridors and wards where the sick were lying.*

Florence Nightingale and her team devoted themselves to nursing the soldiers and to improving the hygiene and dietary standards of the Barrack Hospital in Scutari. In March 1855 a Sanitary Commission was sent out by the British Government to help flush out the sewers, limewash the walls and floors, improve ventilation, and remove dead animals—a horse carcass was blocking one of the water pipes. To what extent these sanitary measures were able to reduce the deaths from diseases such as typhoid, typhus, cholera, dysentery, and the so-called "Crimean fever" remains in dispute. But Nightingale and her "lamp" (which she used to visit the sick at the end of the day) became legendary back in England.

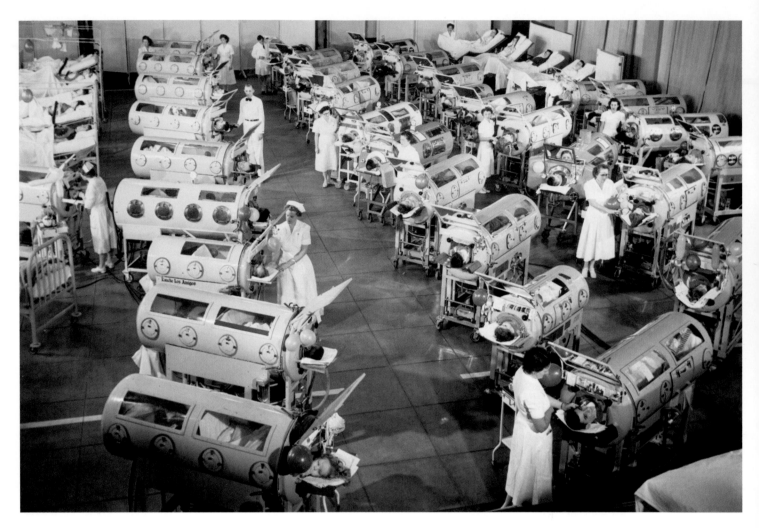

Some of the most poignant scenes of children in hospital are mid-20th-century images of youngsters with polio in iron lungs. These artificial respirators were the first life-support machines.

Another nurse who went off to war was Jamaican-born Mary Seacole (1805–81), or "Mother Seacole" as she was often known. Her application to the British War Office to join Nightingale's nursing team was turned down, but she set off for the Crimea at her own expense and opened the British Hotel near Balaclava in 1855. Using it as a base she would take mules laden with food, wine, and medicines to the battlefield front lines and looked after wounded and dying soldiers on both sides. Her 1857 autobiography, *Wonderful Adventures of Mrs Seacole in Many Lands*, became a bestseller.

Nightingale arrived back in London to set about reforming the military health system, as well as hospital and nursing care and education in London and elsewhere. She campaigned for improvements in workhouse infirmaries, encouraged the importance of district nursing, emphasized the significance of "prevention" rather than "cure," as well as advising on how best to tackle the sanitation and deep-seated roots of poverty in India. And it is those aspects of her life—especially the modernizing of nursing—that created a more lasting, if less dramatic, achievement than that at Scutari.

A new generation of trained "Nightingale Nurses" were slowly put in place; previously they had received no specialist training. In 1860, she set up the Nightingale School of Nursing as part of St Thomas' Hospital in London. The earliest trainee nurses were given a year's instruction and the school is still in existence today. From 1860–1903 the school certified 1,907 nurses, many of whom went on to become matrons or ward sisters elsewhere in Britain, while some founded nursing schools in other countries. By 1900 in the USA there were 432 schools of nursing and a new profession of nursing had been born complete with highly starched uniforms.

Florence Nightingale promoted a healthy, airy style of "pavilion" hospital design. This was highly influential during the 19th century in Europe and the USA. John Shaw Billings designed Baltimore's Johns Hopkins Hospital in the late 1880s on the model of pavilion-style hospitals, inspired by Nightingale's design.

London's specialist hospitals

In Britain, alongside the range of general hospitals—from "cottage" hospitals to "voluntary" hospitals (funded by the rich for the deserving poor) and the notorious Victorian workhouse infirmaries (for "sick paupers")—specialist hospitals developed. By 1860 London boasted 66 specialist hospitals and dispensaries. An article in the 1860 *British Medical Journal* derided such physicians who might hit upon a "striking specialty" such as "inverted toenails or inverted eyelashes'" merely to enhance their own status and cash in on charitable goodwill under the guise of setting up a hospital for the benefit of humanity.

Hospital names reflected their nonreligious and increasingly medical and specialist role as, for example, the Benevolent Dispensary for the Relief of the Poor Afflicted with Fistula, Piles, and Other Diseases of the Rectum in London founded in 1835 (now St Mark's Hospital and still specializing in this area). Charles Dickens went there to sort out his hemorrhoids (piles), the result, he feared, of "too much sitting at my desk."

The list of specialist treatment centers was long, including: an Establishment for Invalid Gentlewomen during Temporary Illness; an Institute for Sick Governesses; the London Infirmary for Diseases of the Legs, Ulcers, and Varicose Veins. Some were short-lived; others lasted. The Dreadnought Seaman's Hospital for the relief of sick and helpless seamen was first established onboard an ex-naval ship in the River Thames in 1821 before moving to dry land as the Hospital for Tropical Diseases, London. The London Homoeopathic Hospital founded in 1849 (now the Royal London Hospital for Integrated Medicine) is a reminder of one of the earliest specialist hospitals for what might today in the West be called "complementary" or "alternative" medicine.

A continuing center of excellence is The Royal Free Hospital in London, which was originally called the London General Institution for the Gratuitous Cure of Malignant Diseases. Its origins date back to a cold winter night in 1828 when William Marsden (1796–1867), a newly qualified surgeon, found a young girl on the steps of the church of St Andrew's, Holborn. She was suffering from TB, starvation, and hypothermia and had been refused admission by three of the city's voluntary hospitals. Marsden recalled that she was "unrecognized by any human being." It was too late to save her life.

> She was suffering from TB, starvation, and hypothermia and had been refused admission by three of the city's voluntary hospitals. It was too late to save her life.

A 1843 survey revealed that, of some 2,400 patients in all the London hospitals, only 26 were under 10 years of age; of the 51,000 people dying in the capital that year, 21,000 were children under 10.

He decided to open a hospital for those who had no letters of recommendation, necessary for admission to the voluntary hospitals. In 1837 the hospital received a royal charter from Queen Victoria (r. 1837–1901) after a cholera epidemic during which the hospital had extended care to many victims. In 1877 it was the first London hospital to provide clinical training for women from the nearby London School of Medicine for Women. Marsden also founded The Free Cancer Hospital in 1851 (later the Royal Marsden Hospital) following the tragic death of his first wife, Betsy Ann, aged 36 from uterine cancer: "I want to found a hospital for the treatment of cancer, and for the study of the disease, for at the present time we know absolutely nothing about it." The Royal Marsden continues to be one of the leading specialist hospitals for cancer.

Another enduring example dating back to the 19th century is the Great Ormond Street Hospital for Children. Charles Dickens, in *Our Mutual Friend* (1864–5), describes how Mrs Boffin persuades an elderly woman to seek good care for an ill child:

"We want to move Johnny to a place where there are none but children; a place set up on purpose for sick children; where the good doctors and nurses pass their lives with children, talk to none but children, touch none but children and comfort and cure none but children."

"Is there really such a place?" asked the old woman with a gaze of wonder.

There was indeed. The first hospital for children in England was The London Hospital for Sick Children, later Great Ormond Street Hospital, which opened in 1852. Its founder was Charles West (1816–98), inspired by children's hospitals on the continent. A 1843 survey revealed that, of some 2,400 patients in all the London hospitals, only 26 were under 10 years of age; of the 51,000 people dying in the capital that year, 21,000 were children under 10. Infant and childhood mortality rates were especially high in the London slums. Diseases such as rickets, scarlet fever, congenital syphilis, whooping cough, diphtheria, and many others, combined with malnutrition, were frequently fatal.

Among the hospital's supporters were Charles Dickens (1812–70) and J M Barrie (1860–1937). Barrie donated the copyright income of his play, *Peter Pan*, in 1929. Queen Victoria sent toys to the hospital. Its first inpatient was Eliza Armstrong, who was suffering from "phthisis (TB) and bronchitis."

The sanatorium

A very different type of hospital—away from the crowded and "pestilential" airs of industrial and metropolitan cities, were the sanatoria for patients suffering from TB. The first sanatorium was opened in 1863 by the physician Hermann Brehmer in Görbersdorf, Silesia (now Poland). Influenced by its ideals and success in treating TB with the "rest cure," Edward Trudeau established the first sanatorium in the USA in 1885—the Adirondack Cottage Sanitarium, at Saranac Lake, New York. Many others followed in Europe and America. Located in isolated mountainous and rural settings, they had bed-lined verandas offering patients "cool and fresh air" for diseased lungs, as well as a regime of good food, rest, and moderate exercise. Health professionals believed that the clean, cold mountain Alpine air of Switzerland was the best treatment for lung diseases and many sanatoria were developed there. One of the most famous was the Schatzalp Sanatorium, in Davos, the setting for Thomas Mann's 1924 novel *The Magic Mountain*. In the USA, warm and dry climates were favored, with California, New Mexico, and Arizona becoming known as the "Lands of the New Lungs" from the early 20th century.

Papworth Sanatorium, near Cambridge, England, developed into a "village settlement" known as the Cambridgeshire Tuberculosis Colony and became famous for its treatments and for helping people to return to work after convalescence. When antibiotics were introduced for curing patients with TB from the 1950s, most of the sanatoria were dismantled or converted into "chest hospitals" treating diseases that replaced TB such as chronic bronchitis and lung diseases. Some, like Schatzalp, became fashionable health resorts.

Papworth became part of the newly founded NHS in 1948 and quickly established itself as one of the country's leading hospitals, initially developing thoracic surgery followed by cardiac surgery and cardiology. The UK's first successful heart transplant operation took place at Papworth in 1979, as well as the world's first heart, lung, and liver transplant in 1986. It continues as a center of expertise and excellence in these fields today.

From "madhouses" and "lunatic asylums" to psychiatric hospitals

I am: yet what I am none cares or knows,
My friends forsake me like a memory lost;
I am the self-consumer of my woes,
They rise and vanish in oblivious host,
Like shades in love and death's oblivion lost;
And yet I am! and live with shadows tost.

John Clare, "I Am" (1848)

The English poet John Clare (1793–1864) wrote his most famous poem, "I Am," while committed to the Northampton General Lunatic Asylum (now St Andrew's Hospital), where he spent his last 23 years. He was encouraged to write by the medical superintendent, Thomas Octavius Pritchard.

The 18th and 19th centuries saw the growth of public "lunatic" asylums in the Western world, as well as private "madhouses," where wealthy patients could stay and be treated by often unqualified "mad doctors" until they "recovered their reason." "Mad" King George III of England (r. 1760–1820) was treated by physician and clergyman Francis Willis at his private asylum. The King was bound in a straitjacket and chained to a chair to control his ravings but also, at times, offered sympathy and patience, making a triumphant, albeit temporary, recovery in 1789 (as featured in the movie *The Madness of King George*, an adaptation of the 1991 play by Alan Bennett). It is now thought that George suffered from a rare blood disorder, porphyria, possibly triggered by arsenic, then widely used in medicines.

More humane and progressive approaches (known as "moral treatment") to psychiatric care—where restraint was minimized and cruelty replaced by kindness and gentleness—were gradually introduced by leading reformers. Physicians grew increasingly involved in neurology and psychological medicine, both in trying to understand causes of mental illness as well as finding the best treatments. By the mid- to late 20th century, the cruel practices of the past

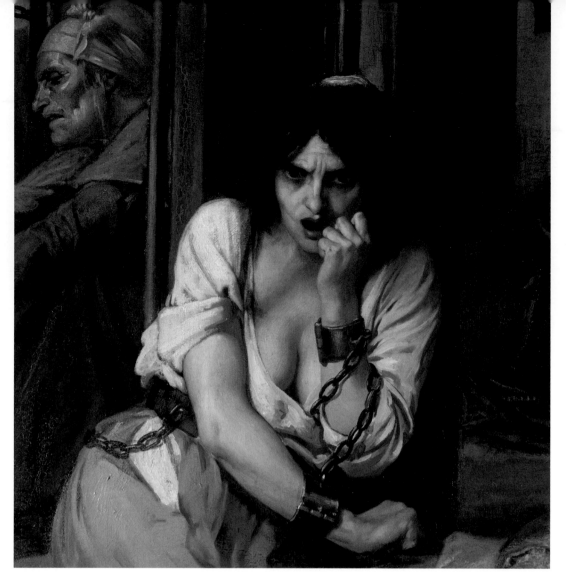

Artists in the 18th and 19th centuries frequently depicted the horrors of "lunatic asylums" where patients were manacled and lived in filth. Reformers, including Philippe Pinel (1745–1826) and Jean-Baptiste Pussin (1746–1811) in Paris, initiated some of the first humanitarian reforms in the treatment of mentally ill people.

had mostly been abandoned along with the transformation of newly modernizing "psychiatric hospitals" supervised by professionally trained psychiatrists. Bethlem Royal Hospital weathered its stormy past and is still in operation today as an outstanding psychiatric hospital, located in Beckenham, Kent, UK. Nevertheless there remains wide variation across the world in hospital and community psychiatric care, and its associated stigma.

"The land that never sleeps"—hospitals in the modern age

Talk of the patience of Job, said a Hospital nurse, Job was never on night duty.
English surgeon Stephen Paget (1855–1926)

The huge transformations that have taken place in medicine—the introduction of anesthesia and antisepsis in surgery; an understanding of anatomy and the causes of diseases; the development of imaging and diagnostic techniques and radiotherapy; isolation wards and barrier nursing techniques to prevent cross-infection; the discovery of antibiotics and methods of pain control; as well as the development of emergency medicine—all have had a major influence on hospitals over the course of the past century. Even such innovations as electricity and telephones have had a far-reaching impact on the modern hospital.

State-of-the-art equipment now used for diagnosing, treating, and monitoring patients has given a completely different focus to the role of hospitals in modern medicine. Bulky, expensive, and complicated machines need to be housed in major hospitals with staff qualified to use them. Many large hospitals have numerous different specialist inpatient wards—from pediatric (children) to geriatric (elderly) wards, isolation to intensive-care units, high-dependency to short-term day-centers, as well as a wide range of outpatient clinics. Surgery plays a major role in the modern hospital. Clinical teaching and scientific research in hospitals are fundamental to the progress of medicine. As Paul Starr wrote in his book *The Social Transformation of American Medicine* (1982):

> *Few institutions have undergone as radical a metamorphosis as have hospitals in their modern history. In developing from places of dreaded impurity and exiled human wreckage into awesome citadels of science and bureaucratic order, they acquired a new moral identity, as well as new purposes and patients of higher status.*

The "failings" of some 21st-century hospitals are, however, commonly highlighted in the media: hospital-acquired "superbugs," misdiagnoses, complex bureaucracy, staff shortages, poor hygiene, as well as unappetizing food. While these can be distressing realities, it is important to remember the incredible lifesaving opportunities that hospitals now offer to the newborn, young, and old. Many dedicated nurses and doctors work long hours, round the clock, to fulfill their expected and desired duties—combining the "art" and "science" of medicine and the "calling" of nursing. As one nurse (Christie Watson) described the expanding role of the nurse: "a nurse is a manager, a leader, a clinical expert, a counselor, a researcher, a carer, a lifesaver, a team-player, and often a friend. In one single shift, I'd use all of these titles." Hospitals are the places where the lights are on 24/7: "the land that never sleeps."

The spiraling cost of high-tech hospital care is a major concern throughout the world. Historian of science and medicine Guenter Risse, in 1999, reminded us that despite being "houses of science and high technology" hospitals "must remember their historical humanitarian mission." Improving hospital provision, alongside the strengthening of local community and primary care, is one of many serious challenges for the future of global health. There are also many people living in poverty, in remote rural areas, in urban slums, or without health insurance in countries with no universal health provision, who may not have the means to be cared for in hospital. Director General of the WHO, Margaret Chan, emphasizes that the ultimate goal is "universal health coverage" for all.

Accident and Emergency medicine

A striking feature of the modern hospital is the Emergency department. This is the focal point of arrival, usually by ambulance, of the desperately sick, dying, or injured. The first mobile ambulances date back to the Napoleonic Wars (1799–1815) when Baron Dominique-Jean Larrey, Napoleon's chief surgeon, introduced covered horse-drawn wagons on the battlefield, known as *ambulances volantes* ("flying ambulances"). He also developed the concept of "triage" to prioritize patient attention and care; this remains vital to modern medicine. Britain introduced 999 as an emergency telephone number in 1938, while 112 is used by 26 countries, and 911 mainly in the Americas.

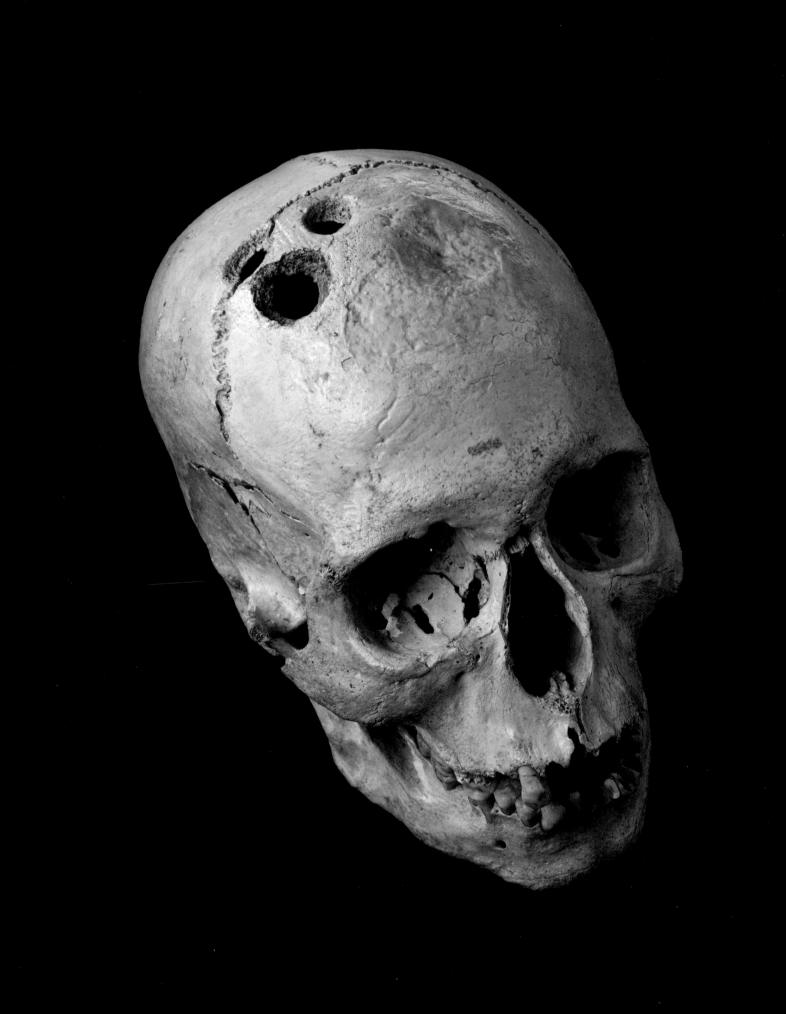

Barbers and Surgeons

There are five duties in surgery: to remove what is superfluous, to restore what has been dislocated, to separate what has grown together, to reunite what has been divided and to redress the defects of nature.

Ambroise Paré (1510–90), French surgeon

Surgery involves suturing wounds; splinting and putting fractured bones together; amputating limbs; as well as cutting out or replacing diseased organs and tissues. Over the centuries, surgery was usually a last resort and for the nonanethetized patient it could be excruciatingly painful and dangerous. There was also a serious risk of infection from the surgeon's knife and amputating saw. The less-reputable barber-surgeons were often described as "knife-cutters" or "Mr Sawbones". Key developments in the 19th and early 20th centuries, such as anesthesia, antisepsis, and "scrubbing up" before (and not just after) an operation, eventually transformed surgery, enabling the patient to be unconscious during the operation and for surgeons to operate in a sterile environment. Today, surgery, including transplant surgery, is a highly sophisticated art.

Ancient surgery

A surgeon should be youthful or at any rate nearer youth than age; with a strong and steady hand which never trembles, and ready to use the left hand as well as the right; with vision sharp and clear, and spirit undaunted; filled with pity, so that he wishes to cure his patient, yet is not moved by his cries to go too fast or cut less than is necessary, but does everything just as if the cries of pain cause him no emotion.

Aulus Cornelius Celsus (25 BC–AD 50)

Trepanation—the drilling of a hole into the head—is, arguably, the oldest surgical procedure in human history, dating back to at least Neolithic times, and still used, in an adapted form, in cranial and neurosurgery today. The practice of "trepanation" (from the Greek *trypanon*,

OPPOSITE This skull, from around 2000 BC, shows evidence of the ancient surgical practice of trepanation, where rings or squares of bone from the skull were cut out. The regrowth of the bone suggests that some people survived this risky procedure.

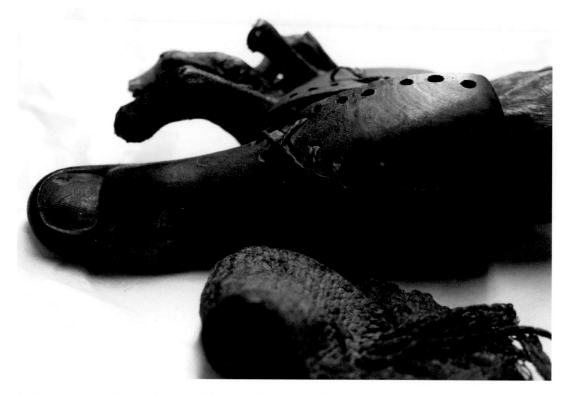

Ancient Egyptian prosthetics. This artificial "Cairo Toe" (now in the Cairo Museum) is made of wood and leather and has three bendable joints. It dates back to 950–710 BC and may be the world's earliest known functional prosthetic.

meaning "a borer"), where rings or squares of bone from the skull were cut out, may have been used following a head injury or to relieve headaches, epilepsy, and even to release tormenting "demons." Over half of Peruvian skulls, for example, show regrowth of the bone, suggesting people survived their ordeal. Archaeological and written records reveal a range of other remarkable ancient surgical practices (without modern anesthesia): removing spearheads, draining abscesses, lancing boils, excising nasal polyps, removing bladder stones, "couching for cataract" (pushing the clouded eye lens of sufferers out of the line of sight with a curved needle).

Surgical instruments such as delicate scalpels, probes, needles, forceps, and knives have been discovered from ancient archaeological sites. The Egyptian Edwin Smith papyrus (c.1600 BC, but believed to be from an earlier version) is one of the most fascinating ancient texts on surgery. It comprises 48 "typical" case reports ranging from gaping head wounds to chest trauma, originally inscribed on a single scroll. The US National Library of Medicine has launched a project, *Turning the Pages*, which allows viewers to see online the Edwin Smith Papyrus, or literally "to unroll the scroll."

Recent anatomical and radiological studies on skeletal and mummified Egyptian remains are shedding insight into ancient surgery, revealing healed fractures and amputation sites. Archaeologists have also found what are thought to be the earliest functional prosthetic "big toes." The famous "Cairo Toe" was discovered in the necropolis of Thebes, near present-day Luxor, on a female mummy identified as Tabaketenmut, the daughter of a priest. It is speculated that she might have had her big toe amputated following gangrene.

In 2011, over 240,000 Americans had a "nose job" for mainly aesthetic reasons, making it one of the most popular cosmetic surgery procedures in the USA. Two thousand years ago, an ancient version of this surgery was carried out for altogether different reasons: the restoration of an amputated nose—a common punishment for crime in the ancient world or the result of battle injury. In India the famous Ayurvedic surgeon Sushruta is believed to be the first person to have written an account of plastic surgery using a technique known later as "rhinoplasty" (Greek, *rhino-*, "nose," and *plassein*, "to form a mold"). The operation used a skin graft either taken from the cheek or the forehead to create a new nose.

British surgeons in the early 19th century revived one of the "Indian methods" of using the forehead flap in rhinoplasty. This involved cutting a leaf-shaped flap of skin from the forehead, making sure the end nearest the bridge of the nose remained attached, and then grafting it over the nose. To keep the air passages open during healing, two polished wooden tubes were inserted into the nostrils. Prosthetic noses were also made of ivory and, in the case of the Danish nobleman and astronomer Tycho Brahe (1546–1601), who lost the bridge of his nose in a duel, silver and gold (or, possibly, copper or brass). Paste or glue were used to keep the nose attached.

Some ancient treatments sounded horrifying, such as this 4th-century BC Hippocratic Corpus text, *On Haemorrhoids*, describing the treatment for piles:

> *Having laid him on his back … force the anus as much as possible with the fingers and make the irons red hot and burn the pile until it be dried up and so that no part may be left behind.*

"Mr Sawbones" and the knife-cutters

The word "surgeon" comes from the Greek *cheir,* "a hand," and *ergon,* "work," via the Latin word *chirurgia*. From ancient Greek and Roman times, there was a, sometimes uncomfortable, division between surgeons (who used their hands—a manual trade) and physicians (who used their heads)—although some, such as Galen, practiced both surgery and medicine. In the Medieval period there were a number of well-known surgeons, including Abu al-Qasim al-Zahrawi (Albucasis) (*fl. c.*AD 1000), who practiced near Córdoba, Spain, and is often called the "father of modern surgery." In his medical texts, Zahrawi describes many surgical instruments, including forceps, specula, and surgical needles. In Italy there were master surgeons trained at universities such as Bologna, Padua, and Naples from the late 12th century onward. They developed an academic surgical body of literature involving surgery and anatomy.

In medieval and early modern northern Europe, however, surgery was considered a "lowly" trade. While physicians were often licensed by universities, surgical skills were learnt by apprenticeship. Surgeons—or "chirurgeons"—were frequently ridiculed by physicians for being "altogether unlearned" and practicing their trade "more by blynde experience than by any science." Surgeons, on the other hand, emphasized the importance of practical experience. In some ways, the differences between physicians and surgeons were perhaps not so great, or as one 17th-century cynic, Maximilianus Urentius, put it: "wherein differs the surgeon

The famous "Cairo Toe" was discovered in the necropolis of Thebes, near present-day Luxor, on a female mummy identified as Tabaketenmut, the daughter of a priest. It is speculated that she might have had her big toe amputated following gangrene.

from the doctor? In this way, that one kills with his drugs, the other with his knife. Both differ from the hangman only in doing slowly what he does quickly."

Surgeons were mostly organized into trade-guilds and were closely linked with barbers. Indeed, for a time many were known as "barber-surgeons" and appeared to have no limits on the range of services they could offer: trimming a beard; removing nits and lice; cutting out bunions and warts; pulling out a tooth; removing a bladder stone; excising cancerous growths; and, with the spread of venereal diseases from the late 15th century, dealing with chancres and sores. As one writer put it: surgeons were pilloried as men who sought the right to "bleed, cut, draw, lance, probe, saw, hack, mangle, tear, blister, burn, embrocate, fumigate, mend-a-pate, potion, lotion, pocket, charge, and kill."

The sight of medical instruments used in the period must have been quite terrifying for the patient—sharp lacerating knives, hot cauterizing irons, pointed lancets, and the amputating saw. Some surgeons earned a reputation as being very skillful in their craft and wrote significant surgical treatises. One of the most famous and innovative barber-surgeons of the 16th century was the Frenchman Ambroise Paré (1510–90) who, while on a military campaign in Italy, ran out of the traditional boiling oil used to treat gunshot wounds. Instead, he made a substitute ointment from egg-yolk, rose-oil, and turpentine that proved more effective and he "resolved never again cruelly to burn poor people who had suffered shot wounds."

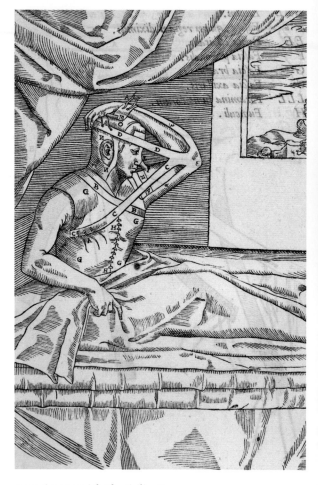

An ancient nose job. The Sicilian Branca family developed a secret method in the 15th century, partially detaching a skin flap from the upper arm and suturing it to the remains of a nose. The arm and nose were attached for two weeks to maintain a blood supply for the graft to take.

Imagine the pain

That morning my Chirurgeon cut off a poore creaturs Leg, a little under the knee, first cutting the living and untainted flesh above the Gangreene with a sharp knife, and then sawing off the bone in an instant; then with searing and stoopes stanching the blood, which issued abundantly; the stout and gallant man, enduring it with incredible patience, and that without being bound to his chaire, as is usual in such painefull operations, or hardly making a face or crying oh.

John Evelyn, Diary, 1672

Operations had to be fast. The patient might be tied down during an operation, sometimes in a chair, with a number of strong assistants to keep them still. It is almost impossible to imagine the excruciating level of pain involved in early surgery, where the patient was fully conscious. Prior to the use of ether and chloroform as anesthetics in the mid-19th century, various "soporific" were used to dull the senses or put the patient to sleep, such as alcohol, henbane, mandrake, opium, and a mysterious herbal concoction called *mafeisan* in China (which has been translated as "cannabis boil powder"). Sometimes these substances were soaked into a "sleeping sponge" and held in front of the patient's mouth and nose. Some surgeons preferred to operate on a sober and awake patient—supposedly easier to handle.

Once the operation had been performed, there was a serious risk of death from postoperative infection, hemorrhage (blood loss), and shock. One common strategy to stop bleeding and prevent fatal infections was to place a red-hot iron, known as a cauterizing iron, on the open wound or gangrenous tissue. As the iron was placed against the flesh, the muscle, blood vessels, and skin were seared together. Stoical patients did, nevertheless, survive to tell the tale. Various methods have been devised over the centuries to "stitch" wounds. In India and South America, termites or beetles were used to bite across the edges of the wound as they were held together by the surgeon. The bodies of the insects were then twisted off, and their jaws, stiffened in death, held the laceration closed like a staple. Catgut, from the intestines of sheep or goats, was (and still is in some parts of the world) a popular material for absorbable sutures.

Survivors of preanesthetic surgery

Surgery has undergone many great transformations during the past fifty years, and many are to be thanked for their contributions – yet when we think of how many remain to be made, it should rather stimulate our inventiveness than fuel our vanity.

Percivall Pott, Surgeon, St Bartholomew's Hospital, London, 1775

By the later 18th and early 19th centuries, as knowledge of human anatomy increased, surgeons were acquiring a newly elevated status. More adventurous operations, including excising tumors, could be performed but the surgeon still had to be quick—the patient, invariably, screaming and struggling, had to be strapped to the operating table or held down by several assistants. The operation would be messy and traumatic.

Scottish surgeon Robert Liston (1794–1847), a towering man of 74 inches (six foot, two inches) in height, was famous for the speed of his operations, when, according to his admirers, "the gleam of his knife was followed so instantaneously by the sounds of sawing as to make the two actions appear almost simultaneous." With students packing the gallery of the University College Hospital, London, operating theater, pocket-watches in hand, Liston would stride across the bloodstained floor, often in Wellington boots, and call, "Time me, gentlemen, time me."

In 1823 he performed an operation that caused a sensation at the time. He removed a large scrotal tumor that measured 42 inches in circumference and weighed 44.5 pounds. Blood loss was likened to a shower. The patient sank off the table, pulseless and flaccid, but with the help of a "cordial" (a pint of good strong whisky) poured down his gullet, he began to show signs of recovery. Three weeks later, he walked out of the hospital.

One of the most graphic descriptions of the pain endured during an operation without an anesthetic was by the novelist and friend of Dr Johnson, Fanny Burney (1752–1840). She underwent a mastectomy for breast cancer, performed by the famous French military surgeon Dominique-Jean Larrey (1766–1842) in 1811. She was lucky to survive the 20-minute operation and later described her excruciating ordeal:

*When the dreadful steel was plunged into the breast – cutting through the veins – arteries –
flesh – nerves – I needed no injunctions not to restrain my cries. I began a scream that lasted
unintermittingly during the whole time of the incision – & I almost marvel that it rings not in
my Ears still! so excruciating was the agony.*

Her surgeon, Larrey, was also traumatized by the suffering he inflicted, as she recalls:

*I then saw my good Dr Larry, pale nearly as myself, his face streaked with blood, its expression
depicting grief, apprehension, & almost horror.*

Another stoic who underwent a bloody and traumatic operation without pain relief was
Mrs Jane Todd Crawford. In 1809 Ephraim McDowell (1771–1830), a US country surgeon
in Kentucky, performed the first successful operation to remove a diseased ovary on Mrs
Crawford using his kitchen table to operate on. The operation took 25 minutes, during which
she recited psalms and hymns—one can only imagine the agony as the surgeon cut through
her abdomen to excise what proved to be a massive tumor (besides which, at one point, her
"intestines rushed out upon the table"). Mrs Crawford not only survived, but lived to the age
of 78. When reports of this and several other daring operations reached the London medical
circle, they responded: "A back-settlement of America – Kentucky – has beaten the mother
country, nay, Europe itself, with all the boasted surgeons thereof in the fearful and formidable
operation of gastrostomy, with the extraction of diseased ovaria."

Putting patients to sleep

*Oh, what delight for every feeling heart to find the new year ushered in with the announcement
of this noble discovery of the power to still the sense of pain, and veil the eye and memory from all
the horrors of an operation ... WE HAVE CONQUERED PAIN.*

The People's Journal of London, 1847

While various narcotics, such as opium, had been used to induce sleep during surgery,
physicians of the 18th and 19th centuries knew they needed new agents. Experiments on both
sides of the Atlantic focused on the effects of a gas called nitrous oxide, known as "laughing
gas." This became a popular recreational drug at parties and was first tried out in dentistry in
the 1840s (see page 113). However, it was the use of the gases ether and chloroform that finally
ushered in a new era of anesthesia in surgery.

The first highly publicized demonstration of using ether as an anesthetic in surgery was
in the USA, at the Massachusetts General Hospital, Boston. At 10 o'clock on October 16 1846,
in the now-famous "Ether Dome," a packed audience of medical students, physicians, and
surgeons waited with bated breath. A young man, Gilbert Abbott, with a benign vascular tumor
of the neck, was strapped down on the operating table, awaiting, not just the surgeon's knife,
but the arrival of 27-year-old William Morton (1819–68). This young dental surgeon had been
experimenting with ether as a way to "diminish the sensibility of pain" for patients. Morton
had tried ether out on himself, on a dog, on his assistants and on his first patient, Eben Frost,
who had a tooth pulled out under the influence of ether saturated into a handkerchief. Abbott's
surgeon, John Collins Warren, had invited Morton to administer his "invention."

At ten minutes past ten, Morton had not appeared. Knife in hand, Warren was going to do his
usual "quick" excision—with the patient conscious, petrified, and awaiting the knife's touch on

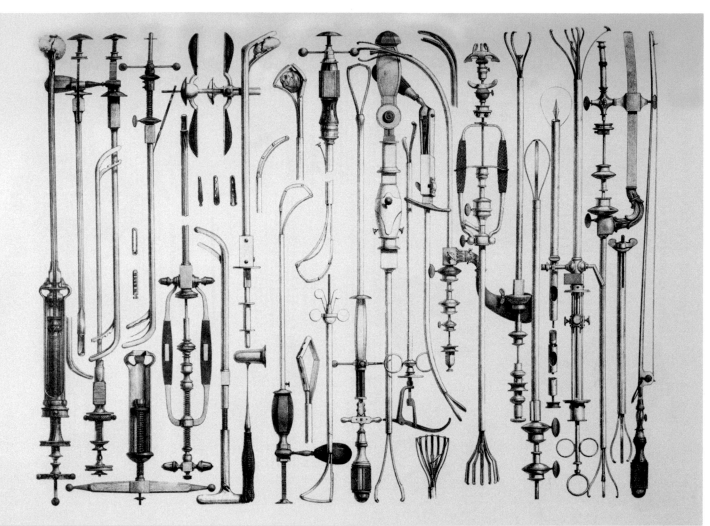

Lithotomy—Samuel Pepys's bladder stone

*The sick creature was strip'd to his shirt, and
bounde arms and thighs to an high Chaire,
2 men holding his shoulders fast down: then the
Chirurgion with a crooked Instrument prob'd til
he hit on the stone, then ... he made an Incision
thro the Scrotum about an Inch in length, then
he put in his forefingers to get the stone as neere
the orifice of the wound as he could, then with
another Instrument like a Cranes neck he pull'd it
out with incredible torture to the Patient.*
(John Evelyn, *Diary*, 1650)

ABOVE As if the thought of unbearable pain was not
enough, patients had to avoid catching sight of the
terrifyingly inventive surgical instruments.

Stones are small mineral masses that can
develop in the bladder, kidneys, or urethra;
a lithotomy was the operation that removed
them. Samuel Pepys underwent this operation
after having suffered violent attacks of pain for
years with his bladder stone "even to the making
of bloody water upon any extraordinary motion."
It was successfully carried out at his cousin's
house by Thomas Hollyer on March 26 1658.
In his own diary, Pepys records that he kept the
stone, which was the size of a "tennis ball." He
held a "solemn feast for the cutting of his stone"
each year on the anniversary of his operation.
An autopsy later revealed seven stones in his left
kidney and a gangrenous bladder.

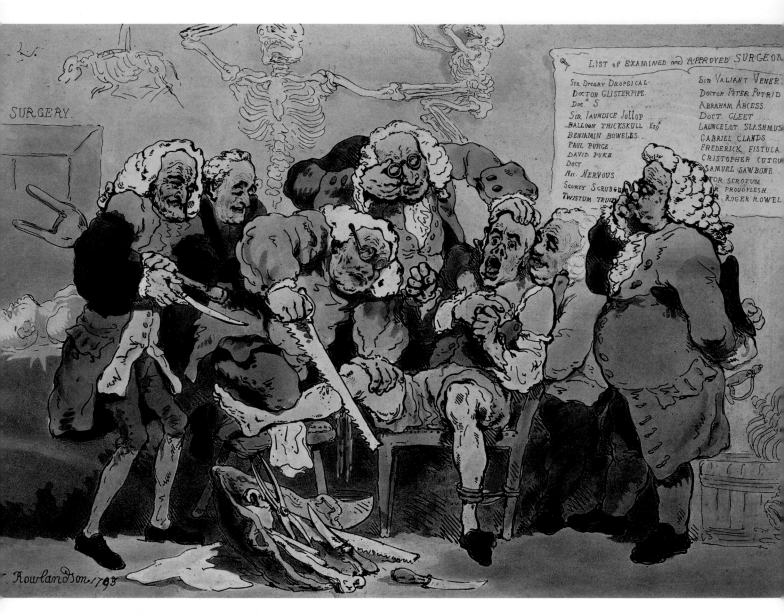

Thomas Rowlandson, *Amputation* (1785), shows the horrors of amputation before the development of anesthetics. Patients would be fully awake and had to be restrained while doctors hastily dispatched a limb.

sensitive nerves. In the nick of time, Morton arrived with a newly modified apparatus in hand for inhaling what he called "letheon" (after the goddess of "oblivion," Lethe). The gas's smell was disguised by orange essence. Morton's wife remembered: "the patient lay silent, with eyes closed as if in sleep; but everyone present fully expected to hear the shriek of agony ring out as the knife struck down into the sensitive nerves, but the stroke came with no accompanying cry."

During the 30-minute operation Abbott was heard to mutter, and said afterward that he had felt some pain, but that it was only as if "the skin had been scratched with a hoe." Warren turned to his awestruck audience and concluded, "Gentlemen, this is no humbug!" Morton revealed that his "ethereal vapor" was ether (also known as diethyl ether) and repeated his "experiment" successfully on a young servant girl, Alice Mohan, who needed a leg amputation. A name for this innovation was suggested by Oliver Wendell Holmes, Professor at the Harvard Medical School: "anesthesia" (Greek *an-* "without" and *aisthēsis*, "feeling or sensation").

After so many centuries of pain and fear for patients, news of this amazing invention spread far and wide. In Britain, a few weeks later, Robert Liston operated on a butler with chronic osteomyelitis of the tibia. A medical student, William Squire, aged 21, was to administer the ether. Liston announced to the packed audience: "we are going to try a Yankee dodge, to-day, gentlemen, for making men insensible." An onlooker that day, Dr F W Cock, recalled:

> He then takes from a long narrow case one of the straight amputating knives of his own invention ... The tube is put into the mouth, William Squire holds it at the patient's nostrils. A couple of dressers stand by, to hold the patient if necessary, but he never moves and blows and gurgles away ... 'Now gentlemen, time me', he [Liston] says to the students. A score of watches are pulled out in reply. A huge left hand grasps the thigh, a thrust of the long, straight knife, two or three rapid sawing movements ... half a dozen (more) strokes, and Ransome (the House Surgeon) places the limb in the sawdust. 'Twenty-eight seconds,' says William Squire.

Chloroform was another anesthetic experimented with. It was successfully pioneered in 1847 by the Edinburgh "accoucheur" (obstetrician) James Young Simpson during the birth of a child. Simpson said that chloroform would "turn the world upside down." A number of chloroform fatalities, however, followed, leading to debates about its risks. But gradually its use was made acceptable in obstetric practice. Queen Victoria was administered chloroform by John Snow for the birth of her eighth child, Prince Leopold, in 1853. She wrote afterward in her journal: "the effect was soothing, quieting, and delightful beyond measure."

Chloroform was also used by some military surgeons for amputations in the Crimean War and the American Civil War as well as by medical missionaries in Africa where it was known as the "sleep medicine" and considered to be "a great wonder." Both ether and chloroform continued to be used in surgery until the 20th century, when safer local and general anesthetics, such as halothane, were introduced.

From sepsis to antisepsis and asepsis

A man laid on the operating table of one of our hospitals is exposed to more chance of death than the English soldier on the field of Waterloo.

James Young Simpson, 19th-century obstetrician

"Conquering pain" for the patient was a radical step forward but there remained the danger of postoperative infection where a neatly dressed stump would start to ooze pus and turn septic in the days following the operation. Some minor wounds, if they were open, might turn septic, necessitating amputation. The foul smell of pus, gangrene, and putrefaction was all-pervading in the surgical wards of the mid-19th century and mortality rates remained high. James Young Simpson had coined the phrase "hospitalism" to cover the outcomes of pyemia ("pus in the blood"), septicemia, erysipelas, hospital gangrene, and tetanus that followed operations. Maggots were sometimes used in the dressings to cleanse the wound and, today, "larvae therapy" using sterilized maggots is making a comeback especially with the rise of antibiotic-resistant infections.

The year 1865 was to be another milestone in the history of surgery. On August 12 1865, James Greenlees, aged eleven, was run over by a cart. He was admitted to the Glasgow Royal Infirmary, Scotland, with a compound fracture of the left leg and a nasty open wound where the broken bone had perforated the skin. The usual procedure for compound fractures was amputation (to save a life, if not the limb). The boy's surgeon was Joseph Lister (1827–1912), Professor of Surgery at Glasgow University, who would become known by many of his followers as the "greatest surgical benefactor to mankind."

Lister was intrigued by the ideas published between 1857 and 1860 of the famous French chemist Louis Pasteur—in particular, his ideas that microscopic living organisms, carried from place to place by the air, caused putrefaction. He wondered, by analogy, whether surgeons could find a way to stop open wounds from putrefying. He had heard about the use of carbolic acid in the treatment of sewage during a typhoid epidemic in Carlisle, England, which had seemed to "disinfect" it. He reasoned that a chemical used to destroy microorganisms in sewage might also be used to act as a chemical barrier between the wound and the air. He was able to test his ideas on James Greenlees.

The boy's leg was splinted and Lister directed his house-surgeon to dress his wound with lint soaked in carbolic acid (in the form of "German creosote") and to cover it with a sheet of "block tin" (tinfoil), followed by applications of (diluted) carbolic acid over the ensuing weeks. The wound did not putrefy and, after six weeks, James walked out of the hospital on both legs.

Lister's carbolic-acid "antisepsis" (Greek *anti-*, "against" and *sēpsis*, "putrefaction") resulted in many successes, and he constantly experimented with different antiseptics and their application to sutures and ligatures, wound dressings, and drainage tubes. He also developed an aerosol spray of carbolic acid to use throughout the operating theater. Two years after James's operation, Lister could confidently declare:

> Since the antiseptic treatment has been brought into full operation, my wards have completely changed their character; so that during the last nine months not a single instance of pyaemia, hospital gangrene or erysipelas has occurred in them.

Lister's ideas soon spread to other countries through the medical practice of his students. Surgeons from overseas visited to observe his "antiseptic system." But some were not convinced by the "antiseptic" methods of using chemicals in operations, preferring water to clean wounds and the Nightingale principle of keeping hospitals clean and well ventilated. It took, as Professor Harold Ellis, a British surgeon and leading authority on surgical history, notes: "a full two decades of patient experiment, demonstrations, lectures, and learned articles in the journals ... before surgeons were entirely won over to Lister's ideas."

As an understanding of germ theory spread among a new generation of bacteriologists, surgeons eventually accepted that bacteria in wounds were the cause of suppuration and infection. This also encouraged the principle of "asepsis" (Greek *a-*, "without" and *sēpsis*, "putrefaction"), with the aim of excluding germs in the first place without skin irritation of chemical antiseptics. Dramatic blood-encrusted frock-coats were gradually abandoned in favor of clean surgical gowns, caps, gloves, and masks and the steam sterilization of surgical instruments and dressings. Surgical gloves, now routinely used in the operating theater to protect both the patient and theater staff from cross-infection, were introduced in the late 1880s by US surgeon William Halsted, originally to protect his theater nurse (later his wife) from antiseptic skin irritation.

Following Lister, generations of brilliant surgeons pioneered new surgical techniques—

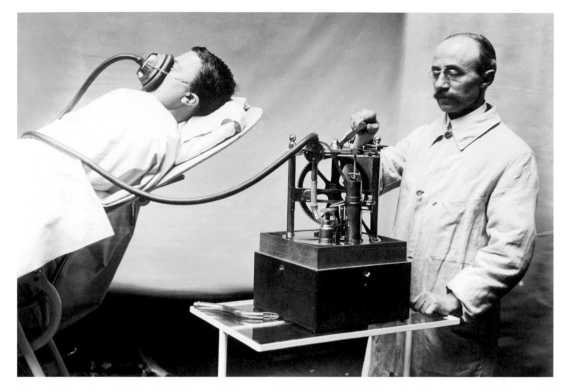

This early form of anesthesia, a chloroform machine, was called the Dubois inhaler (*c.* 1905) and was operated using a crank.

becoming bolder and braver in their efforts. The newly sterile, well-equipped operating theaters of the late 19th century encouraged increasingly ambitious operations. These included removal of an entire lung (pneumonectomy); operations on brain tumors; and radical mastectomy for breast cancer in which the breast, all the lymph glands in the nearest armpit, and the muscles of the chest wall are removed. Patients of leading US brain surgeon Harvey Cushing (1869–1939) bequeathed him their brains. There are over 500 of these perfectly preserved brains, each labeled with case details. They can be seen today in his archive at Yale University.

The early 20th century witnessed rapid changes in surgery and better survival rates. The motorized bone saw replaced the handsaw for amputations. The US Mayo Clinic in Minnesota saw a massive increase in the number of operations carried out: at the end of the 19th century, over 3,000 operations; by 1924, 23,628—and with over 60,000 patients on their books. Analgesics (painkillers), including morphine, played a key role in pain control for pre- and postoperative patients. Infections following surgery did continue to be a problem in the preantibiotic days.

Surgical innovations during the First and Second World Wars

Over the centuries, surgeons on the battlefield have been faced with appalling conditions and terrible injuries, including those caused by a new generation of weaponry used in the First and Second World Wars. The challenges of dealing with these situations hastened the development of innovative techniques, as well as progress in the use of blood transfusion and the principles of emergency medicine. Devastating injuries led to the invention of evermore sophisticated forms of plastic surgery, rebuilding disfigured faces and bodies. In 1917 Harold Delf Gillies (1882–1960) established the first hospital of reconstructive plastic surgery (The

The "-ectomies" and the "-ostomies"

Many surgical procedures end in "-ectomy" (Greek *ek*, "out" + *-tomē*, "a cutting"), as in nephrectomy—removal of the kidney (Greek *nephros* for kidney)and hysterectomy (*hystera*, "womb"). Medical terms ending in "-stomy" (Greek *stoma* for "mouth" or "opening") usually refer to the surgical opening of that part of the body, such as tracheostomy (opening of the trachea or windpipe) or gastrostomy (opening of the stomach, from *gastro*—the Greek for "belly," not to be confused with gastronomy!)

The Agnew Clinic by Thomas Eakins (1889) shows Dr Agnew (on the left with a scalpel) performing a partial mastectomy in a medical amphitheater.

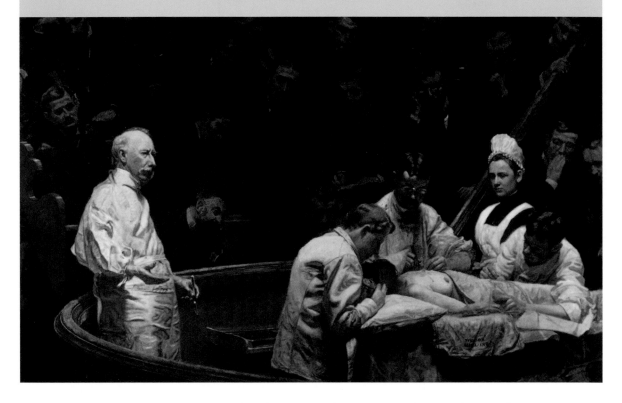

Queen's Hospital, Sidcup, England). A harrowing, but remarkable, set of pastel drawings, by the artist-surgeon Henry Tonks, captured before and after images of surgery on soldiers.

In Germany, Otto Bock responded to the large number of injured veterans by founding a prosthetics company in 1919. Many of the modern prosthetics, such as the C-leg, a computerized knee that adaptively varies its passive resistance to suit the patient's walking gait, have been made by his company.

The Second World War saw further techniques that included rebuilding entire limbs, extensive skin grafts, microsurgery, and increased knowledge about tissue health. Lifesaving penicillin was introduced during the Second World War (see pages 187–8). One of the most incredible stories was that of the neurosurgeon Ludwig Guttmann (1899–1980). A German-Jewish refugee, Guttmann was appointed by the British Government in 1944 to run a spinal injuries unit at Stoke Mandeville Hospital (today, it is a leading international center), in Aylesbury, England, for injured British soldiers returning from the battlefields of the Second World War. Patients were heavily sedated with morphine, desperately ill with life-threatening infected bed sores, and most had given up hope of ever returning to normal life. Guttmann was determined to give them a second chance. He concentrated on physical, emotional, and mental rehabilitation and encouraged his bedridden patients to take an active role in sport—mobilizing them in wheelchairs. His inspiration and vision led to the idea of the Paralympics.

The first organ transplant

Surgeons had long dreamed that it might be possible to remove a healthy organ from one human being and transplant it into a sick patient in place of the diseased or damaged one. Various experiments, mostly using animal models, had been tried over the centuries. The French surgeon Alexis Carrel (1873–1944) won a Nobel Prize in 1912 in recognition of his work on "vascular suture and the transplantation of blood vessels and organs." Carrel, who had learned the art of stitching from a French lacemaker to improve suturing techniques, conducted numerous experiments mostly on cats and dogs while working in the USA. He recognized the practical difficulties of applying his organ-transplantation techniques to humans. In the absence of immunosuppressants, transplanting living tissue from one human being to another inevitably failed, due to the rejection of the transplanted tissue by the recipient's immune system.

The dream of organ transplantation, however, became a reality on December 23 1954. Identical twin brothers, Richard and Ronald Herrick, were 23 years of age. Richard had been admitted with severe kidney failure to the Peter Bent Brigham Hospital in Boston, under the care of John Merrill (1917–84), a nephrologist. Richard's identical twin had the same blood group, identical eye colors, and even the same fingerprints—a perfect match. Genetic identity was established by reciprocal skin graft. Richard was put on a kidney dialysis machine (invented in the late 1940s) until the surgeons were ready to go ahead with a kidney transplant operation.

The surgeons, Joseph Murray (1919–2012) and Hartwell Harrison (1909–84), were to perform the operation simultaneously in two adjacent theaters. A normal, healthy left kidney was removed from Ronald and grafted into the right lower abdomen of Richard. By the time the operation was over, three and a half-hours later, the transplanted kidney had turned a healthy pink and a clear urine flowed copiously from the "donor" kidney. The operation was a major surgical breakthrough. Richard married his nurse and they had two children. Tragically, he died eight years later from a recurrence of kidney disease, while Ronald lived to the age of 79. Murray shared the Nobel Prize in Physiology or Medicine in 1990 with the bone marrow transplant pioneer E Donnall Thomas (1920–2012).

Replacing a broken heart

The heart had long been a no-go area. As Stephen Paget had written back in 1896: "surgery of the heart has probably reached the limits set by nature to all surgery; no new method and no new discovery, can overcome the natural difficulties that attend a wound of the heart."

The first half of the 20th century saw developments in diagnostic tools for heart disease, including the electrocardiograph (ECG/EKG) in the early 1900s. A key innovation for open-heart surgery was the heart-lung machine, invented by US surgeon John Gibbon (1903–73), and used from the late 1950s. This technology, along with body-cooling techniques, enabled surgeons to "bypass" the heart, maintaining circulation and respiration artificially, while surgery was conducted on the stopped heart. By the 1960s, surgical techniques were developed to relieve obstruction of the coronary arteries.

For some, the heart was beyond repair. Christiaan Barnard (1922–2001) performed the first —very daring—heart transplant in 1967 at the Groote Schuur Hospital in Cape Town, South Africa. Bernard described the condition of his patient:

> Louis Washkansky's heart came into full view – rolling in a rhythm of its own like a separate and angry sea, yellow from the storms of half a century, yet streaked with blue currents flowing from its depths – blue veins drifting across the heaving waste and ruin of a ravaged heart.

Bernard sewed the heart of a young woman, who had died in a car crash, into his patient. Sadly, Washkansky died of pneumonia 18 days later, and the operation caused both sensation and controversy. The first successful heart transplant in Britain was performed by South African-born Terence English (b. 1932) at Papworth, near Cambridge, in 1979.

Artificial organs and stem cells

The development of immunosuppressive drugs, which have played a major role in organ transplants preventing transplant rejection, started with the first, 6-mercaptopurine (Purinethol), in the 1950s, followed by the development of the more effective cyclosporin in the early 1980s. New ways of working—of researching—internationally and collaboratively have driven innovations in the field of organ transplants as many distinguished scientists, immunologists, pharmacologists, physicians, and surgeons have worked together for a common goal.

By the mid-1980s hundreds of successful transplants, from heart to lungs and liver, were being conducted, with recipients surviving over five years. Today, heart surgery is routine and around 5,000 heart transplants are performed worldwide each year in 225 specialist centers. Recently, hand and face transplants have made the headlines.

A problem, however, is not always the technology, but an imbalance between the supply (of suitable donor organs, which is low) and demand (which, with increasing referrals, is high). Exciting advances are being made to overcome the shortage of donor organs. Artificial hearts powered by pumps can now keep a patient alive while awaiting a donor, and artificial organ transplants, using a patient's own stem cells grown on an artificial scaffold, remove the need for a donor organ or antirejection drugs.

In 2011 a major new breakthrough in transplant surgery was announced when an international team of surgeons in Stockholm, Sweden, led by the Italian Paolo Macchiarini, performed a synthetic windpipe (trachea) transplant on a young man suffering from an inoperable tracheal tumor. The patient's own stem cells (from his bone marrow) had been seeded onto a plastic scaffold built from nanofibers to create the world's first artificial organ. The patient's tumor and diseased windpipe were removed and replaced with the tailor-made replica—an extraordinary feat.

This novel surgical operation was made possible by advances in both nanotechnology and medical research. We now know that stem cells are unspecialized cells that can renew themselves indefinitely and develop into specialized more mature cells. For example, embryonic stem cells give rise to blood, skin, liver, muscle, and a variety of other tissues and organs. Scientists are also able to "reprogram" (by introducing a few genes) mature adult

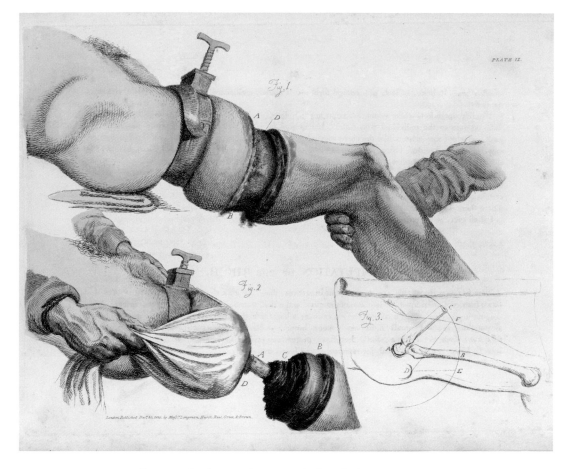

Leg amputation in an 1821 illustration by the Scottish surgeon Charles Bell. The tourniquet was there to numb the pain and reduce blood flow, but this could also lead to serious tissue damage.

cells to become immature stem cells capable of developing into all the specialized tissues of the body. These can then be used, in turn, to replace diseased or damaged tissue. This discovery has been likened to turning the "developmental clock" backward.

The potential of stem cell therapy is huge, and in 2012 the Nobel Prize in Physiology or Medicine was awarded to two scientists, John Gurdon from Cambridge, England, and Shinya Yamanaka from Kyoto, Japan, whose research and discoveries have led the way in this field.

From keyhole to the future: robotic- and tele- surgery

Conditions requiring surgery—such as benign and malignant tumors, heart defects, traumatic injuries, worn-out hips and knees—have benefited from advances in technology as well as the skills of surgeons. Robotic surgery enables surgeons to perform delicate and complex operations through a few tiny incisions with increased vision, precision, and dexterity. While X-rays, first discovered in 1895, remain useful for detecting some problems, such as broken bones, hospital staff can now use powerful noninvasive imaging techniques developed over the past few decades to "see" inside the body and locate and record with precision any abnormalities prior to an operation. It is even possible for a patient to swallow a tiny capsule with a remote-controlled camera, which, as it moves through the digestive system of the body, can transmit images of the gastrointestinal tract to a screen.

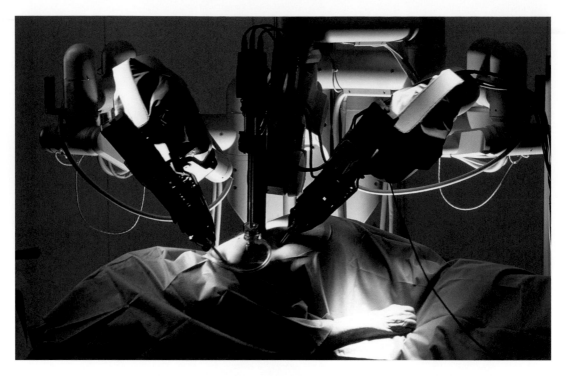

This *da Vinci* "robot surgeon" performs minimally invasive surgery on a patient's heart—one of the latest cutting-edge methods of operating. The surgical tools, on the ends of the robot arms, are controlled by a "real surgeon" who views a live 3D image of the operation site from an endoscope on one of the robot's arms. The *da Vinci* system allows precise control of surgical tools through tiny incisions, just ½ inch wide.

Surgeons' tools are infinitely more refined than the old scalpels and saws of the "knife-cutters." Keyhole (minimally invasive) and laser surgery are now routine. Natural orifice transluminal endoscopic surgery is an emerging surgical technique in which surgeons go through a natural orifice (the mouth, rectum, or vagina) instead of making an incision on the outside of the body. Robots, such as the *da Vinci* Surgical System, first introduced in the 1990s for minimally invasive surgery, are still relatively new on the scene (and expensive) but will increasingly be used to "cooperate" with surgeons and improve their diagnostic and operating techniques in the coming decades. Robotic-assisted surgery will also help develop the field of "telesurgery"—an operation carried out by a remote surgeon communicating with robotic tools using internet technology, first performed in 2001.

The 21st-century surgeon

In a compelling book, *Direct Red* (2009), a female surgeon, Gabriel Weston, takes us behind the scenes of a 21st-century surgeon's life in a London hospital:

> *I still see the beauty of surgery all around me when I'm at work ... In clear diagnosis. In methodical procedure. In the rudimentary environment of the operating theatre. In the rigorous magic performed by surgeons on patients, whose diseases are often cured by going under the knife.*

But surgery can also be ugly and brutal, and Weston relates those darker aspects with honesty. There are desperate times when things go wrong. She writes candidly of the mistakes made by herself and other hospital staff.

In so many ways, Gabriel Weston's story reflects the dilemmas of surgery's successes and its limits. It also heightens our awareness that only a minority of surgeons worldwide are women (women account for around 7 percent of consultant surgeons in Britain), although numbers are increasing.

Global surgery: some patients are more equal than others

It is estimated that nearly 250 million surgical procedures take place globally each year. Of these procedures, only a quarter are performed in low- and middle-income countries where nearly three-quarters of the world's population lives. The poorest 35 percent receive only 3.5 percent of all surgery. Sub-Saharan Africa has approximately 1 percent of the number of surgeons available in the USA, as well as extreme shortages of nurses trained in anesthesia and surgical care.

Conditions that need surgery—including complications of childbirth and traumatic injuries—are common in developing countries and contribute significantly to the burden of disability and mortality. Various organizations are working to reduce this by improving emergency and essential surgical care. The Bellagio Essential Surgery Group (BESG), set up in 2007, includes experts in surgery, anesthesia, and obstetrics and aims to increase access to surgical services in sub-Saharan Africa. Charities such as Chain of Hope (for heart surgery) work with leading surgeons to treat children in war-torn and developing countries and can make a vital difference to the lives of the most vulnerable.

As an editorial in *The Lancet* (January 2012) entitled "Global surgery – the final frontier?" reminds us, "reducing the disparities in surgery between developed and developing countries will take a massive, co-ordinated, worldwide effort." Surgery has the power to transform lives in the modern world; it is hoped that advances can be offered to many more in the future.

A 41-year-old man having a hernia operation in Warri Central Hospital, Nigeria. The hospital has limited surgical equipment, no intensive-care unit, a 30-year-old anesthesia machine and a nonfunctioning X-ray machine.

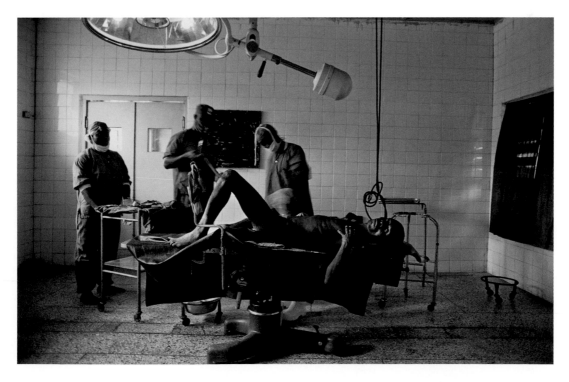

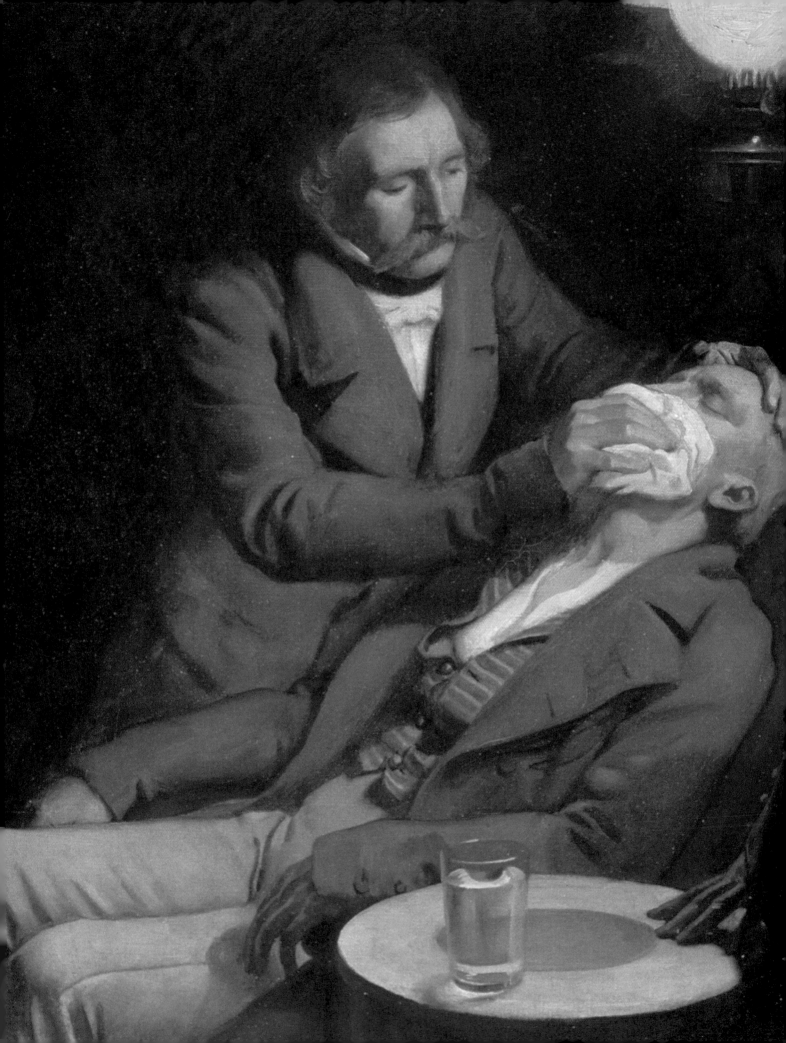

Tooth-drawers and Dentists

Dental tools are simply copies in miniature of articles used in the Spanish inquisition and on refractory prisoners in the Tower of London. There are monkey wrenches, raspers, files, gouges, cleavers, pickes, squeezers, drills, daggers, little crowbars, punches, chisels, pincers, and long wire feelers with prehensile, palpitating tips, that can reach down through the roots of a throbbing tooth and fish up a yell from your inner consciousness.

Chicago Herald, 19th century

Dentistry is a branch of medicine that has only in the recent past assumed professional status. Yet, the search for solutions to dental problems—loss of teeth, toothache, and even bad breath—dates back to ancient times. All sorts of ideas were suggested for the cause of dental decay, including "tooth worms." Tooth decay became especially serious in Europe from the 16th century onward, primarily as a result of the newly widespread consumption of sugar. A group of practitioners, known as "tooth-drawers" or "tooth-operators," offered their services (for a fee) to remove and replace rotten teeth—an agonizing procedure for the majority of patients. The first book entirely devoted to "the teeth" was published in 1530; the term "dentist" was becoming popular by the late 18th century. The introduction of general and local anesthetics from the second half of the 19th century, and antibiotics from the mid-20th century, transformed dentistry. Today, it is a highly sophisticated skill and most of us in the developed world are lucky to be able to smile without showing blackened, decayed, or missing teeth. Poor oral health, however, is a much-neglected problem for children and adults in less affluent parts of the world.

Tooth worms and the first "dentists" in the ancient world

There is a long tradition, continuing right up to the 20th century (albeit one that was debunked many times over the centuries), that "tooth worms" caused holes in the teeth, which subsequently rotted and decayed. "Smoking" worms out of the cavities, using a mixture

OPPOSITE It was in dentistry, rather than surgery, that the trials of nitrous oxide and ether were first performed. This painting by Ernest Board shows William Morton using ether as an anesthetic in dental surgery for the first time in 1846.

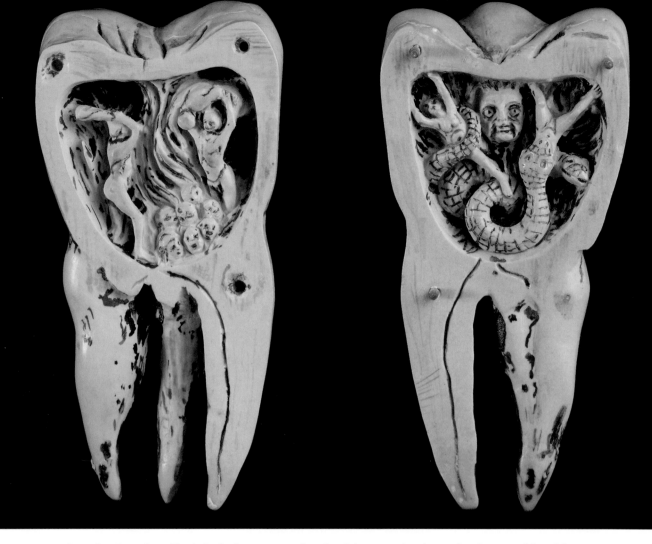

An ancient Sumerian tablet dating back to *c.* 5000 BC describes *Zahnwurm* or (tooth worm) as the cause of dental decay. This 18th-century carved ivory image of a human tooth shows a demonic worm inside it.

of henbane seed and beeswax, heated over a piece of iron, was used as long ago as the 3rd millennium BC. Some ancients also believed in demons and spirits as the cause of toothache, while the Greeks and Romans wrote extensively on the role of morbid humors.

The ancient Egyptians' teeth were ground down, often to the sensitive pulp, most probably as a result of the large amounts of sand, dirt, and grit in their food. Numbers of skulls show multiple abscess formation, indicative of the severity of the problem.

Some of the first records of dental care date back to the dawn of civilization in Mesopotamia and the Nile Valley, where scholars have identified tablets that describe methods of dealing with toothache, falling out or stained teeth, gums, and bad breath. A hieroglyph of an eye over a "tusk" in ancient Egypt denotes "one who deals with teeth" and in 2006 a tomb was found with graves of three royal dentists dating back over 4,000 years, suggesting their prominent status. The earliest recorded named "dentist" not only in Egypt but in the world is thought to be Hesy-Re who lived about 2660 BC. An inscription on his tomb includes the title "the greatest of those who deal with teeth, and of physicians." Scholars believe that the ancient Egyptian dental practitioners were more likely to have treated dental disease with pharmaceutical preparations rather than operative techniques.

The Etruscans in central Italy, *c.*8th–6th centuries BC, even produced gold splints to put around loose teeth. They also, occasionally, if a tooth was missing or worn down, inserted an artificial tooth carved from an ox tooth—the ancient equivalent of braces and false teeth.

Cleaning the teeth

If in your teeth you hap to be tormented
By meane some little worm therein to breed
This pain if heed be ta'en may be prevented
By keeping clean your teeth whenas you feed
Take Francomsense, a gum not evil scented
Put henbane unto this and onion seed
And with a tunnel to the tooth that's hollow
Convey the smoke thereof and ease shall follow.

From the 12th–13th centuries, "Regimen Sanitatis Salernitarum," (17th-century translation by Kenelm Digby)

Keeping teeth clean was as much a preoccupation in ancient times as it is today. Toothpicks in vanity sets made of gold have been found from 3500 BC , indicating the importance of dental hygiene over 5,500 years ago.

Tooth powders, known as dentifrices, and used for rubbing or polishing teeth, were, for centuries, made up from all sorts of materials usually with some abrasive content, such as ground cuttlefish, eggshells, chalk, animal hooves, or even ground china. An advert, in the *Daily Courant*, 1717, for an early tooth powder claimed: "it at once makes the teeth as white as ivory, tho' never so black or yellow, and effectually preserves them from rotting or decaying, continuing them sound to exceeding old age."

Who invented the modern toothbrush?

Toothbrushes have been in use for centuries. Around the 11th–15th centuries, the Chinese made toothbrushes with bristles from the necks of long-haired hogs or used horse-tail hairs on a cattle-bone stick. In Europe the French, in the mid-17th century, produced innovative "little brushes for making cleane of the teeth."

In the late 18th century, William Addis (1734–1808) of England created the first mass-produced toothbrush, founding a company, Addis, in 1780; he soon became very wealthy. While in prison (charged with causing a riot) he decided that the usual method of rubbing a rag on your teeth with salt and soot could be improved. Adopting materials he acquired from a prison guard, he devised a toothbrush using a small animal bone and bristles from horsehair.

The Addis company supplied British troops with toothbrushes during the First World War, creating a new national "habit" of teeth cleaning; and by the 1920s Addis was producing 1.8 million toothbrushes a year. The iconic "Wisdom" brand was launched by the company in 1940 with the first synthetic toothbrushes with plastic handles and nylon bristles. Electric toothbrushes started to be marketed in the 1960s and have become increasingly popular for domestic use.

Sugar, syphilis, and scurvy: the rot sets in

Sugarcane originated from the South Pacific and spread along human migration routes to South Asia and Southeast Asia over two thousand years ago. It reached the West via the Middle East during the medieval period as Crusaders brought it home after campaigns in the Holy Land. There they had encountered caravans carrying what they called "sweet salt." It was not, however, until the 16th century that refined sugar became a popular part of the European diet. Following the discovery of the New World in 1492, Europeans saw the possibilities of introducing sugarcane cultivation into the Americas—especially Brazil and the Caribbean. This policy had disastrous results for Africans, who were transported to the West Indies and elsewhere in the New World to work as slaves on the sugar (as well as tobacco) plantations.

For the wealthy elite, who found a new taste—a "sweet tooth"—for sugary cakes, marzipan sweetmeats, candied fruit, jams, as well as sugar in the newly popular coffee, tea, and chocolate, tooth decay became a major scourge that could be relieved only by extraction. Queen Elizabeth I (r. 1558–1603) suffered from the effects of overindulging in sugar. A German visitor to her court in 1598 reported: "her lips are narrow and her teeth black, a defect that the English seem subject to, from their great use of sugar."

A drawing (1888), showing the effects of syphilis on the teeth of an 11-year-old who had inherited the disease. The notching of the incisors is typical.

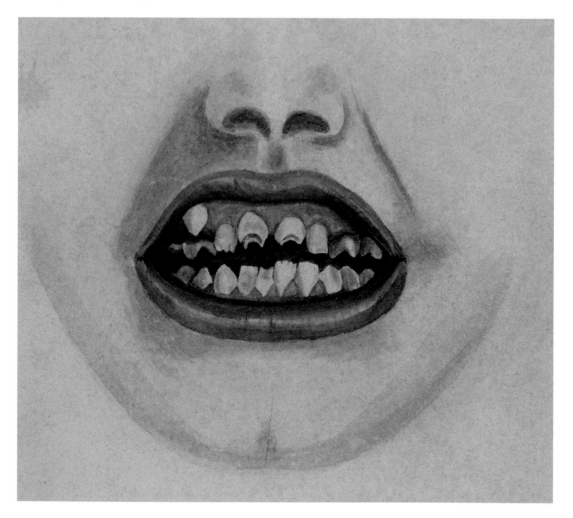

One New Year's day, the court laundress, Mistress Twist, presented Queen Elizabeth with "four tooth-cloths of coarse Holland wrought with black silk and edged with bone lace for rubbing her teeth clean." Her teeth eventually became so bad and blackened that, to conceal both the decay plus her missing teeth, it was said that "when she cometh in public she putteth many fine cloths into her mouth to bear out her cheeks." Evidence from excavations of burial sites dating from the 18th century shows that the majority of people had cavities—reflecting the rise in sugar consumption after the price dropped during that period.

Another major cause of tooth loss in early modern Europe was syphilis. In addition to the gross pustules that erupted over the entire body, this also caused abscesses to eat into the bones (seen in skeletons from the time), and teeth to fall out. The disease was often treated with mercury and this merely contributed to further dental erosions, destruction of the bone and soft tissues of the palate and nose. Children born to syphilitic mothers were often infected in the womb, later developing various deformities, including blindness, deafness, and characteristic "peg-shaped" teeth.

Sailors were exposed to another disease that affected teeth. Between the 15th and 19th centuries, it is estimated that as many as 2 million European sailors succumbed to scurvy. Away at sea for months on end, sailors had to put up with filthy, cramped living conditions, and a barely nutritious diet of foul water, rancid salt meat, seabirds, "moldy maggoty biscuits," and the occasional rat. In 1596 the English naval surgeon William Clowes described the symptoms:

> Their gums were rotten even to the very roots of their teeth, and their cheeks hard and swollen, the teeth were loose neere ready to fall out ... their breath a filthy savour. Their legs were feeble and so weak, that they were not scarce able to carrie their bodies. Moreover they were full of aches and paines, with many blewish and reddish staines or spots, some broad and some small like flea-biting.

Many other accounts tell of the spongy and purple gums, and fetid breath of scurvy sufferers, which affected not only sailors but also soldiers, prisoners, adults, and infants whose diet lacked the essential vitamin C.

Tooth-drawers and quackery

As toothache and rotten teeth became commonplace, an opportunity arose for would-be practitioners to make a living charging a fee to offer assistance. The most notorious of these were the flamboyantly dressed traveling "tooth-drawers," complete with a necklace of human teeth. Often accompanied by jugglers and chattering monkeys, they would set up their stage in the marketplace and encourage all those who needed dental assistance to pay for extracting a rotten tooth. It is said that they would also offer to get rid of "tooth worms."

The tooth-drawer would perform public extractions—first fumigating and then removing the "tooth worms" along with the rotten tooth. There were various cunning ploys to extract the "tooth worms." Pods of henbane, which, when heated, burst open and produced seeds might be craftily hidden in the operator's hand who would then "painlessly" pretend to extract a tooth from the accomplice and pass off the seeds as maggots of the worm.

The "instruments of torture" that tooth-drawers used were gruesome and, undoubtedly, unwashed between patients. One such instrument was the "pelican" described by one contemporary as "brutal, horrific, and not infrequently fatal." Forceps, used to extract teeth, were also known by such names as parrot's beak or crow's bill. Some tooth-drawers used red-hot irons to stop excessive bleeding and gumboils. The "dental key" was popular with tooth-drawers in the 18th century. It was clamped over the tooth, which was first loosened by an "elevator," and turned like a key in the door. Infection usually followed tooth extraction in the preantibiotic era and could prove fatal.

By the 17th century, the term "tooth-operators" came into parlance, defined as "one skilled in drawing teeth and in making artificial ones." Barber-surgeons could also offer tooth-drawing. One popular and larger-than-life tooth-operator was "le Grand Thomas," or "Fat Thomas." He kept a regular spot on the Pont-Neuf in Paris and for nearly half a century, from the 1710s, he pulled out teeth and plied his dental wares and "secret" medicines.

From tooth-drawers to dentists

He had the calm, possessed, surgical look of a man who could endure pain in another person.

Mark Twain on his dentist, Dr Riggs

The English word "dentist" was first used from the late 1750s. It came from the French word "dentiste" (Latin, *dens*, for "tooth"). The adoption of the word "dentist" was at first ridiculed as in the *Edinburgh Chronicle* of September 15 1759: "*dentist* figures now in our newspapers, and may do well enough for a French puffer; but we fancy Rutter [Samuel Rutter, Master of the Barber Surgeons] is content with being called a *tooth-drawer*." The French led the way in "opening up" the field of dentistry.

Pierre Fauchard (1678–1761), often known as the "father of modern dentistry," published *Le Chirurgien Dentiste* (1728), setting out for the first time current knowledge about dental disease. Chapters covered scaling the teeth, filling them, false teeth, extraction, and moving teeth. He also noted that sugar damages gums and teeth, and he shared some of his own inventions. One of his aims was to expose the tricks and practices of itinerant tooth-drawers. Fauchard coined the term "chirurgien-dentiste" (surgeon-dentist) to establish a "new" scientific profession.

Following Fauchard, at least 740 books on dentistry were published up to 1800. The surgeon and anatomist John Hunter wrote widely on the subject, writing *The Natural History of the Human Teeth, Explaining Their Structure, Use, Formation, Growth and Diseases* (1771), with its supplement, *A Practical Treatise on the Diseases of the Teeth* (1778). This gave a scientific basis to dental anatomy and included numerous meticulous illustrations.

Dentists on both sides of the Atlantic in this era, however, generally remained untrained in a formal sense. They picked up tips on the job or learned the trade as an apprentice. Some were watchmakers or pharmacists who recognized a lucrative business opportunity when it presented itself. Paul Revere, best known for his famous "Midnight Ride" from Boston to Lexington on the night of April 18/19 1775 to warn about the approach of British soldiers, was a silversmith and a dentist—as well as a patriot of the American Revolution. Perhaps less well known is the fact that he was a pioneer of postmortem dental forensic science! His friend, Dr Joseph Warren, a Major General during the Revolution, was killed at the Battle of Bunker Hill. Warren was buried in an unmarked grave. Some ten months later, Paul Revere visited the site and although Warren's face was unrecognizable, Revere was able to identify Warren's body on the basis of the bridge of hippopotamus ivory and silver wire that he had inserted to replace his friend's missing teeth.

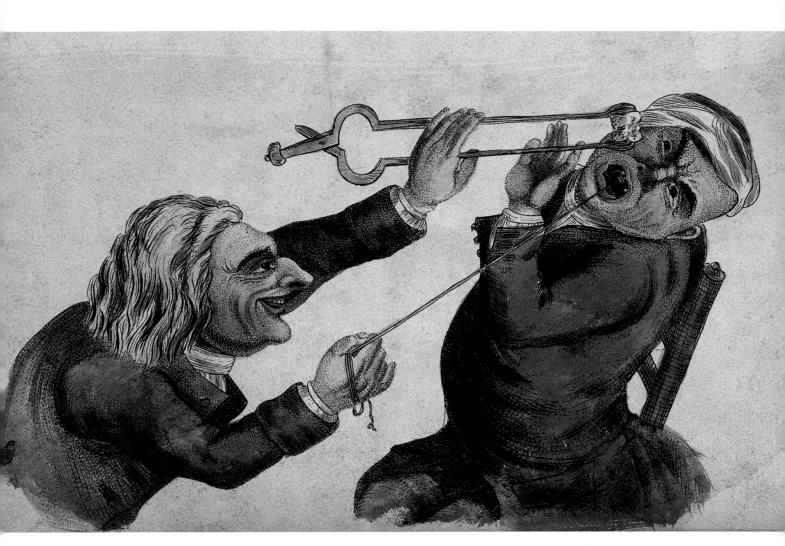

The Tooth-drawers (c. 1810). Audiences were initially fooled by fake—seemingly painless—removals on accomplices, only to suffer agonizing torture from the removal of their teeth without any anesthetic.

It remained difficult to distinguish the quacks from the experts. Some certainly continued to promise near-"miracles," as one 18th-century French "dentist," Sieur Roquet, practicing in the USA, boasted in a newspaper advertisement:

> He also cures effectually the most stinking Breaths, by drawing out, and eradicating all decayed Teeth and Stumps, and burning the Gums to the Jaw Bone, without the least Pain or Confinement; and putting in their stead, an entire Set of right African Ivory Teeth, set in a Rose-colour'd Enamel, so nicely fitted to the Jaws, that People of the first Fashion may eat, drink, swear, talk Scandal, quarrel, and shew their Teeth, without the least Indecency, Inconvenience, or Hesitation whatever.

"Waterloo teeth": gappy mouths

Transplanting teeth from animals or humans attracted the attention of the dental world in the later 18th century, especially after John Hunter performed an important experiment. He placed a human tooth into the comb of a cockerel, which became firmly implanted. Some were convinced that this would work for humans. Poor children were paid to have their healthy teeth removed, which would then be transplanted into the gums of wealthy adults. Once implanted, the new tooth was tied to the neighboring teeth until the transplant stabilized.

An advert in New York's *Independent Journal* of 1783 requested "Any person disposed to part with their front teeth may receive Two guineas for each Tooth, on applying at No. 28 Maiden Lane." Transplantation was the most expensive dental procedure money could buy. It was, however, rarely effective and most still resorted to the good old-fashioned removable dentures.

By the early 19th century, graveyards, mortuaries, dissecting rooms, and battlefields were being ransacked for the corpses' teeth. The term "Waterloo teeth" came into being after the Battle of Waterloo in 1815. The teeth of the dead soldiers were seen, by the victorious British, as a rich source of "false" teeth for those back home. As late as the 1860s, human teeth obtained from the battlefields of the American Civil War were being shipped to Europe for sale.

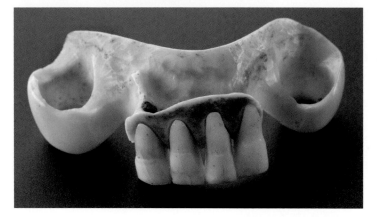

"Waterloo teeth." A 19th-century lower denture carved from hippopotamus ivory with human teeth fixed into it.

The main problem was getting the teeth to fix into a denture base. The most favored material was made from hippopotamus ivory into which the teeth would be riveted. Finally, in the 1850s, vulcanite, a hardened rubber, invented by the US Goodyear family in Cleveland, Ohio, was introduced into dentistry. This was a material that could be molded to fit a person's gums providing an ideal and inexpensive base for dentures. A popular 21st birthday present for young ladies was the extraction of all the teeth (to save later agonies of tooth decay) and replacement by a set of dentures.

George Washington (1732–99) had dentures made of gold, hippopotamus ivory, and lead —together with human and animal teeth. Springs helped them open, and a hole in the left lower plate created a snug fit over his last remaining tooth. In Britain, Winston Churchill wore gold-plated dentures to help disguise a lisp during his inspirational Second World War speeches. In 2010 part of one set sold for $23,870. Today we can have plastic dentures or individual implants fitted, the latter being very complicated and therefore expensive.

Amalgam fillings

Scientists have recently analyzed a 6,500-year-old human mandible (lower jawbone) from Slovenia whose cavity in a cracked tooth bears traces of a filling with beeswax. For the very rich, gold foil, or gold leaf was used for centuries to fill holes or caries. An amalgam of mercury and silver fillings had been tried in China in the 11th and 12th centuries and, again, in France in the early 19th century—using melted-down silver coins.

Controversy surrounded the use of mercury and in the 1840s, during what became known as the "amalgam war," it was thrown into disrepute by the Crawcour brothers from Paris. It turned out they were flogging a replacement, traveling first to London and then to America, where, in 1833, they introduced their own filling material "Royal Mineral Succedaneum." This dodgy amalgam was thumbed into cavities without removing the decay, ultimately causing tooth damage. As they were rumbled and returned to Europe, amalgam was left with a bad reputation. In 1843 the American Society of Dental Surgeons forced members to pledge not to use amalgam, describing it as "malpractice."

From the late 19th century an improved amalgam convinced practitioners that this was suitable as a filling material. Today, more expensive white fillings are made of composite resins. Prompted by attacks on empirics and charlatans, and especially by the fight against the Crawcour brothers, dentistry increasingly became more regulated. The world's first dental college, the Baltimore College of Dental Surgery, was founded in 1840, followed by others on both sides of the Atlantic. In Britain a leading figure in the professionalization of dentistry was John Tomes (1815–95). The London dental schools created some of the first clinical training establishments for dental students and also provided places for the poor to receive free treatment.

Laughing gas: the end of pain

The pain of having a tooth extracted or even a whole set of rotten teeth pulled out with little in the way of general or local anesthetics must have felt like torture, as well as being bloody. It was also nerve-racking for the patient, and even for the dentist. According to one famous anecdote, King George III was awaiting a tooth extraction and feigning fear he asked the dentist to present him with a glass of brandy before the operation. The King then declined to take the glass, saying: "I have no need of it; but was merely anxious to observe if your hand was steady."

While all sorts of concoctions, including opium and various narcotics and alcohol, as well as Chinese acupuncture, had been tried down the centuries to help the patient be oblivious to the pain of an extraction, it was the introduction of a number of inhalation gases that eventually transformed anesthesia in dentistry.

The story of "modern" anesthesia dates back to the late 18th century when the British scientist Humphry Davy (1778–1829), best known for his invention of the Davy lamp for miners, began to experiment with nitrous oxide (N2O) at Thomas Beddoes' Medical Pneumatic Institution in Bristol, England. Originally discovered in the 1770s by the British chemist Joseph Priestley (1733–1804) and known as "dephlogisticated nitrous air," Davy in the late 1790s explored its intoxicating effects of making people laugh, hence its nickname of "laughing gas." The poet Samuel Taylor Coleridge described it as "great ecstasy." Robert Southey, another Romantic English poet, imagined that "the atmosphere of the highest of all possible heavens must be composed of this gas." It became very popular at wild parties. Doctors and poets alike recorded the amazing sensations when they inhaled the gas through silken or "Paradise" bags.

On one occasion, the young US dentist-physician Horace Wells (1815–48) was fascinated by a laughing gas display at Hartford, Connecticut. It had been advertised as an exhibition of "Nitrous oxide, exhilarating or laughing gas! ... It [makes] people Laugh, Sing, Dance, Speak, or Fight, etc. according to the leading trait of their character.'"

Wells noticed how a man under its influence seemed impervious to the pain of an injured leg sustained while frolicking around. Wells was so impressed he decided to try it out in his private dental surgery. Administering the gas from an animal bladder through a wooden tube placed in the mouth, he found it was successful in deadening the pain during tooth

Cocaine (from the South American coca plant) was introduced as a local anesthetic in dentistry in the late 19th century. Apart from being highly addictive, it was soon found to damage the tissues of the mouth.

extractions. He even used it to have one of his own teeth pulled out painlessly, exclaiming "it is the greatest discovery ever made! I didn't feel it so much as the prick of a pin!"

Fired with enthusiasm, Wells gave a public demonstration of dental extraction under nitrous oxide at the Massachusetts General Hospital in Boston, in January 1845. According to the story, the operation was deemed a failure—the patient, a Harvard student, cried out during the extraction and Wells was booed out of the room amid cries of "humbug." Wells was humiliated by his apparent failure. Tragically, he later committed suicide. He did, however, receive posthumous recognition for his contribution to conducting dental operations without pain and nitrous oxide was "reintroduced" into dentistry in the 1860s and later became popular in combination with oxygen as "gas and air" for childbirth.

Shortly after Wells's attempt to anesthetize a dental patient, William Morton (Boston dentist and former partner of Wells), on September 30 1846, used another gas, ether, to successfully induce unconsciousness while extracting the infected tooth of Eben Frost. Morton is also now generally credited—although there was much disagreement at the time about this—with introducing anesthesia to surgery.

Cocaine (from the South American coca plant) was introduced as a local anesthetic in dentistry in the late 19th century. Apart from being highly addictive, it was soon found to damage the tissues of the mouth. Chemists in Germany searched for a better alternative and succeeded in synthesizing a new drug called procaine (Novocain) in the early 1900s, which remained the main local anesthetic for a further 40 years.

Transforming dentistry

Over the course of the 19th century, the wealthy began to pay more attention to their teeth. Respectable dental practices started to hire female dental assistants and "Lady in Attendance" signs were routinely seen in windows of dental offices. Their duties included chair-side assistance, instrument cleaning, appointments, bookkeeping, and reception. Toothbrushes became increasingly popular—at least among the rich—and many expensive versions were made. Some were part of elaborate traveling sets that included tooth-powder boxes and tongue scrapers.

Toothpicks might also be fashioned in gold or silver, enriched with precious stones, and even hung on a chain around the neck. Levi Spear Parmly, a New Orleans dentist in the early 19th century, recommended the use of "waxen silken thread passed through the interstices of the teeth" and is credited with inventing dental floss.

Newly styled forceps that had beaks anatomically shaped to fit the crowns of the teeth were introduced. These helped to prevent slippage of the instruments on the teeth and to stop the terrible damage to the surrounding gums and bones that had been so common with the pelican and key. Toothpastes of various kinds were developed in the 19th century and by the 1890s they came in a soft metal tube. False teeth began to be made with porcelain, replacing the traditional animal and human teeth, and by the mid-19th century porcelain sets were being produced in large numbers.

Although the state of many people's teeth still remained pretty deplorable in the early and mid-20th century, further key advances for the dental profession were underway. The discovery of bacteria in the later 19th century led to a new understanding of the cause of dental decay.

In the late 1880s, W D Miller (1853–1907), a US dentist working in Koch's laboratory in Berlin, developed the "chemico-parasitic" theory in which he showed that caries were caused by the initial action of acids resulting from fermentation of food, followed by the action of bacteria on softened tissue. He published his findings in 1890 in a book entitled *The Micro-Organisms of the Human Mouth*. In modern terms, this concept focuses on what is now called "plaque," a soft sticky yellow film that adheres to teeth and is composed mostly of bacteria which live on the dissolved sugars from things we eat and drink. The acid produced by the bacteria then corrodes the enamel and dentine of teeth. Bacteria also release toxins, which can cause inflammation of the gums, leading to the breakdown of the fibers and bone that support the teeth.

The arrival of X-rays at the end of the 19th century was a huge advantage for dentists, enabling them to visualize all sorts of problems within the jaw. Indeed, one of X-rays' first clinical applications was in dentistry. Electrical lighting also enabled dentists to get a brighter image of the teeth, and the use of electric drills, which followed on from Morrison's foot-treadle dental engine (invented in 1871), as well as the first dental chair in 1867 (reclining dental chairs came into use in the late 1950s), were just some of the scientific and technological innovations that combined to advance the dental profession and improve the patient experience. Indoor plumbing was a tremendous help as was the new understanding

"You won't feel a thing!" A dentist anesthetizes his patient with "laughing gas" (nitrous oxide). By the 20th century, dental surgeries catering for the wealthy were kitted out with all the latest (if quite frightening-looking) equipment—from X-ray machines to electrical drills.

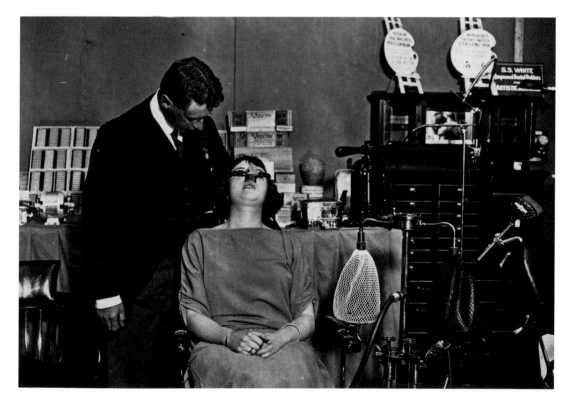

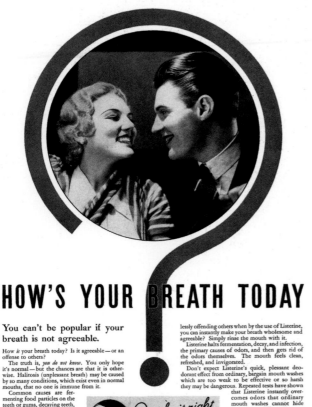

HOW'S YOUR BREATH TODAY

You can't be popular if your breath is not agreeable.

How *is* your breath today? Is it agreeable—or an offense to others?

The truth is, *you do not know.* You only hope it's normal—but the chances are that it is otherwise. Halitosis (unpleasant breath) may be caused by so many conditions, which exist even in normal mouths, that no one is immune from it.

Common causes are fermenting food particles on the teeth or gums, decaying teeth, leaky fillings, unwise eating and drinking, and infections of the mouth, nose, and throat. But 90% of all cases are caused by food fermentation.

Why take the risk of need-

lessly offending others when by the use of Listerine, you can instantly make your breath wholesome and agreeable? Simply rinse the mouth with it.

Listerine halts fermentation, decay, and infection, the primary causes of odors, and then gets rid of the odors themselves. The mouth feels clean, refreshed, and invigorated.

Don't expect Listerine's quick, pleasant deodorant effect from ordinary, bargain mouth washes which are too weak to be effective or so harsh they may be dangerous. Repeated tests have shown that Listerine instantly overcomes odors that ordinary mouth washes cannot hide in 12 hours. When you want to be *sure,* use Listerine, the safe antiseptic and quick deodorant.

Lambert Pharmacal Company, St. Louis, Missouri.

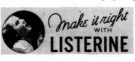

make it right WITH **LISTERINE**

A 1930s magazine advert for Listerine. This mouthwash was promoted to improve oral hygiene and tackle "bad breath"— a shrewd commercial move.

of the importance of antisepsis and sterilizing dental instruments.

An American dentist, Alfred Civilion Fones (1869–1938), led the dental hygiene movement in the USA (and created the name "dental hygienist") with the first course in 1913 and the first license in 1917. A key figure in Britain in introducing "oral hygiene" into schools was the Cambridge dentist George Cunningham (1852–1919). A survey in 1891 revealed the appalling state of children's teeth in Britain and, in 1907, Cunningham opened the Cambridge Dental Institute, the first British children's clinic. He campaigned vigorously, even setting up "Toothbrush Clubs," to encourage schoolchildren to brush their teeth. Cunningham also recognized the appalling state of the teeth of military recruits with his warning: "You can't fight if you can't bite." One of the greatest changes for the dental health of the British nation followed the introduction of the NHS in 1948, providing free dental care for all. Within nine months, 33 million individual artificial teeth had been supplied!

Fluoride in the early 20th century was recognized to be beneficial for teeth in preventing dental caries. It occurs naturally in some fresh waters but in some countries additional fluoride is added to public water supplies. The addition of fluoride to toothpastes began in the 1950s and most toothpastes on the market now contain this. In the early 1920s, mouthwash company Listerine introduced the word "halitosis" to describe bad breath (and sell new products). Traditional solutions for this had included gargling urine, wine, and herbs, or chewing betel nuts, fennel seeds, or cinnamon sticks. The US public today spends about $1–3 billion a year on breath fresheners and oral health products.

The discovery of antibiotics to fight infection was a major boon for dentists and toothache sufferers in the second half of the 20th century. New safer and more effective local anesthetics were also introduced into dentistry, including lidocaine in 1949. Today, most dentists will numb the patient's mouth, often with an injection using a local anesthetic; the injection might be briefly painful but not nearly as excruciating as feeling the dental drill.

Dental specialists

Dentists are highly trained general practitioners, handling a variety of dental needs. Most modern dental surgeries are fitted out with the latest high-tech equipment enabling effective management of individual dental health. Some dentists also practise in one of the specialist areas of which orthodontists—who straighten teeth with dental braces and other appliances

—are the largest group. Periodontists are trained to deal with the supporting structures of teeth and conditions such as gingivitis (inflammation of the gum) and the more serious periodontal diseases that can lead to destruction of the supporting bone around natural teeth with consequent tooth loss.

Oral and maxillofacial surgeons are usually trained in both medicine and dentistry, enabling them to operate in hospitals on a range of pathological conditions of the mouth, jaw and face, notably facial deformities, oral cancers, and oral-facial trauma. Many dental practices today also have dental hygienists (98 percent worldwide are female) to "scale and polish" teeth as a preventive measure and advise on brushing and flossing. Cosmetic and aesthetic dentistry, including teeth whitening, is increasingly popular.

"Please help this child to smile": global dental health

The latter part of the 20th century saw a transformation in both general health and oral health unmatched in the history of the Western world. The gleaming smile that many of us aspire to is, sadly, not always an option for everyone, especially in the world's poorest and marginalized communities. Indeed, oral diseases are one of the greatest health burdens for low-income countries, while the increase in sugar, tobacco, and alcohol consumption that has accompanied modernization in emerging economies is bad news. Oral cancers (often tied to the consumption of tobacco products) are the eighth most common cancer globally, and in Southeast Asia, cancer of the oral cavity ranks among the three most common types of cancer.

There is also a serious shortage of dentists in certain parts of the world, and some African countries, like Sierra Leone and Rwanda, have just ten dentists for the whole population. Meanwhile, in Britain, there is one dentist to every 2,100 people.

In poverty-stricken communities, orofacial congenital clefts occur in about one per 500–700 births. In areas with no surgeons, dentists, and anesthesia providers, many children are denied corrective surgery, leading to feeding and speech problems. Noma (also known as cancrum oris or necrotizing ulcerative stomatitis) is an appalling disease linked to extreme poverty, profound malnutrition, seriously weakened immune systems (following a disease such as measles or HIV/AIDS), inadequate sanitation, and poor dental hygiene. It was once prevalent in the Western world, dating back to antiquity, but is now mostly confined to the developing world, especially the very poor savannah region directly south of the Sahara desert—which is known as the world's "noma belt." This bacterial infection can lead to the destruction of the periodontium (the tissues that surround and support the teeth) and necrosis of the tissues in the cheeks, lips, and bones of the jaw. The pain and suffering of those affected is indescribable. At least 140,000 cases occur each year and over 80–90 percent of children with untreated noma die following the onset of sepsis.

A number of charities, such as Smile Train, Operation Smile, and Facing Africa—Noma, send volunteer dentists and surgeons to treat infants and children suffering from these conditions, and the WHO has begun to make "oral health" part of its mission to improve "global health."

Listerine introduced the word "halitosis" to describe bad breath (and sell new products). Traditional solutions for this had included gargling urine, wine, and herbs.

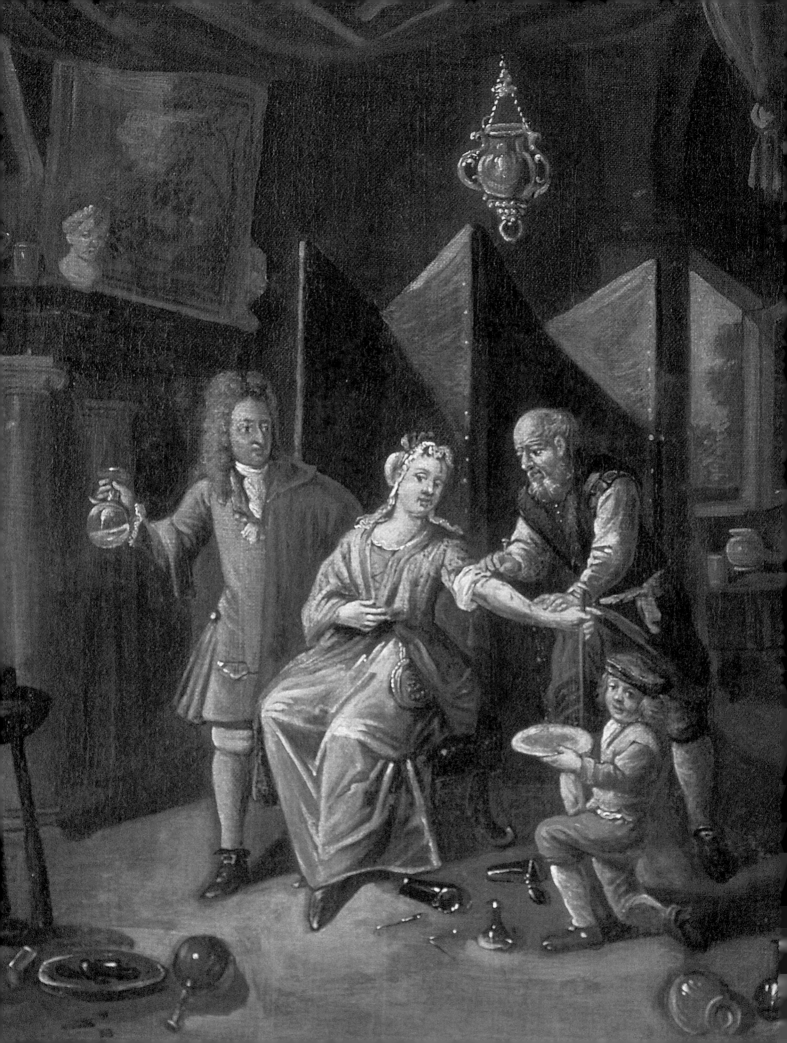

Bloodletting and Purging

If anybody comes to I,
I physics, bleeds and sweats 'em;
If, after that, they like to die,
Why, what care I, I lets 'em.

"On Dr Lettsom," Anonymous

Of all the curious remedies for treating ill-health down the ages, one of the most intriguing is bloodletting. This withdrawal of often considerable quantities of a patient's blood was thought to cure or prevent disease. Bloodletting was practiced by the ancients and continued to be recommended by barber-surgeons and doctors, though the efficacy and dangers of such "heroic" treatments began to be questioned by herbalists and homeopaths who favored more natural methods of healing. Forms of purging the body have included laxatives or enemas for flushing out the bowels and emetics to induce vomiting. Many people treated themselves and their families with home remedies. Some of the old "cures," such as drinking one's own urine, may seem bizarre to modern practitioners and patients; some, like arsenic and mercury, were downright dangerous; while others such as honey may well have been beneficial.

Bloodletting and deathbed scenes

Raymond Crawfurd (1865–1938) recreated the scene of treating King Charles II (r.1660–85) on his deathbed:

> Sixteen ounces of blood were removed from a vein in his right arm with immediate good effect.
> As was the approved practice at this time, the King was allowed to remain in the chair in which
> the convulsions seized him. His teeth were held forcibly open to prevent him biting his tongue ...
> Urgent messages had been dispatched to the King's numerous personal physicians...
> They ordered cupping-glasses to be applied to his shoulders forthwith, and deep scarification
> to be carried out, by which they succeeded in removing another eight ounces of blood ... Strong
> purgatives were given, and supplemented by a succession of clysters [enemas]. The hair was
> shorn close, and pungent blistering agents were applied all over his head. And as though this was
> not enough, red-hot cautery was requisitioned as well.

The King graciously apologized for being "an unconscionable time a-dying."

OPPOSITE A surgeon letting blood from a woman's arm, and a physician with a urine-flask, in an 18th-century Flemish painting. Diagnosing disease by "looking at" the color of a patient's urine (uroscopy) and relieving symptoms by removing quantities of blood (bloodletting) were two of the most common and iconic medical procedures for hundreds of years.

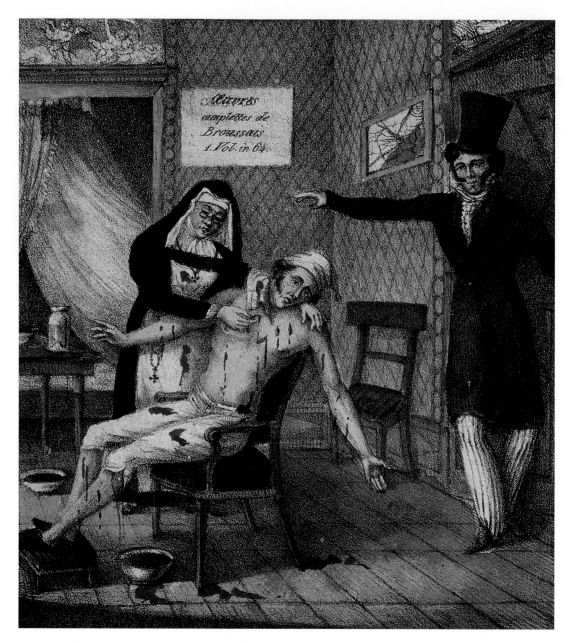

The French physician Broussais—a notorious "bleeder" whose views dominated medicine in 19th-century Paris—instructs a nurse to carry on bleeding a pallid, blood-besmeared patient.

A century later, on December 13 1799, George Washington (1732–99), the first US President, went out riding in cold weather. By the next morning he was suffering from a severe sore throat, "hoarseness," and chills. The usual solution: "bleed him." Washington's personal physician, two other doctors, and a lay phlebotomist ("bloodletter") were sent for. Over the next 12 hours, several pints of blood were taken. He was also given various doses of calomel (a mercury-based laxative) to evacuate the bowels, and blisters of cantharides (dried beetles) were applied to his neck to draw the infection away from the throat. Perhaps unsurprisingly, by the end of the night, he was dead. Did he die from his distemper or was he literally bled to death? Washington was just one of generations of patients over the past three millennia whose illnesses were treated by removing frequent and often large quantities of blood.

"To breathe a vein": lancets and leeches

Bloodletting, also known as phlebotomy (Greek, *phlebo-*, a "vein," and *tomē*, "a cutting") and venesection (Latin, *vena* for "vein" and *secare*, "to cut"), describes the practice of making an incision or puncture into a vein to permit the outpouring of blood ("to breathe a vein"). Bloodletting from a patient to cure or prevent illness dates back many centuries and has an extremely wide geographical distribution, having been practiced by the ancient Mesopotamians, Egyptians, Greeks, Mayans, and Aztecs. It fitted in with early ideas of disease causation relating to "imbalances" and "blockages," as, for example, the "humoral" theory of the Greeks and Romans.

Galen thought that blood was the dominant humor that needed to be brought into balance and developed complex guidelines on how much blood should be drawn, while also advising which blood vessels should be used depending on the condition. Historians have noted that the popularity of bloodletting was that it could be seen to "work" as it produced a visible response: a flushed face becomes paler and the delirious patient may faint, calm down into sleep, and apparent comfort.

There were (and still are in some parts of the world) various methods of bloodletting. One technique might involve tying a bandage tightly round the arm above the elbow to make the veins in the forearm swell up so that the barber-surgeon or physician could then cut into the vein. The lancet (after which the internationally famous British medical journal *The Lancet* was named) was one of several instruments used to open up the vein and draw out the blood, which would then spurt out into a receiving bowl. In medieval England, most abbeys had a "flebotomaria" or "bleeding house" in which the monks underwent "minutions" or bleedings at stated periods of the year for general maintenance of health. Doctors devised elaborate charts indicating the most favorable astrological conditions for bleeding. Another popular practice was to use leeches, the freshwater bloodsucking creatures that secrete chemicals in their saliva which block the natural clotting mechanism and keep the blood flowing from the capillaries. Sometimes, leeches would disappear up or down an orifice—a nostril, anus, or throat. To prevent this, the practitioner might draw bits of thread through their tails. The French "sanguinary" physician François-Joseph-Victor Broussais (1772–1838) often used up to fifty leeches at a time, all over the skin. He treated typhoid fever, syphilis, smallpox, worms, tuberculosis, or mental diseases by applying leeches to the abdomen. In recent decades, sterile leeches have been "reintroduced" into modern plastic and reconstructive surgery to help restore blood flow.

Another traditional way of drawing out impurities with centuries of history behind it is cupping. A flame is used to produce a vacuum in a cupping vessel, which is then applied to the skin. "Dry" cupping uses only the heated cup to bring blood to the surface of the skin, while "wet" cupping is a form of bloodletting in which the skin is scarified (cut) and blood drawn from the wound by

Leeches

These slithery sluglike creatures (Latin: *Hirudo medicinalis*) would be first starved before being put on the skin. Their minuscule teeth would puncture the skin and they would greedily suck up the blood of a patient. Once gorged and swollen to six or seven times their original size, they would drop off. The demand for leeches became so great that in the early 19th century France imported around 40 million leeches a year. Leech farms were set up to feed the demand; a new profession of women collectors waded into ponds to attract the leeches to their bare legs.

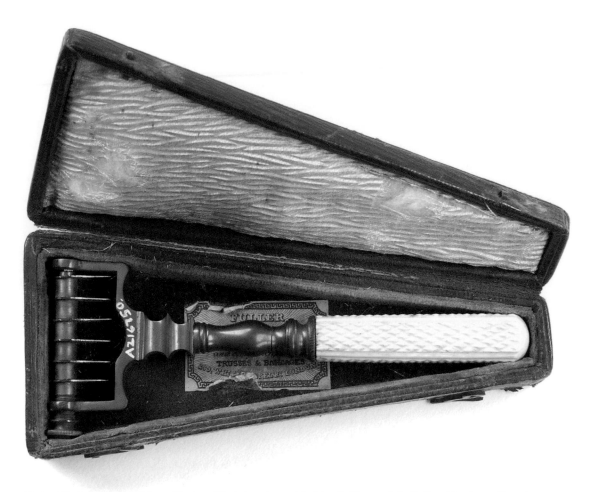

Tools of the trade: an English scarificator with six lancets used for bloodletting made by Fuller of London, 19th century.

suction. One instrument used in "wet" cupping was the scarificator, which was first developed in the 1600s. This had blades that cut into the skin when a trigger was released.

Depending on where in the world they were being used, cups could be made from buffalo horn, bamboo, glass, bronze, or tin. In Europe, cupping was often performed by female lay practitioners and used for a wide range of conditions including chest pains, indigestion, muscular problems, and colds. Within the Chinese medical tradition, cupping was described as early as 281 AD and is a practice still used in Traditional Chinese Medicine to aid the circulation of stagnant *qi* energy and remove toxins from the body. It is sometimes used in conjunction with acupuncture and moxibustion.

The French physician Pierre Louis (1787–1872) was one of the first to apply group comparisons and numerical methods to assess the value of various therapies and he conducted a systematic study of the practice of bloodletting. His results were published in *Researches on the Effects of Bloodletting in Some Inflammatory Diseases* (1835). He was equivocal about the virtues of bleeding to treat fever, but it continued to be a mainstay of therapeutics until the mid-19th century. The new "alternative" practitioners in Europe and America, such as the homeopaths, rejected this "heroic" practice, favoring natural ways of healing (see Complementary and Alternative Medicine). Today, therapeutic phlebotomy is still used in Western medicine for certain disorders: to reduce iron overload in hemochromatosis, to remove excess red blood cells in polycythemia vera, or to reduce toxic levels of porphyrin in porphyria.

Flushing out the system

A range of methods and ingredients were used to "flush out" or purge the system. Those that caused diarrhea were laxatives, cathartics, or purges, depending on their ferocity. Sudorifics made patients sweat. Stimulants woke them up. Enemas (liquids of various concoctions injected into the rectum through the anus for stimulating evacuation of the bowels) were routinely given and were recorded as far back as ancient Assyria, Babylonia, and Egypt. These were considered such an essential component of good health that the Pharaohs, supposedly, had their own so-called "Guardian of the Anus." Like bleeding and cupping, the enema was touted as a cure-all. In pre-Revolutionary France, it is said that more people probably had daily enemas than brushed their teeth.

Emetics were used to induce vomiting. The root of the hellebore plant was said to "procureth vomite mightily ... and by that meanes voideth all superfluous slime and naughtie humours." Diuretics—substances or drugs to increase the discharge of urine—were, likewise, popular. Sweating to remove excess moisture was also thought to cleanse the body of impurities. Samuel Pepys started the year 1663 "drunk" in a coffeehouse until almost sick. He then suffered a blistered lip, followed by itching (which he thought was caused by the bite of two lice), and inflammation, due, he suspected, to the cold, and, next, great pain in his stomach and a fever. He sought expert opinion:

Cupping is an ancient practice used in many cultures to "draw out" impurities in the blood and treat a range of conditions. It is still practiced today, as this contemporary (2004) image from South Korea illustrates.

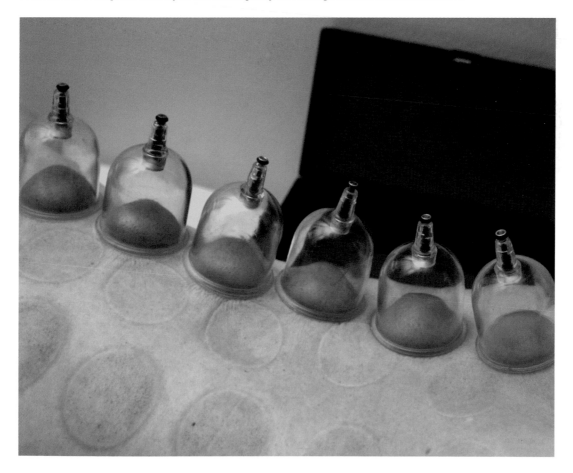

And by the apothecary's advice, Mr Battersby, I am to sweat soundly and that will carry all this matter away; which nature would of itself eject, but this will assist nature – it being some disorder … [of] the blood; but by what I know not, unless it be by my late great Quantitys of Dantzicke-girkins that I have eaten.

The 17th-century English herbalist Nicholas Culpeper (1616–54) was highly critical of both bloodletting and purging and wrote a diatribe against the Royal College of Physicians:

They are bloodsuckers, true vampires, have learned little since Hippocrates; use bloodletting for ailments above the midriff and purging for those below. They evacuate and revulse their patients until they faint. Black Hellebor, this poisonous stuff, is a favourite laxative. It is surprising that they are so popular and that some patients recover. My own poor patients would not endure this taxing and costly treatment. The victims of physicians only survive because they are from the rich and robust stock, the plethoric, red-skinned residents of Cheapside, Westminster and St James.

Bowel movements were a major obsession in Victorian England. A condition called intestinal autointoxication—self-poisoning from one's own retained wastes—was widely diagnosed, especially in young women. It was thought that the colon leaked toxic matter into the bloodstream, which caused sufferers to feel weak and depressed.

The public became prey to marketers of anticonstipation remedies such as an everlasting pill made out of antimony that entered the gut to cause vomiting and diarrhea. The pill, itself, went straight through so it could be used again and again!

The American doctor John Harvey Kellogg (1852–1943), brother of Will of cornflakes fame, practiced colonic washing as he believed the lower bowel to be a sewer of autointoxication,

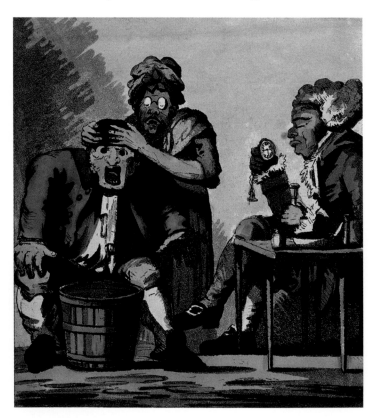

full of poisonous metals. He used an enema machine that could run 15 gallons of water through the bowel in a matter of seconds. Afterwards, half a pint of yogurt was eaten and half given by enema to restore intestinal flora. Nowadays, there is a flourishing field of research on the complex mixture of microorganisms that make up the human "gut microbiota" and its influence on host systems such as the immune system and neurological function. "Probiotics"—live microorganisms taken to alter the composition of the gut microbiota—are now popular products.

A doctor waiting for his patient to vomit after administering an emetic (colored aquatint by G M Woodward, 1800). A range of methods and ingredients were popular to "flush out" or purge the system including emetics (to induce vomiting), enemas (to evacuate the bowels), and diuretics (to increase the discharge of urine).

"One night with Venus and a lifetime with Mercury"

A disease which is so cruel, so distressing, so appalling that until now nothing so horrifying, nothing more terrible or disgusting, has ever been known on this earth.

Joseph Grüenpeck, on syphilis, 1503

Many Arabic and European alchemists, from the medieval to the early modern period, pioneered the use of metals, minerals, and chemicals in medicine. New substances, including mercury, sulfur, and antimony became the wonder drugs of the late Renaissance. In the early 16th century, Girolamo Fracastoro recommended mercury ("quicksilver") to treat the "new" European epidemic of syphilis spread through sexual intercourse.

Syphilis patients were shut up in a "stew," a small steam room, often for 20 or 30 days at a time. Wrapped in blankets, they were left to sweat in a hot tub or by the fire and given mercury, either as a drink or as an ointment for their suppurating sores. Another method involved locking the patient in a box in which mercury was heated until it vaporized so that the patient breathed in its fumes. These methods induced sweating and salivation. It was said that the patient needed to produce at least three pints of saliva for the poison to be expelled from the body. During the treatment disgusting secretions issued from patients' mouths and noses; sores filled their throats and tongues; their jaws swelled and often their teeth fell out. Everything stank.

One physician even marketed underwear coated inside with a mercury ointment. Like bloodletting, the dramatic effects of mercury may have given credence to the idea that this treatment worked. The German syphilis sufferer Ulrich von Hutton (1488–1523), however, was so appalled at the outcome of his years of mercury treatment that he advocated a far more gentle remedy called guaiacum or "holy wood," a decoction made from a tree native to the West Indies. Large quantities of the wood were imported into Europe and the syphilitic rich drank guaiac cocktails.

We are reminded of the dangers of mercury in the phrase "mad as a hatter." Mercury was, later, used in the process of curing felt in some hats and hatters and mill workers often suffered poisoning from the fumes, causing neurological damage, including confused speech.

Kitchen remedies

Bloodletting and mercury were among the more spectacular purges and potions of the past. But the sick would try anything—and there were plenty of physicians and quacks eager to meet their needs. Many people over the centuries also relied on their own home remedies before seeking medical help. Oral traditions have played a major role in hand-me-down remedies and we can all cite many old-wives' tales of cures used by our mothers and grandmothers. Some would be collated into handwritten "recipe" (or "receipt") books. Often the remedies were based on herbs and plants that might be found growing in fields, meadows, hedgerows, and orchards, or in kitchen gardens. Others, including foreign imports, could be obtained from apothecaries, grocers, spicers, and traveling drug sellers.

An insight into just what a home kitchen might contain for everyday and emergency needs is documented in the story of Elizabeth Freke (c.1641–1714), an elderly gentlewoman living in Norfolk, England. In the fall of 1711, Elizabeth busied herself planning a trip to London. At the age of 69, she decided to make an inventory of "some of the best things" in

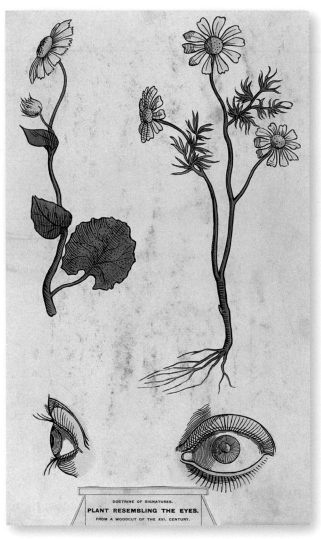

Doctrine of signatures. In this colored ink drawing (c. 1923), after a 16th-century woodcut illustration, a plant with flowers resembling the human eye is described as having properties for healing the eye.

her house, just in case she did not return. The room-by-room inventory was written into her notebook of "remembrances and culinary and medical recipes." Included among her more obvious precious items of jewelry and furniture, she listed the contents of five locked cupboards!

In these Elizabeth kept a whole variety of medicinal potions, syrups, cordials and cure-alls (including her *elixir salutatis* and *aqua mirabilis*), designed to deal with every sort of ailment from common complaints to severe diseases, such as agues, fevers, and smallpox. Rosemary water, lemon water and brandy, tincture of lavender, syrup of saffron, and tincture of nutmegs contained just a few of the herbs and spices that went into her healing remedies. Among her worldly goods, she also owned brass and metal skillets, chaffing dishes, mortars and pestles, and distillation equipment, all of which she could use to make up her medicinal waters, syrups, juleps, and salves. There were times, however, when Elizabeth sought a cure from another practitioner—in one case, the local vicar. When, in 1708, she was suffering from a head ailment and a "tissick," it was the Revd Edward Smith who "let her blood and cut her hair."

Some home remedies, as well as those prescribed by apothecaries, were based on the principle of the "doctrine of signatures." Paracelsus believed that the universe (macrocosm) and the body (microcosm) were interlinked—that man and nature were locked into one interacting world. His "doctrine of signatures" linked macrocosm and microcosm by identifying the curative power of plants through their similarity to parts of the body. For example, a walnut resembling a skull might be good for skull fractures; the leaves of lungwort (*Pulmonaria officinalis*) resembled lungs and were used for chest diseases; the root of the orchid looked like a testicle and could cure testicular ailments; yellow plants such as saffron were remedies for jaundice; spotted plants cured spots, and so on. This might also apply to the use of animals. Oil of earthworm was applied to bruises as the skin of earthworm looks like a bruise.

Other complaints might, by contrast, be treated not with "similars" but with "contraries." A chilling disease was thus treated with heat and a dry one with moisture. These ideas fitted in with various religious beliefs that for every disease God sent a cure in nature. Sometimes, the remedy was found adjacent to the "cause." Dock leaves grew next to nettles because they took away the sting of nettle rash. Willow bark treated ague and fevers because the trees grew in marshy places where such fevers were common. This was part of a general idea that the world was made for the benefit of humanity.

From folk healing to fantastic cures

The story of digitalis from the foxglove plant is an interesting example of the value of herbal remedies. William Withering (1741–99), a doctor practicing in Birmingham, England, was given a recipe for treating "dropsy" by an old lady. "Dropsy" is a medical term that is now obsolete but means an excess of fluid, and may have been applied to a number of diseases in which an abnormal accumulation of fluid in the body could lead to death.

The recipe given to Withering contained a concoction of different plants, but Withering worked out that the vital ingredient was the purple foxglove (*Digitalis purpurea*), which, if used carefully and in small doses (for it is extremely toxic), can act as a powerful stimulant on the heart, as well as increasing urine flow and reducing edema (the accumulation of fluid in the tissues). Withering published reports on his trials and notes on the medicinal virtues of the foxglove in 1785. When he died, his friends carved a bunch of foxgloves on his memorial. Digitoxin and digoxin—the active substances, respectively, of the purple foxglove and the woolly or Balkan foxglove (*Digitalis lanata*)—are still used today to improve the speed and force of cardiac contractions.

Other remedies, based on plants and herbs such as the opium poppy, and the barks of the cinchona and willow trees, were also found by the modern era to contain active medicinal compounds—yielding morphine, quinine, and aspirin, respectively. New drugs derived from some of the old remedies, as well as their synthetic equivalents, now play a major role in medicine. (See Opium, Morphine, and Heroin and New Drugs from Old Remedies).

Cures and curiosities

One of the curious aspects of the history of medicine is to look back at some of the old "cures," which, if they can be believed, might seem bizarre, although in some cases they were, indeed, based on pragmatism. Here are just a few fascinating highlights.

Blood was taken out but according to historical anecdotes, vampire-like, it was seen as a rejuvenating force. The ancient Egyptians supposedly bathed in blood to "resuscitate the sick and rejuvenate the old and incapacitated." It is said that the Romans drank the blood of newly wounded gladiators to give them strength and courage; Europeans collected precious drops of warm blood as it spilt from executed felons.

Numerous recipes down the ages contained urine, human feces, or animal dung. The Romans whitened their teeth with fresh urine. A Saxon leech book recommended "against shoulder pain, mingle a turd of an old swine, which be a field goer, with old lard, warm it, lay it on, that is good for shoulder pain and side pain." The French customarily soaked stockings in urine and wrapped them around their necks in order to cure sore throats.

Ingredients entering some of the formulae in the early 17th-century *London Pharmacopoeia* were the excrements of human beings, dogs, mice, geese, and other animals, while it was not unknown for nail parings, earwax, and sweat to be used in medical recipes. A folk remedy for smallpox involved chewing powdered horse manure. Thomas Beddoes in the 18th century tried curing his consumptive patients with the hot breath of cows, which, he claimed, "is the most delicious thing imaginable." Delicate children in rural England in the early 20th century were sent to stay on farms because "the smell of manure" gave them strength (it may well have worked wonders!).

The root of the orchid looked like a testicle and could cure testicular ailments.

Ambergris, produced in the digestive system of sperm whales, was called "dragon's spittle fragrance" by the ancient Chinese. During the Black Death, Europeans believed that carrying a ball of ambergris could prevent them getting the plague. Known also as "whale vomit," ambergris remains an extremely expensive ingredient in perfumes.

One of the most prized ingredients in European medicine came from human remains. An extract of mummified corpses dug from ancient Egyptian tombs was considered a powerful remedy for many different conditions. Demand for "mummy" became so great by the mid-16th century that counterfeit substitutes, such as the flesh of beggars or camels, were often given instead. By the late 18th century, however, hostility to corpse medicine became widespread.

Tobacco from the "New World" was praised by some as a treatment for toothache, chilblains, headaches, cramps, worms, even bad breath. Culpeper described it as a "universal medicine made for all diseases ... as of any thing in the world, the *Philosophers Stone* excepted." During the Great Plague of London of 1665–6 a schoolboy at Eton College in England is recorded as being "never whipped so much in his life as he was one morning for not smoking"—tobacco being regarded as a way of preventing infection. Others, however, such as King James I of England (1566–1625) described tobacco smoking as "a custom loathsome to the eye, hateful to the nose, harmful to the brain, [and] dangerous to the lungs."

The King organized the first public debate on the effects of tobacco at Oxford and, to make his point, he displayed black brains and black viscera, allegedly from the bodies of smokers. In the early 20th century, many medical practitioners smoked and even Richard Doll, who in the mid-1950s conducted the first epidemiological study to establish a link between smoking and the rising rates of lung cancer, was, initially, skeptical that tobacco played a role. Another use of tobacco was in resuscitation. For example, in 1767 the Dutch Humane Society published guidelines for resuscitation of victims of drowning, stating: "keep the victim warm, give mouth-to-mouth ventilation, and perform insufflation of smoke of burning tobacco into the rectum." Tobacco resuscitator kits were built by the leading makers of scientific and medical instruments of the day. In the 1780s the Royal Humane Society in England stationed boxed tobacco resuscitators at points along the Thames to assist in reviving people pulled from the river after nearly drowning.

Liver—human or animal—was frequently used in medicinal recipes. The Egyptians treated eye diseases with liver. In fact, raw liver in the early 20th century was found to be a remedy for a debilitating and ultimately fatal disease, pernicious anemia. In a poor Irish community in Boston, a patient with pernicious anemia appeared to be surviving

The top ten drugs/ treatments used in the late 18th and first half of the 19th centuries

1. Opium
2. Venesection, blisters, and cupping
3. Senna
4. Aloes
5. Tartar emetic
6. Cinchona/quinine
7. Licorice
8. Calomel (mercury)
9. Ipecac
10. Jalap

Before the first decade of your life as a practitioner has passed, perhaps before you have made a year's acquaintance with the sick room, you will have learned that though Senna will purge, and Ipeacac vomit, and Calomel salivate, and Opium stupefy, yet that neither Senna, Ipeacac, Calomel or Opium will cure disease except in rare instances.
(Edward Clarke, Harvard University, advising his medical students, 1856–7)

because he loved raw liver. Dogs, bled to make them anemic, were fed raw liver to test, and confirm this idea. Raw liver became a lifesaving therapy to ward off pernicious anemia but it meant an intake for sufferers of one pound of raw liver a day. Later an extract was made and it was eventually discovered that the disease is a deficiency of vitamin B_{12} due to lack of an "intrinsic factor." Those with a B_{12} deficiency can now be given cyanocobalamin by intramuscular injections.

> Tobacco from the "New World" was praised by some as a treatment for toothache, chilblains, headaches, cramps, worms, even bad breath.

Cod liver oil was a 19th- and 20th-century treatment for rickets and it became a "cure-all" for children in the post-Second World War era. A description of the process in late 19th-century Norway notes how the cods' livers are left to "putrefy" in barrels over several months until the walls of the hepatic (liver) cells burst, releasing the raw medicinal oil, which rises to the top of the barrels.

Peter of Spain (13th century) had a recipe for loss of eyebrows: "tried and true: lizards of the walls are cooked three times in oil and (when removed) from the oil are smeared on the eyebrows." From lizards to snake venom, from fermented mashed viper's flesh (the basis of theriac) to poisonous toads and toxic tarantulas, various creatures and their venom have provided ingredients for traditional medicines around the world. Such remedies may sound speculative today. But some modern pharmaceuticals are still based on these sources.

Controlling infections

Anecdotes about the benefits of molds to control infections go back centuries. The ancient Egyptian Ebers Papyrus describes the use of moldy bread applied to wounds, and in other cultures and eras moldy bread was a traditional folk remedy for surface wounds. Other "moldy" medicinal preparations include a mash of mouldy corn, mouldy starch poultices, wet bread mixed with spider's webs, moldy milk, cheese, jam, soybeans, fruit, vegetables, and rotten meat. The mold (usually a greenish color) was scraped off the food stuff or whatever substrate was used and applied to the wound. John Parkington, London apothecary and King's herbalist, advised in 1640 that molds have a curative effect when applied to infections. The widespread reference to "mold therapy" in many cultures in the "preantibiotic age" (penicillin was first derived from a mold and statins originated from *Penicillium citrinum*, a mold isolated from a rice vendor in Japan) provides at least circumstantial evidence for its effectiveness.

Fly larvae (maggots) have been used by many different cultures for treating wounds throughout history. Their use by Central American Mayan Indians, Australian Aborigines, and Chinese and Burmese hill people is well documented. The application of larvae in Western medicine came about after observations made on the battlefields of the Napoleonic, American Civil, and First World Wars. With the increased availability of antibiotics during the 1940s and 50s, larvae therapy fell out of favor. However, the increasing incidence of antibiotic resistance has renewed interest in this therapy over the past few years. Recently, manufacturers have begun producing sterile larvae, primarily of the common green-bottle fly, which may be used in the management of wounds complicated by MRSA (Methicillin-resistant *Staphylococcus aureus*) bacterial infection.

Honey, with its antioxidant properties and antimicrobial action, has been used for thousands of years to treat wounds and infected ulcers, and to treat coughs. In ancient Egypt half a human brain was added to honey to make an ointment for a damaged eye, while a cure for blindness was a mixture of mashed pig's eyes, honey, and red ocher, poured into the ear of the patient. It was thought that the benefit of sight would then pass from the pig to the patient. Honey is mentioned in about 500 of the prescriptions in the Ebers Papyrus. A leaf from an Arabic translation of *De materia medica* of Dioscorides (AD 1225, Baghdad, Iraq) shows the preparation of medicine from honey. Manuka honey is now being introduced to combat some of the most hard-to-treat surface infections, such as festering wounds, that are resistant to powerful antibiotics. The latest laboratory work shows that honey can make MRSA more sensitive to some antibiotics (such as oxacillin)—effectively reversing antibiotic resistance.

Trying and exchanging different therapies

It is easy in hindsight to wonder about the effectiveness—or otherwise—of treatments such as bloodletting and boiled dung. But it is also important to remember that in different societies and periods of history, remedies were (and still are) sought and selected according to ideas about what caused disease, which diseases were prevalent, and what medicinal "ingredients" were known and available at the time. Whether it was demons, spirits, humoral imbalances, or breathing "bad airs" that were believed to cause disease, people down the ages have tried to find remedies to prevent and cure plagues, poxes, and pestilence and to restore sick bodies back to health.

Moreover, in the past as today, patients might well have tried out a variety of different therapies and pondered their relative virtues. When Pepys, to his surprise, ended the year 1664 in "good health" he wondered: "But I am at a great loss to know whether it be my Hare's foote, or taking every morning a pill of Turpentine, or having left off the wearing of a gowne." Pepys's turpentine pill was probably a herbal-based remedy from pine resin. He tells us how he was recommended this: while at a dinner party served with a hot pie made of swan, he had discussed the "Disease of the Stone" (from which he had suffered horribly and had, already, had his "stone" surgically removed, see page 93) with one of the guests who happened to be a doctor. Over the dinner table, the doctor had extolled the benefits of turpentine, which he assured Pepys could be taken in pills with great ease. Meanwhile, Pepys had also purchased a hare and tried out wearing a "hare's foot," presumably as an amulet to prevent his usual bouts of illness. Again, he relates how various "discourses" with his friends and colleagues had attracted him to this idea.

The *Gentleman's Magazine*, first published in 1731 in London and running continuously into the early 20th century, provided a good opportunity for lay readers to swap remedies. Hundreds of folk and herbal recipes were sent in by subscribers—cures for colds and coughs, for the bloody flux, for seasickness, for worms, for scalds, for the stone, gout, and asthma. There was even an equivalent of an "agony aunt" exchange in which readers could ask other readers for medical advice: How do you cure corns? How do you purge worms? Treat viper bites? What do you do after swallowing arsenic poison? Sometimes what was sought was not a remedy but rather an explanation: why is it believed that a good antidote to excessive water retention is to apply a live toad to the region of the kidneys?

For Pepys and others, exchanges of ideas about remedies were everyday topics of conversation and interest while religion, magic, medicine, diet, and personal behavior, invariably, coalesced for therapeutic purposes.

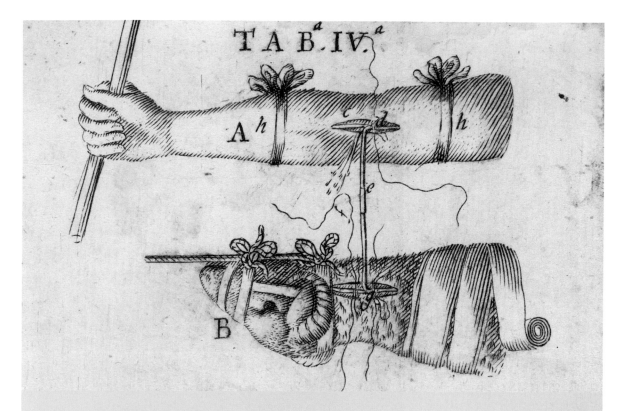

Blood transfusion

While for centuries blood was removed from people as a supposed therapy, one extremely important lifesaving medical technique is blood transfusion. Today, every two seconds in the USA, someone needs blood. From the 17th century, scientists began to experiment with the possibility of transfusing blood between animals and humans. Samuel Pepys described one of the first attempts, in 1667, to transfuse blood from a sheep into a man from Cambridge called Arthur Coga. It was hoped that the transfusion would have "a good effect upon him as a frantic man by cooling his blood." Coga claimed to feel better, although Pepys wrote in his diary "he is cracked a little in the head." Shortly thereafter, following further experiments and a fatality in France, blood transfusion was forbidden throughout most of Europe and the practice fell into disrepute for more than a century and a half.

With the discovery by Austrian Karl Landsteiner (1868–1943) and others of different blood groups in the early 20th century and the recognition of the need for compatibility of blood type between donor and recipient, real progress was made. By the First World War, arm-to-arm transfusions were performed on soldiers with severe blood loss. Further developments included the addition of citrates to prevent blood clotting, and refrigeration— both of which enabled blood to be stored and "banked." While blood transfusion can be a lifesaving operation, tragically there have in the past half-century been cases when blood contaminated with viruses such as hepatitis B and C, and HIV, as well as a few rare cases of vCJD (variant Creutzfeldt-Jakob disease), has been used. Screening, as well as typing, of blood is an essential safety procedure in the 21st century.

ABOVE Enterprising scientists in the 17th century tried experimenting with blood transfusion, as shown in this 1668 Italian image.

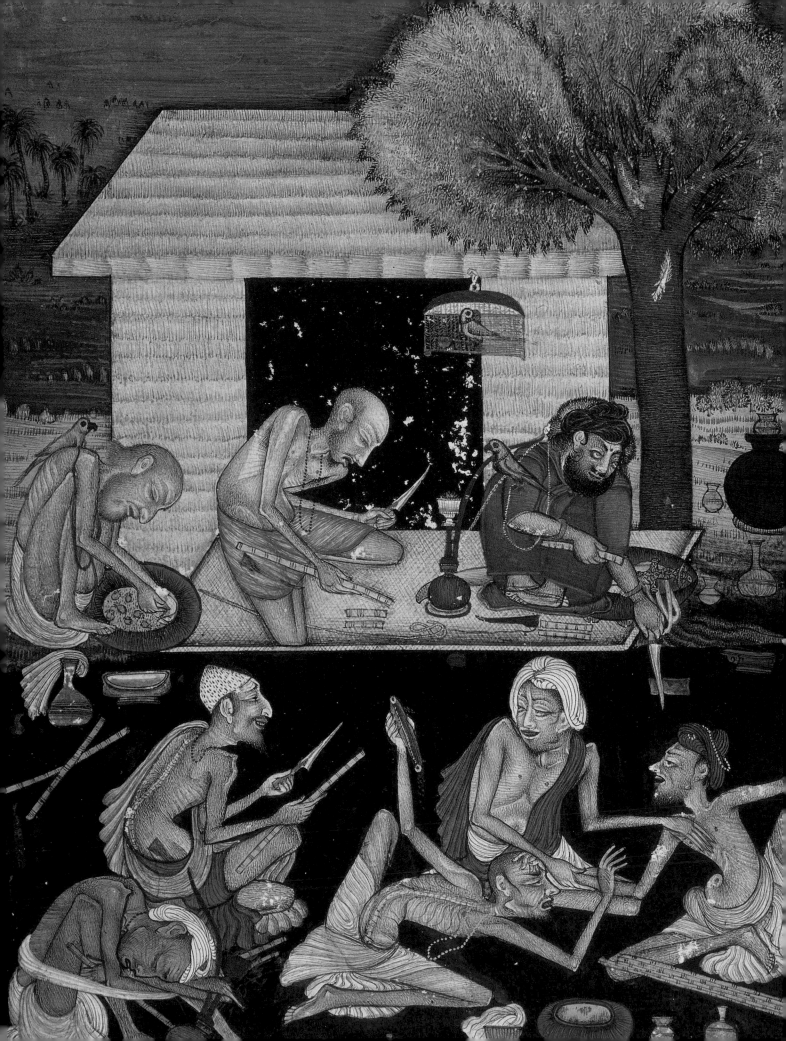

Opium, Morphine, and Heroin

Not poppy, nor mandragora,
Nor all the drowsy syrups of the world,
Shall ever medicine thee to that sweet sleep.

Shakespeare, *Othello*, Act III, Scene 3

Opium, from the white poppy, is one of the oldest of all drugs known to humankind and has played a major role in medical practice and in self-medication throughout history. It has been consumed or inhaled in its raw form since ancient times as a painkiller and sleep-inducing soporific and was combined with alcohol as "laudanum" in the early modern period. Opium was seen as both a wonder drug for medicinal purposes as well as a dangerous narcotic for those who became opium addicts. In the first decade of the 19th century, morphine was isolated from opium and introduced into medicine as a powerful painkiller and remains in use today. Heroin, a semisynthetic derivative of morphine, was briefly used in medicine in the early 20th century but its addictive and dangerous effects were soon recognized.

"Poppy juice"

Opium ... beyond all other agents made known to man, is the mightiest for its command, and for the extent of its command, over pain.

Thomas de Quincey, *Confessions of an English Opium-Eater*, 1821

The opium poppy is arguably the oldest medicinal plant in history. Part cure, part poison, opium's paradoxical effects, ranging from pleasure to pain; stimulation to narcosis; euphoria to despair; and paradise to imprisonment, have been well documented. When, where and how the medicinal use of "poppy juice," containing opium, was first discovered remains a mystery, although its use certainly dates back to the earliest civilizations of Babylonia and Egypt, and the Greek and Roman Empires. Fossil remains of poppyseed cake and poppy pods have been found in Neolithic Swiss lake dwellings dating from over 4,000 years ago. Language can give us

OPPOSITE Ascetics preparing and smoking opium outside a rural dwelling in India, *c.* 1810. Opium, from the white poppy, was used for centuries as a painkiller and a narcotic stimulant.

The principal source of opium is the dried sap of the seed capsules of the white poppy, *Papaver somniferum* (the plant's name is from the Latin *papaver*, "poppy" and *somniferus*, "sleep-bringing").

clues: Sumerians of the 5th century BC referred to the opium poppy as *hul gil*, "the plant of joy." An early written inscription describing the painkilling virtues of "poppy juice" is found in the Egyptian Ebers Papyrus where "Isis brought juice from the 'berry-of-the-poppy plant' and [the great Sun-God] Ra was instantly cured."

The ancient Egyptians also used poppy juice to stop infants crying and help them to sleep; and, sweetened with honey, it was a remedy for looseness of the bowels and many other ailments. The famous poppy fields around the ancient Egyptian city of Thebes were a source of immense wealth to the pharaohs. The Greek poet Homer alludes to it in his epics, the *Iliad* and *Odyssey*. The principal source of opium is the dried sap of the seed capsules of the white poppy, *Papaver somniferum* (the plant's name is from the Latin *papaver*, "poppy" and *somniferus*, "sleep-bringing"). Celsus, the Roman encyclopedist, known for his medical work *De Medicina*, described one of the methods of preparing opium and its varied uses:

> Take a handful of poppy when it is ripe for taking its tears, put it into a vessel, add enough water to cover it, and cook it. When it is well cooked, squeeze out the mass of poppy into a vessel before discarding it, and mix with the fluid an equal quantity of raisin wine. Boil it until it thickens, then cool it and make it into pills about the size of domestic beans.

Galen prescribed a treatment called "Olympic Victor's Dark Ointment" containing opium for injured athletes. The Greek physician, Dioscorides, who produced one of the first significant pharmacopoeias, *De materia medica*, gave detailed descriptions of hundreds of medicinal plants of which one-third (including the poppy) were designed to alleviate pain. Arab physicians used opium extensively. One of the best-written descriptions of the nature and methods to relieve pain is by the physician Ibn Sina, who said that potions must accomplish three roles: they must alleviate pain; they must calm the mind; and they must induce restful sleep. He recommended opium in a variety of forms—as a "cake," a poultice, an infusion, a suppository, a plaster, or an ointment.

Poppy cultivation and the production of opium (*afyun*) continued to flourish in the medieval Arab world. Traders carried the raw opium to India, Indonesia, China, and along the North African coast into Moorish Spain. Medieval Europeans learned of opium's value for eliminating physical pain and mental anguish from the Arabs, following the Crusades of the 11th–13th centuries. Opium was imported from Persia through the Italian port of Venice; travelers in the Middle East recounted meeting caravans of 50 or more camels laden with nothing but opium destined for the West progressing in stately file across the desert.

"Sleepy sponges" in surgery

Another use of opium was as an "anesthetic" during surgery to calm frightened patients. Sleepy sponges, or *spongia somnifera*, were first described and used by the Arabs for this purpose in the medieval period. The practice was then introduced into Europe so that a patient might be "insensible to any cutting."

"Screaming with pain": the mandrake plant

And shrieks like mandrakes torn out of the earth,
That living mortals, hearing them, run mad.
(William Shakespeare, *Romeo and Juliet*,
Act IV, scene 3)

Mandrake (*Mandragora officinarum*) is part of the belladonna family with a root that contains the alkaloids hyoscine and hyoscyamine. It was used as a powerful painkiller as well as a soporific in sleeping sponges prior to amputations and surgery. It was also given as a purgative, emetic, and ointment for ulcers. The plant was believed to give off a shriek when plucked from the ground. Medieval texts offered advice on how to pick mandrake and avoid the resulting insanity believed to take place. Mandrake's mystical power even permeates modern literature. J K Rowling's *Harry Potter and the Chamber of Secrets* (1998) includes a scene in which the eponymous hero and his friends are in a greenhouse, taking instruction in their herbology class from Professor Sprout on the rerooting of mandrakes. To protect them from the mandrakes' cries, the class is equipped with earmuffs.

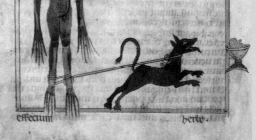

Medieval illustration showing the mandrake plant being torn out of the earth by a dog so that the dog, rather than a person, will suffer the ensuing madness.

These were prepared by soaking sponges in a range of potent narcotic and aromatic extracts, including poppy juice, hemlock, henbane, mandragora, mulberry, wild lettuce, ivy, and alcohol. The sponges were then dried, soaked in hot water, and applied to the mouth and nostrils of the patient undergoing surgery. To what extent the patient was really "insensible" as the surgeon's saw cut through flesh and bone hardly bears thinking about. Another problem was whether the comatose patient would wake up again.

Paracelsus and his "secret" painkiller—laudanum

My mother began to suffer from the exercise or fatigue of travelling, and she was a good deal indisposed ... [she] received much comfort from a mess of broth and the sight of Mr Lyford, who recommended her to take twelve drops of laudanum when she went to bed as a composer, which she accordingly did.

Jane Austen, writing to her sister, Cassandra, about their mother, October 27 1798

Laudanum became one of the most widely used medicines for a whole range of ailments, especially during the 18th and 19th centuries. It contained powdered opium diluted with

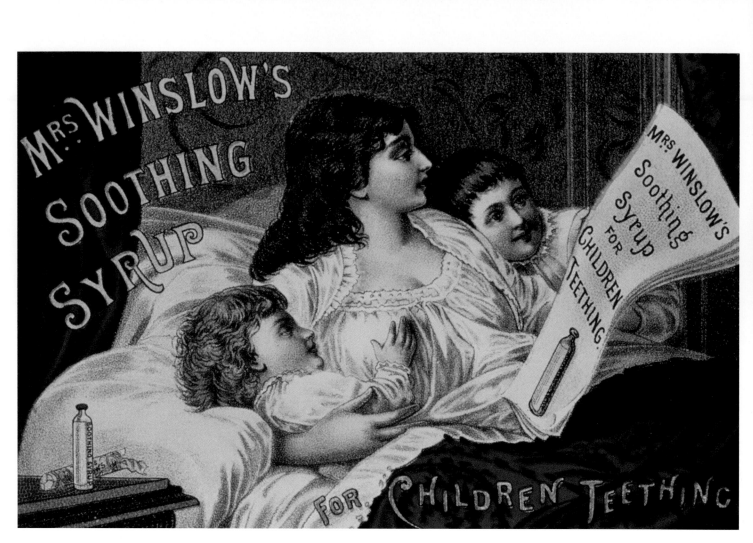

Mrs Winslow's Soothing Syrup was created by a Mrs Charlotte N Winslow and marketed heavily in the USA and Britain from 1849 for teething and colicky babies. It contained morphine and alcohol and claimed it was "likely to soothe any human or animal."

alcohol, and many became addicted to the relief from pain that this bitter-tasting tincture brought. The word "laudanum" was introduced in the 16th century by the famous Swiss physician-alchemist Paracelsus, who claimed he had a secret remedy that he considered *laude dignum*, "worthy of praise." In the 1660s, Thomas Sydenham popularized his own version of laudanum for a range of painful complaints—and for the suppressing of coughing. He praised the wonder drug: "of all the remedies it has pleased almighty God to give man to relieve his suffering, none is so universal and so efficacious as opium." His own tincture was made of:

> *One pint of sherry wine, two ounces of good quality Turkish or Egyptian opium, one ounce of saffron, a cinnamon stick and a clove, both powdered. Mix and simmer over a vapour bath for two to three days, until the tincture has a proper slightly viscid but still easily poured liquid consistence, easy and pleasant to administer.*

Sydenham, like many others of this time, extolled the virtues of opium, claiming "medicine would be crippled without it; and whoever understands it well, will do more with it alone than he could hope to do with any other single medicine."

John Jones, a Welsh physician, wrote one of the first medical monographs about opium,

The Mysteries of Opium Reveal'd (1700), warning of its addictive nature and the depression caused by withdrawal. He was also clear about the many benefits, noting that it:

> *Causes a brisk, gay and good Humour ... prevents and takes away Grief, Fear, Anxieties, Peevishness, Fretfulness ... causes Euphory, or easie undergoing of all Labour, Journeys etc.*

Opium was available over the counter in various forms besides laudanum, as pills or penny sticks. There was also a growing sector of patented commercial medicines containing opium. These preparations of opium were sold under various names, including the famous Dover's Powder prescribed for gout by Thomas Dover, a pupil of Sydenham's. Dover claimed that, if drunk in wine before going to bed "all pain will vanish by next morning." There were also children's opiates such as Godfrey's cordial (mixed with blackstrap molasses and spices) and Mrs Winslow's Soothing Syrup. Chlorodyne—a concoction of chloroform, ether, opium, cannabis, alcohol, and syrup devised by Dr John Collis Browne (1819–84), an army surgeon, was a popular patent medicine for cholera and a host of diseases in the 19th century. Others, such as Perry Davis's opium-based Universal Pain Killer, were advertised as cure-alls.

The wonders of using such drugs as opium to deaden physical pain or enliven the spirit, as well as the euphoria associated with the consumption of alcohol, were well known. But so, too, were the dangers of overimbibing, self-poisoning or the side effects of habitual use and the sudden withdrawal.

Confessions of an "opium-eater"

One of the most powerful revelations describing the ease with which the use of opium, as a painkiller, could lead to an addiction is Thomas de Quincey's *Confessions of an English Opium-Eater* published in the early 1820s. Opium in this period was still the "drug of choice" for deadening and relieving pain. It was relatively cheap to buy from any chemist and grocery store. De Quincey (1785–1859) describes his journey from young Oxford undergraduate to a chance recommendation of opium for his severe toothache. He purchased some from a London apothecary:

> *I have often been asked – how it was, and through what series of steps, that I became an opium-eater ... Most truly I have told the reader, that not any search after pleasure, but mere extremity of pain from rheumatic toothache – this and nothing else it was that first drove me into use of opium.*

De Quincey then recalled its wonderous effects:

> *In an hour, O heavens! what a revulsion! what a resurrection, from its lowest depths of the inner spirit! what an apocalypse of the world within me. That my pains had vanished was now a trifle in my eyes; this negative effect was swallowed up in the immensity of those positive effects which had opened before me, in the abyss of divine enjoyment thus suddenly revealed. Here was a panacea ... for all human woes; here was the secret of happiness.*

De Quincey soon became "habituated" (addicted) to opium—in the form of laudanum. His *Confessions* were presented in two sections: "The Pleasures of Opium" and "The Pains of Opium." In the second part he examines how, because of the constant pain of a gastric condition, he was forced to consume ever more of the drug, eventually becoming unproductive, depressed, and moreover suffering terrifying visions:

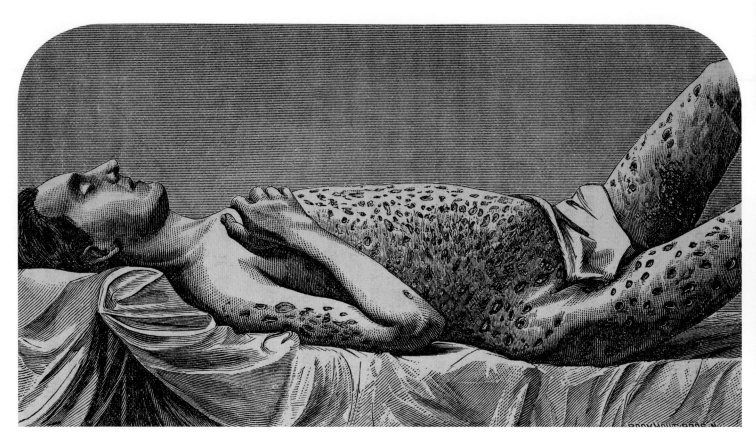

"Drugs that enslave: opium, morphine, and hashish." An 1881 image showing a body marked from repeated subcutaneous injections of narcotic drugs.

My dreams were accompanied by deep-seated anxiety and funereal melancholy ... I seemed ... to descend ... into chasms and sunless abysses, depths below depths, from which it seemed hopeless that I could ever re-ascend.

Toward the end of his life he was spending much of his income on 1,200 drops of laudanum a week.

Likewise, his friend, the English Romantic poet Samuel Taylor Coleridge (1772–1834), turned to opium in the late 18th century for pain relief, quickly becoming dependent on its life-enhancing effects. Opium promotes vivid dreams and rich visual imagery and is said to have inspired many of the Romantic poets. Coleridge's poem *Kubla Khan* was begun "in a sort of Reverie brought on by two grains of Opium, taken to check a dysentery."

Coleridge spent the last 18 years of his life living with a general practitioner, James Gillman, in Highgate, London, with the avowed intention of seeking help in "breaking" his opium habit. But he never succeeded in giving up completely and, surreptitiously, managed to obtain laudanum from the local chemist.

There were many other well-known opium and laudanum users, whether for medicinal or recreational purposes, in the artistic world. The English novelist Wilkie Collins (1824–89) took laudanum originally to deaden the pain of gout and a rheumatic complaint, and continued taking it for the rest of his life. Toward the end of his days, in almost constant pain, he carried his supply of laudanum in a silver flask wherever he went. In his novel *Armadale* (1866), Miss Gwilt writes in her diary:

Who was the man who invented laudanum? I thank him from the bottom of my heart ... I have had six delicious hours of oblivion; I have woke up with my mind composed ... I have dawdled over my morning toilet with an exquisite sense of relief – and all through the modest little bottle of Drops, which I see on my bedroom chimney-piece at this moment. Drops, you are darling! If I love nothing else, I love you!

The stories of opium use (and abuse) by writers, poets, musicians, artists, and monarchs, to ease pain or relieve the symptoms of chronic disease, especially the excruciatingly last stages of tuberculosis, are well-publicized instances of the increasing dependency on opium in the 18th and 19th centuries. But the popular usage was far more extensive than even these well-known "confessions" portray.

The poppies of the English Fens

By the mid-19th century, opium had permeated all layers of society. Between 1825 and 1850, imports to Britain rose from 51,400 to 304,200 pounds a year, much of it coming from Turkey as this was more potent than the Indian variety. About a third was reexported, mainly to the USA. Such was the demand for opium that white poppies were grown in the Fens of Eastern England. These low-lying marshlands of Cambridgeshire, Lincolnshire, Huntingdonshire, and Norfolk had by the 19th century become known as "the Kingdom of the Poppy." In these backwaters, opium had initially been used as "an antidote to the effect of the noxious vapors." The Fenland folk, like inhabitants of other marshland areas in Europe, were frequently stricken by "agues" and "fevers"—most probably malaria.

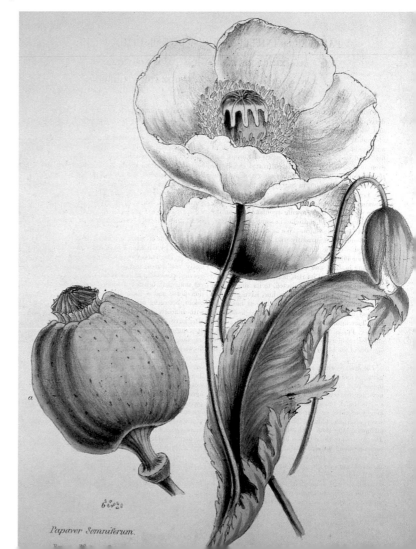

Opium was said 'to prevent shiverings in Ague fits if given in due time and quantity'. Mothers would often leave their babies to be nursed by a sibling or neighborly baby-minder while they worked in the fields. It was all too easy to dose a cranky child with an opium-based tincture. Early versions of Gripe Water for a "griping" child with "fen fever" contained "garden poppy syrup" and spearmint. Opium-eating youngsters were clearly recognizable. They were described as "wasted," and some said they "shrank up into little old men."

Even though malaria was declining in the region by the 19th century, the drug had become in time both a habit as well as a necessity. The infant mortality rates in the

The white opium poppy (*Papaver somniferum*; 1853 print). The poppy-seed capsules yield opium and other alkaloids used in medicine. The use of opium was completely unrestricted—as, for example, in England until the first Pharmacy Act of 1868, which made the sale of opium illegal by anyone other than a registered chemist.

Papaver Somniferum.

Fens were on a par with, if not greater than, the worst slums of industrial cities, with one in four infants dying before their first birthday. In the cathedral city of Ely, in the heart of the region, there was no need to ask for a stick of opium or an ounce of laudanum in the stores. A coin laid on the counter meant only one thing. As a Fenman explains to a visitor in *Alton Locke* (1850) by the English writer Charles Kingsley:

> Oh! Ho! Ho! – you goo into the druggist's shop o' market day, into Cambridge, and you'll see the little boxes, dozens and dozens, a'ready on the counter, and never a venman's wife go by, but what cals in for her pennord o' elevation, to last her out a week. Oh! Ho! Ho! Well it keeps womanfolk quiet it do; and it's mortal good agin the pains ... Opium, bor alive, opium!

A local doctor explained the popularity of the drug: "their terrible lives could be temporarily brightened by the passing dreamland vision afforded by the poppy."

Opium smoking and opium dens

The Mystery of Edwin Drood (1870) was the last and unfinished novel by Charles Dickens (who was taking heavy doses of laudanum in the later months of his life). Set in Rochester, a port close to the malarial marshes of north Kent, it described the scene of opium smoking (another way of imbibing the substance) in its first chapter:

> Shaking from head to foot, the man whose scattered consciousness has thus fantastically pieced itself together, at length rises, supports his trembling frame upon his arms, and looks around. He is in the meanest and closest of small rooms.

"Gripe Water"

Gripe Water was formulated in 1851 by William Woodward and registered as a trademark in 1876. In the 19th century people in Eastern England were afflicted by a condition known as "fen fever" (malaria). Woodward noted that their local treatment formula was also an effective "soother of fretful babies" and helped with gastric problems ("gripes"). Woodward's original Gripe Water contained alcohol, dill, oil, sodium bicarbonate, sugar, and water. It was initially marketed with the slogan "Granny told mother and mother told me" and achieved huge commercial success. Its composition now varies according to the country of manufacture and in Britain, following public pressure, alcohol was removed—but not until 1992.

With him are "a Chinaman and a Lascar" in a stupor. A haggard woman "blows at the pipe as she speaks, and, occasionally bubbling at it, inhales much of its contents." She reminds the man that he has smoked "as many as five since ye come in at midnight." The few small opium dens in the East End of London were akin to a Chinese social club and probably not as mysterious and threatening as fictional accounts and images made out. One visitor to a Chinese den found it clean and tidy and admired the skill with which opium was prepared for smoking, adding: "It might be useful if the subject were investigated by medical men, to see if opium smoking might not be found a convenient way of administering the drug to patients who otherwise cannot take it without the stomach being upset." There was, however, an increasing antiopium movement, which helped perpetuate the myth of the sordid dens.

In China, itself, opium was culturally acceptable and the smoking of opium became popular among the leisured classes, although its use had officially been banned there in the early 18th century. In addition to considerable domestic production, by the 19th century

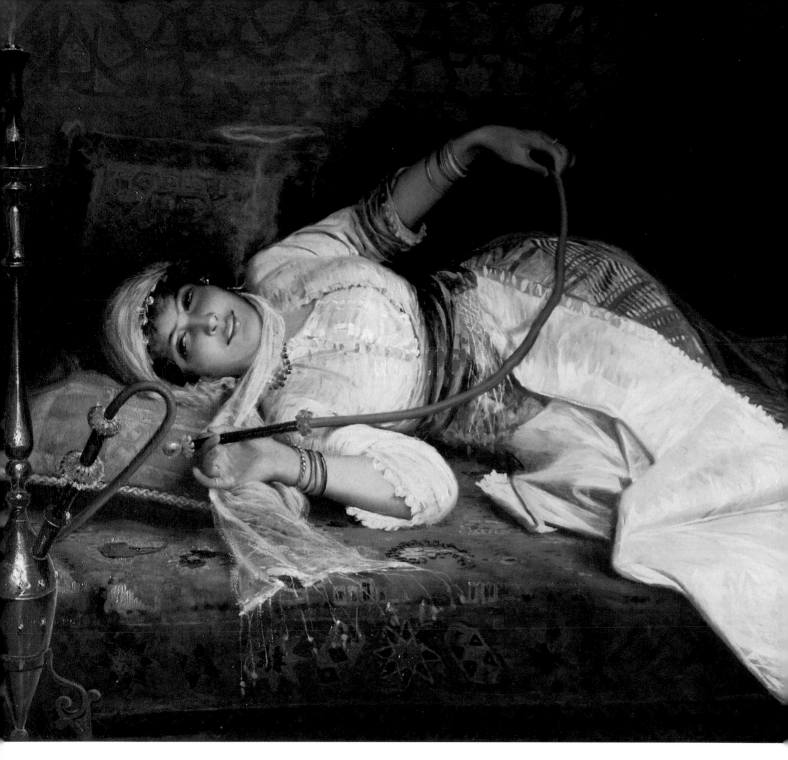

The Opium Pipe, by Leon Herbo (1850–1907), a Belgian painter who specialized in Asian scenes. In this image he captures the romantic and exotic perception of opium smoking.

much of the opium in China was coming from India. The British imported large amounts of Chinese goods and solved the resulting balance of payments deficit by exporting or smuggling Indian opium into China. The Chinese authorities, however, tried to suppress the trade, leading to the two Opium Wars (1839–42, 1856–60) in which Britain used force against the Chinese. The resulting Treaties led to the opening of trading ports and the legalization of the import of Indian opium. The traffic peaked toward the end of the 19th century and declined thereafter, ending in the early 20th century.

From opium to morphine and beyond

Take all the morphine (or other forms of opium if that disagrees) you want, and don't be afraid of becoming an opium drunkard. What was opium created for except for such times as this.

William James advising his sister, Alice, after she was diagnosed with incurable breast cancer in 1891

In the early 19th century, a young German pharmacist, Friedrich Sertürner (1783–1841), isolated a raw crystalline alkaline substance from opium, which he initially called "principium somniferum," then "morphium"—later to be known as morphine. The origin of the word "morphine" has long been disputed—though some suggest that Sertürner named his alkaloid after the name of the Roman god of dreams—Morpheus. It was not only the first alkaloid to be extracted from opium, but the first ever alkaloid to be isolated from any plant. For a time, Sertürner's morphine, which was more concentrated than raw opium, was not widely used, though Sertürner, himself, tested it on numerous occasions. He discovered its effects, from euphoria to depression, from nausea to constipation and, most strikingly, its capacity to dull pain. He even realized that morphine did not so much suppress pain as to make the sufferer "beautifully indifferent to it." In the 1820s, Merck of Darmstadt, Germany, pioneered commercial manufacturing of morphine for an expanding global market.

With the introduction of the hypodermic syringe and hollow needle, developed initially by the French surgeon Charles-Gabriel Pravaz and, subsequently, by the Scottish physician, Alexander Wood in the mid-19th century, a new way of injecting morphine (subcutaneously) was offered to those who could afford to purchase the small syringes. Even doctors taught their patients how to inject themselves and, though more expensive than raw opium or laudanum, morphine was easily administered and able to bypass the gut and avoid some of the unpleasant gastric effects of opium.

Injecting oneself unobtrusively in public was acceptable, and rich users were delighted to receive gold or platinum syringes in vanity cases initialled by famous jewelers. Doctors were happy to offer it to patients for any number of painful complaints. The therapy became so woven into the fabric of daily medical practice that, as one author of a standard British medical textbook, William Aitken, proclaimed in 1880, "the hypodermic syringe and the morphia solution are now almost as indispensable accompaniments of the physician as the stethoscope and thermometer." The American Civil War (1861–5) was the first war in which morphine was administered on a massive scale to alleviate the pain of wounds.

By the end of the 19th century, around half the habitual morphine users were health professionals who had easy access to the drug. Florence Nightingale was an invalid and in chronic pain for much of her life after returning from the Crimean War. She remarked on the benefit of the "curious little new fangled operation of putting opium under the skin," which gave her pain relief for 24 hours. Morphine was used as a symptom-and pain-relieving substance rather than as a curative medicine. It was, however, also offered as a "cure" for opium addiction!

Morphine and another opium derivative, codeine, isolated by the French chemist Pierre Robiquet (1780–1840) in 1832 are still widely used today in various safe forms for medically prescribed pain control.

> Injecting oneself unobtrusively in public was acceptable, and rich users were delighted to receive gold or platinum syringes in vanity cases.

Heroin: sold as "a safe family drug"

While morphine and codeine have brought great benefits to humankind, another drug, heroin, has had a much more disturbing effect on society. In the later 19th century, with the growing concern about the habit-forming nature of opium and morphine, the search was on to find an equally effective but nonaddictive alternative analgesic.

The answer, or so it seemed at the time, was a morphine derivative, diacetylmorphine, which was originally synthesized in 1874 by C R Alder Wright and then "rediscovered" by Felix Hoffmann (1868–1946) in 1897, just two weeks after he had synthesized another compound —acetylsalicylic acid (ASA) or aspirin (see New Drugs from Old Remedies). Hoffmann worked for the German Bayer Company. Originally founded as a dye company, by the 1880s it had expanded to support two key scientific departments—pharmacology and pharmaceuticals. Hoffman was in the former under the leadership of Arthur Eichengrün (1867–1949) whose aim it was to come up with ideas for new drugs. The head of the latter was Heinrich Dreser (1860–1924) and it was his role to test all new products.

Dreser initially tested diacetylmorphine on frogs and rabbits, then on himself and then on a few local workers. After a limited number of so-called human "trials," the potential of the drug seemed boundless. It was decided to call it "heroin" because all who tried it felt positively "*heroisch*" (heroic, strong). The head of research, Carl Duisberg (1861–1935), was caught up in the excitement. It was said to be ten times more effective as a cough medicine than codeine and, at a time when TB, whooping cough, and pneumonia were leading causes of death, even routine coughs and colds could turn out to be serious chronic and painful infections. Its most popular form was the pastille. "Heroin cough lozenges" were sold by the million. Heroin was also, initially, advertised as a "cure" for morphine and opium addiction.

The true habit-forming nature of heroin, however, increasingly became apparent and by the early 20th century, serious concerns were being voiced over the addictive nature of this so-called "safe" opioid and cough remedy. People started taking heroin not just as a medicine but also in search of thrills. In 1913 there was a rash of bad publicity when heroin-related admissions mushroomed in hospitals across the east coast of America. Reluctantly, Bayer decided to stop making the drug and within five years it had been declared an illegal substance in much of the world.

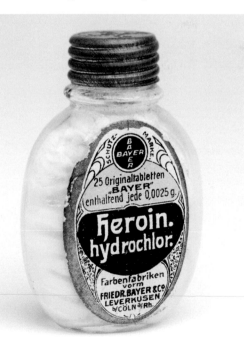

Increased regulation of all manner of narcotics began to be introduced over the course of the 20th century. Opium and heroin control remains a central and complex issue in national and international policy-making in the 21st century.

Bayer introduced heroin in 1898 as a cough suppressant. It was quickly recommended and marketed as "completely nonhabit forming" and "a safe family drug." Aspirin was produced in the same Bayer laboratories and released to the public in 1899.

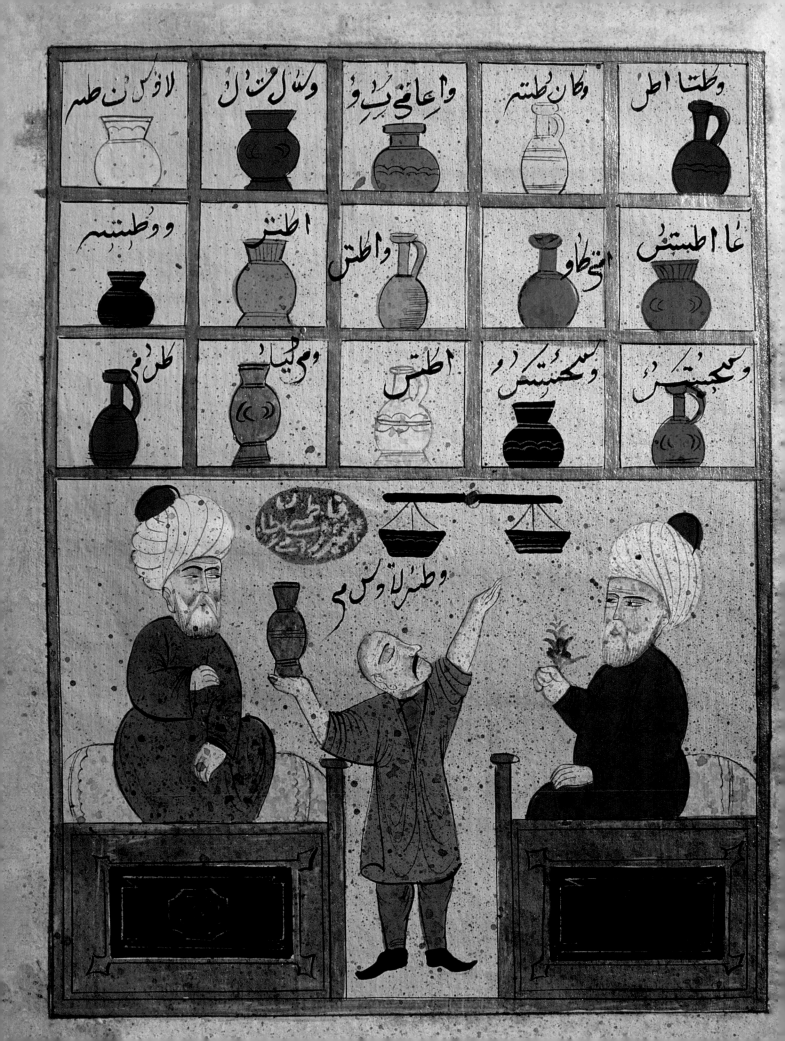

Pharmacy and Patent Medicines

There is only one cure for grey hair. It was invented by a Frenchman. It is called the guillotine.

P G Wodehouse, 1881–1975

Pharmacy derives its name from the Greek root *pharmakon* or "a drug." The Greek term was used to designate remedies, as well as charms and poisons. Practitioners from ancient times have prepared numerous medicinal remedies. Many were based on plants, including the opium poppy; some were concocted from animal products, as well as from metals, minerals, and stones. The remedies and prescriptions for their use were often recorded in pharmacopoeias and herbals, as well as in domestic manuals to be used in the home. Apothecaries began to play a role in dispensing and selling drugs in the medieval Arabic world. In Europe in the early modern period they were joined by itinerant quacks selling all sorts of potions to their clients. The modern-day pharmacy store began to flourish in the 19th century. Pharmacists soon began to buy "patent" or "proprietary" medicines, often from commercial salesmen, leading to regulation in the late 19th and early 20th centuries to prevent the sale of poisonous and ineffective medicines.

Herbals and pharmacopoeias

In the days before any physician or pharmacist dreamed of being able to produce a little white pill or synthesize drugs, medical practitioners, apothecaries, folk healers, and "wise women" must have scoured the countryside in search of herbs, roots, seeds, leaves, bulbs, barks, vegetables, flowers, and fruits that could form the basis of medicinal remedies. Gardens were also established to plant and propagate native or imported species of medicinal value. Some of the remedies were written down or collated into illustrated "herbals" and "pharmacopoeias" (an authoritative list of drugs, their components, and preparation) to be read and used by others.

OPPOSITE Ottoman manuscript showing two doctors in a pharmacy. From ancient times, all sorts of ingredients went into the making up of medicines, from herbs and spices to minerals and animal products. Ideas and ingredients were exchanged across the globe and adapted to local settings.

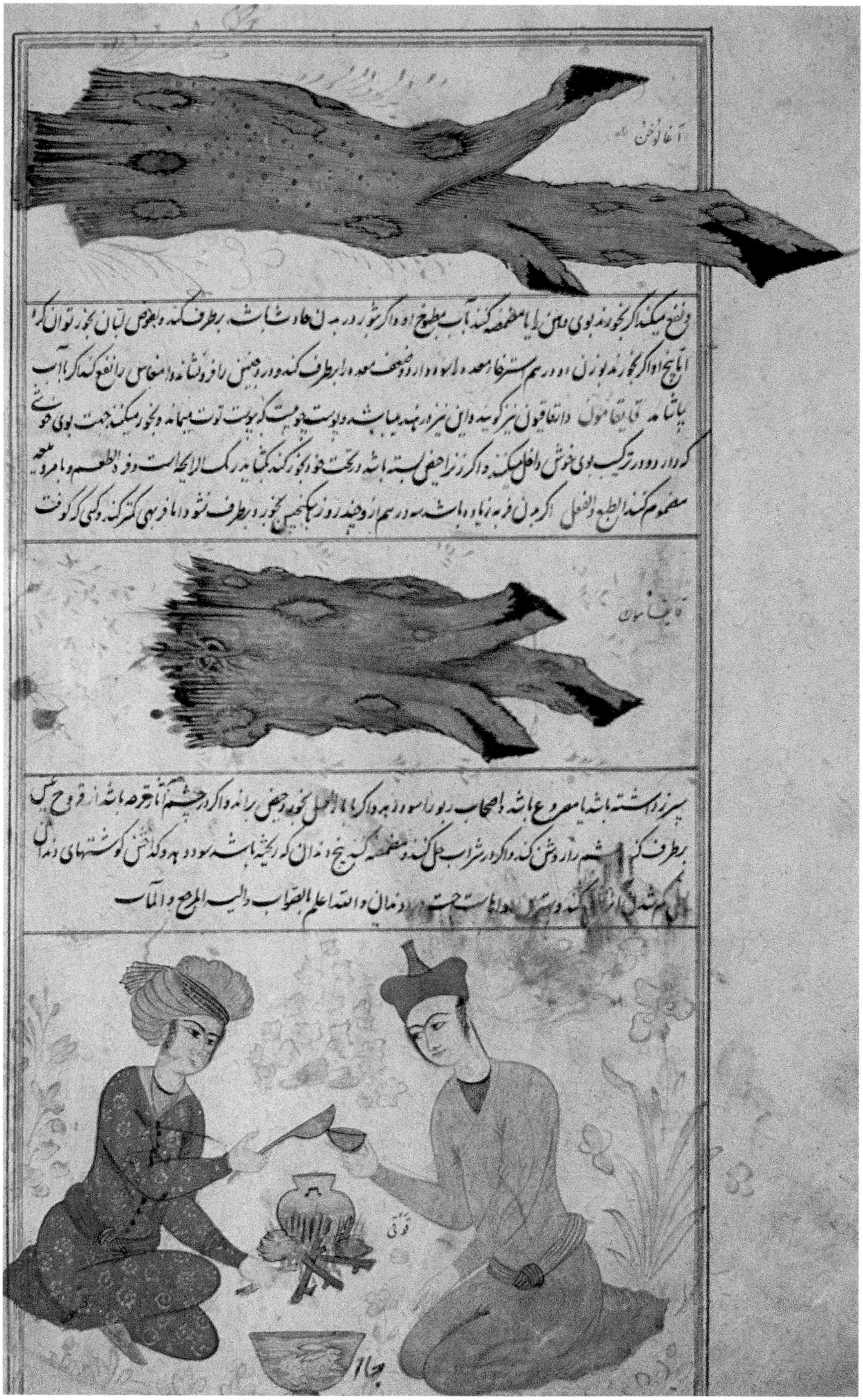

آغاز ادحمل

فنفع میکند اگر بجوشد بوی دهن را بامعطر کند و آب مطبوخ او اگر در مدل عادت باشد بطرف که بعوض اللسان بخور نوال کرد... بآیچ او اگر کم زور باشد هم مستفاد معده و اگر ضعف معده باشد بطرف که در روشن راو و بیش رانفع کند که کار بآب بیاشامد... قای بقانون داناقانون نیز کوسیده وان نیز زرمند بیاش بدوست و...

قایف سوس

سبز رسته باشد باسو ع بایشد و اصحاب رو راسود و بهد و راسه ال الحل بجو دحبش بر آینده و اگر در چشم آنجوره باشد...

TREATMENTS AND THERAPIES

The medical papyri of ancient Egypt are some of the oldest written documents containing medical prescriptions and their ingredients. The Ebers Papyrus, for example, includes over 800 prescriptions and 700 drugs. Eye diseases and disorders were among the most prevalent ailments in the hot and dusty climate of Egypt and the medical papyri detail different lotions and salves used as treatment, containing substances such as antinomy, goose grease, fried ox liver, myrrh, and honey.

A great many of the medications and plants used in ancient Egypt found their way into the herbals of Theophrastus, Galen, and Pliny. One of the most famous pharmacopoeias of the Roman Empire was written by the Greek physician Pedanius Dioscorides (*fl.* AD *c*.40–*c*.90), a military surgeon who served for a time in the Roman Emperor Nero's army. The five volumes of his groundbreaking *De materia medica* (medical substances) contained detailed descriptions of the preparation and uses of over 300 medicinal plants, including the opium poppy, as well as chapters on metals such as copper and lead; minerals, such as sea salt; and various spices. It was the most influential book in this field for 1,400 years.

Arabic translations during the 8th to the 12th centuries incorporated additional new medicinal drugs from the Islamic world. With their advanced development of chemistry, Islamic physicians were the first to extract effective substances from their natural sources rather than using the whole plant. They developed methods of distillation and extraction and introduced the use of "mercurial ointments" as well as developing apparatuses such as mortars, flasks, spatulas, and phials.

The ancient Greek and Roman, and medieval Arabic, pharmacopoeias were inherited by the Europeans. Dioscorides's magnificent text was translated into Latin and various European languages, becoming the physician's bible during the Renaissance. Official pharmacopoeias were also published that set out to standardize drug formulations. The first was produced in Florence, Italy, in 1498. *The Pharmacopoeia Londinensis*, with 2,000 "recipes," was issued by the College of Physicians of London in 1618. As these pharmacopoeias have been updated over the centuries, such ingredients as dried viper lozenges, foxes' lungs, wolf oil, crabs' eyes, spider's webs, and moss from human skulls have, not surprisingly, dropped off the list. The first *US Pharmacopoeia* was published in 1820, printed in both Latin and English. An *International Pharmacopoeia* (Ph. Int.) was first published in 1951 and is the most authoritative source internationally.

Pharmacopoeias and herbals were, likewise, produced by physicians in Asia. During the Ming Dynasty in China, Li Shizhen (1518–93) wrote his *Bencao Gangmu,* a compendium of *materia medica*, summarizing herbal medicine knowledge up to the late 16th century. It described in detail more than 1,800 plants, animal substances, minerals, and metals, along with their medicinal properties and applications. Traditional Chinese Medicine in the 21st century continues to base many of its therapies on these natural products.

> As these pharmacopoeias have been updated over the centuries, such ingredients as dried viper lozenges, foxes' lungs, wolf oil, crabs' eyes, spider's webs, and moss from human skulls have, not surprisingly, dropped off the list.

OPPOSITE 17th-century Persian medical manuscript showing a remedy made from bark extract. Willow bark contains the basis of one of the most popular painkillers of all time, aspirin.

Medicinal plants and exotic spices, as well as formulae for their preparation, were also exchanged and traded across the world. From East to West and West to East, traders from different nations bought and sold their products, across the Indian Ocean and along the "Silk Road" and overland caravan routes. Ginseng came from Korea; musk from Tibet; camphor, cardamom, and cloves from Southeast Asia; anise, saffron, frankincense, and myrrh from Persia and Arabia. With the opening up of the "New World" in the late 15th century, a new route of exchange began, with a number of medicinal plants—sassafras, ipecacuanha, cinchona, and guaiacum wood—as well as potatoes and tobacco traded across the Atlantic to Europe and beyond.

Physic and botanical gardens

During the Renaissance in Europe, physic gardens began their contribution to a deeper scientific curiosity about plants. On the continent, the first formal physic or medicinal garden was founded in Pisa in 1543. Similar gardens were established in other European cities, often alongside university schools of medicine—such as Oxford and Cambridge. Botany was a standard subject in medical education until about 1900.

Today, you can wander round London's Chelsea Physic Garden, established in 1673, and the Royal Botanic Gardens at Kew, created in 1759. Physician Hans Sloane (1660–1753) came up with a recipe for milk chocolate (from cacao) while in the West Indies and his vast collection of plants, insects, and other curiosities became the foundation of the British Museum. He was closely connected with the Chelsea Physic Garden. His collection of pressed plants was relocated to the Natural History Museum in London and is still used as a reference source. The botanist and explorer Joseph Banks (1743–1820) was also influential in obtaining exotic plants from many parts of the world for the Chelsea Physic Garden. One of the new species introduced in the 18th century was *Vinca rosea*, now known as *Catharanthus roseus* (Madagascar periwinkle), which is the source of the modern anticancer drugs vincristine and vinblastine. It can still be seen growing in the greenhouses just off the King's Road in London, where the Pharmaceutical Garden displays plants that are the origin of many of the drugs used in contemporary medicine, including chemotherapy. Worldwide there are now over 1,800 botanical gardens attracting millions of visitors each year.

The search for indigenous plants with medical potential, especially in Asia, Africa, and South America, continues to this day. It is estimated that while 70 percent of the world's population relies on traditional plant remedies for medicine, only one in five plant species has been screened. Conserving and screening plants for possible future cures is a major focus of Kew Gardens' Millennium Seed Bank Project, located inside the Wellcome Trust Millennium Building at Wakehurst Place in Sussex.

"Domestic medicine" and self-help manuals

"Domestic medicine" was defined by William Buchan in the mid-18th century as: "an attempt to render medical art more generally useful by showing people what is in their own power, both with respect to the prevention and cure of diseases."

While physicians wrote their erudite texts on diseases and drugs or set up specialist botanical gardens, for the majority of the population treating sickness often started (and, indeed, often ended) in the home (see "Kitchen remedies," pages 125–6). To assist lay (and literate) people, astute physicians published guides as to what might be useful for growing, purchasing or keeping in the domestic "medical cabinet." Razi in the 9th century, for example, wrote a home medical manual, *Man la Yahduruhu Al-Tabib* ("Who has no Physician to Attend Him") for the general public in which he described dietary and drug components that could be found in apothecary stores, the marketplace, or well-equipped kitchens.

The 13th-century scholar-physician Peter of Spain (d. 1277), following in this tradition, wrote his *Thesaurus Pauperum*. This "Treasury of the Poor" contained descriptions of a range of diseases—arranged in descending order from head to toe—with advice on methods of treatment. Its English translator noted in his introduction:

The Genizah medical collection: scrapheap to treasure trove

Sacred documents no longer in use were consigned to a Genizah or depository within a Jewish synagogue. The dry climate of the Middle East and North Africa has preserved this discarded "rubbish" over the centuries. The Taylor-Schechter Collection, from the Cairo Genizah, is the largest worldwide and was shipped to the University Library, Cambridge, in the late 19th century. Since then, scholars have been painstakingly putting together the scraps, translating and archiving the material dating from the 9th century. Over 1,800 fragments deal with medicine, ranging from merchants' letters and trading books, to alchemical recipes and medical prescriptions. The latter detail 242 different substances and of these, 195 are of plant origin, 20 from animals and 27 are minerals. Almonds from the Levant were prescribed for migraine and dressing bites, while arsenic was used as a depilatory for hairy women. Pharmacists who made up the prescriptions had their stores in the lanes and alleys of the medieval Jewish quarter of Cairo.

Fragment of a medieval prescription from the Cairo Genizah hoard, for a syrup, probably a purgative, since it contains purging cassia, rhubarb, and senna.

This lytle treatyse which was gathered out of the workes of the most noble and auncient phicicions, Hipocrates, Galene, Dioscordes, and Avicen by one Petrus Hispanus whyche (although he chaunced in a barbarous and rude tyme) was a man of great knowledge and large practyce.

In the early modern period from the 16th–18th centuries, books such as Thomas Elyot's *Castel of Helth*, *The Queens Closet Opened* (by one "WM"), John Wesley's *Primitive Physic*, Samuel-Auguste Tissot's *Avis au peuple sur sa santé*, John Tennent's *Every Man His Own Doctor*, and William Buchan's *Domestic Medicine* were designed to be read by the literate public, offering readers an assortment of medical information from the theoretical to the practical. They taught how to treat ills with the aid of simple kitchen ingredients like onions and honey; licorice for a consumptive cough; toasted cheese for binding on a deep cut. Leonard Meager's *The English Gardener, or, A Sure Guide to Young Planters and Gardeners* gave advice on the different types of medicinal herbs suitable for the domestic herb or home physic garden.

The *English Physician* (1652) and the *Complete Herbal* (1653) written by the botanist, herbalist, physician, and astrologer Nicholas Culpeper were some of the most famous British herbal texts of the 17th century, containing a rich store of knowledge of medicinal herbs. Culpeper published his works in English as self-help medical guides for use by the poor who could not afford the medical help of expensive physicians.

Women also collected and developed medicinal recipes and often published their work. Some were specifically for the "lady" of the house: Hannah Woolley's *The Ladies Directory*, *The Cooks Guide*, and another based on her work called *The Accomplisht Ladies Delight: In Preserving, Physick, Beautifying and Cookery*, and Eliza Smith's *The Compleat Housewife, or Accomplish'd Gentlewoman's Companion*. Foods and medicines were often one and the same. Besides numerous culinary recipes, Eliza Smith's book, which is known as the first US "cookbook" (first published in America in 1742), contained "nearly two hundred family receipts of medicine; viz. drinks, syrups, salves, ointments, and many other things of sovereign and approved efficacy in most distempers, pains, aches, wounds, sores, etc. never before made publick in these parts; fit either for private families, or such publick-spirited gentlewomen as would be beneficient to their poor neighbors." Indeed, as many domestic manuals attest, housewives and housekeepers were expected to possess basic medical skills and knowledge of the body for assisting family, friends, and neighbors in times of need.

Inside an apothecary's store

Some of the earliest "apothecary stores" were in the Middle East and were strictly regulated to prevent adulteration. Abu al-Muna al-Kuhen al-'Attar, a Jewish pharmacist working in Cairo, wrote a handbook in 1259 entitled *The Management of an Apothecary Shop*. The term "apothecary" (Greek for a "storehouse") is associated with someone who formulates and dispenses medicines. In Shakespeare's play *Romeo and Juliet*, Romeo on hearing and believing that his beloved Juliet is dead, seeks out a local apothecary in the Italian town of Mantua:

> *I do remember an apothecary –*
> *And hereabouts he dwells, – which late I noted*
> *In tatter'd weeds, with overwhelming brows,*
> *Culling of simples; meagre were his looks,*
> *Sharp misery had worn him to the bones:*

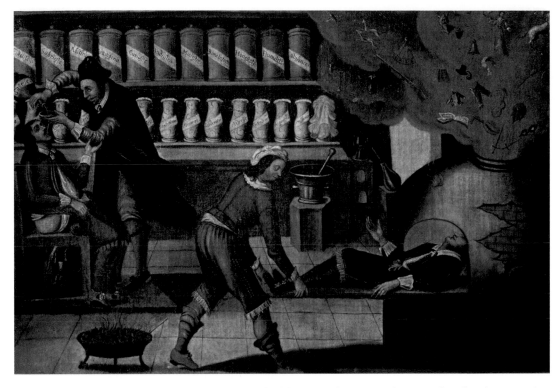

Pharmacy stores, such as this 17th-century French example, didn't just make purges and potions, they also administered them to a steady stream of patients who did not have the benefit of those personal physicians used by the wealthy.

And in his needy shop a tortoise hung,
An alligator stuff'd, and other skins
Of ill-shaped fishes; and about his shelves
A beggarly account of empty boxes,
Green earthern pots, bladders and musty seeds,
Remnants of packthread and old cakes of roses,
Were thinly scatter'd, to make up a show.

While against the law in Mantua, Romeo persuades the apothecary to sell him a "dram of poison" to end his life: "My poverty, but not my will, consents," says the apothecary, to which Romeo replies: "I pay thy poverty, and not thy will." Romeo ends his life with the words: 'Here's to my love! O true apothecary! Thy drugs are quick. Thus with a kiss I die." Romeo's apothecary was poor and his store bare. Other apothecary stores might be filled with a whole eclectic range of potions.

Apothecaries often had their own herb garden behind their stores. Larger apothecary stores in early modern Europe also served as repositories for medicines and spices brought from the Arab world and Far East. The mortar and pestle for grinding and mixing the ingredients was a symbol of the apothecary store. Scales for weighing the ingredients, too, were vital for the apothecary (or druggist, as they were also known). Jars containing leeches were commonly on display and a heady mix of fragrant floral smells and pungent spices filled the air.

Some of these old stores can still be visited today. The "Spezieria All'Ercole d'Oro" in Venice, Italy, dating back to the late 17th century, is a magnificent room that contains its original elegant furnishings and the jars for drugs and medicines. It was frequented by learned patricians, clergymen, and scholars, who treated it more like a coffee shop, a place for erudite conversation. One of its most popular pills was a laxative preparation known as "Santa Fosca purgative pills" or the *pillule del piovan*. Tradition had it that the remedy was first concocted by a parish priest (*piovan*) who lived in the area. A curious speciality was *Olio di Scorpioni* ("Scorpion Oil"), which was used to treat wounds and was produced by drowning some hundred live scorpions in two quarts of olive oil. Specializing in the preparation of more unusual drugs, this apothecary store had its own *Sala dei Veleni* ("Poison or Venom Room") where rare herbs and medicines, often from overseas, were stored.

Venice was a major European trading and maritime center and the Venetians imported many items of value to pharmacy from the Islamic world and beyond. They became most famous for their *Teriaca* (or theriac) and *Mithridato* (mithridatium), the "mother of all antidotes," named after King Mithridates VI of Pontus in Asia Minor (*c*.132/4–63 BC), who was known for his supposed immunity to poisons. This was a concoction of herbs and *castoreum* (an oily extract from the sexual glands of the beaver). Theriac was a universal panacea said to cure any number of ailments and was produced in Venice by the apothecary (*spezier da medicine*) and used far and wide. Depending on which of the many recipes was followed, theriac contained up to seventy ingredients, including roasted and fermented mashed flesh of vipers and opium. Its origins are legendary. Theriac was possibly first concocted by Mithridates and was popular in Roman times, and was "perfected" by Andromachus, physician to the Roman Emperor Nero, in the 1st century AD. Galen devoted a whole book to theriac. It was produced in many parts of the world, including China and India, and disseminated along the Silk Road. By the Renaissance in Europe, the Venetians had a monopoly on its production and trade and it was known in England as Venice treacle ("treacle" is a corruption of theriac). This was one of the most expensive of all medicines, with apothecaries in Venice being licensed to produce it. The recipe was made public by the French apothecary Moyse Charas (1619–98), thereby ending the Venetian monopoly on manufacture.

Traveling salesmen and quack remedies

So they [the common people] were as mad upon their running after quacks and mountebanks, and every practising old woman, for medicines and remedies ... who fed their fears and kept them always alarmed and awake on purpose to delude them and pick their pockets.

Daniel Defoe, *A Journal of the Plague Year, 1722*, describing the Great Plague of London, 1665–6

Quacks took advantage of other people's fears and were the first on the scene during times of deadly epidemics with their "nostrums." During the great plague epidemics of the 17th century a "flock" of such characters was said to have descended on London. Each claimed to be the sole producer of a nostrum that could cure victims of the plague, establishing proprietorship, as well as flaunting a knowledge of Latin. As Defoe conjured up the scene:

> *The posts of houses and corners of streets were plastered over with doctors' bills and papers of ignorant fellows, quacking and tampering in physic, and inviting the people to come to them for remedies, which was generally set off with such flourishes as these, viz. 'Infallible preventive pills against the plague' ... 'Sovereign cordials against the corruption of the air' ... 'The only true plague water'.*

Indeed, Defoe said there were so many claims for these pills, potions, and preservatives that

"I could fill a book" of them. Most, he believed, poisoned the unfortunate bodies with their "odious and fatal preparations."

Other quacks made fortunes out of useless nostrums (their "own" remedies) for common aches and pains or by selling "panaceas" or "cure-alls" for every illness. The poor and disabled were most susceptible to the lure of these "nostrums." The public, who often had no knowledge of the ingredients, effectiveness, or safety, used these remedies faithfully according to the indiscriminate dosage prescribed. Elixirs and tinctures were marketed under hundreds of different trade names and for a host of, often unrelated, indications. Many of the potions also contained known poisons such as arsenic and mercury. Goddard's Drops were made in England during the 17th century by a "Dr Goddard" from a concoction of human bones and skulls to create "a medicine beyond all comparison." A surprising number of so-called "quacks" gained favor with the royal families of Britain and Europe, leading the medical profession to despise them (the quacks!) even more.

Patent and proprietary medicines

The drugstore, as we know it today, began to flourish in the 19th century. Those owning and running pharmacies, like the traditional apothecaries, continued to make up many of their potions in their store but they also now began to buy "patent" or "proprietary" medicines

Beecham's Pills

Thomas Beecham (1820–1907) in the 19th century used a variety of techniques to promote his products, including his famous laxative, Beecham's Pills, but his main success was a result of widespread advertising. It is said that a vicar from a local English church needed some money to buy new hymn books and asked Beecham if he would oblige in exchange for printing an advert inside them. When the books arrived the vicar saw no sign of any advert. However, on a Sunday just before Christmas the congregation found that they were singing rather different words:

Hark the herald angels sing
Beecham's Pills are just the thing
For easing pain and mothers mild
Two for adults and one for a child.

Thomas Beecham denied the story but his "reps" were trained to go around the country humming the tune.

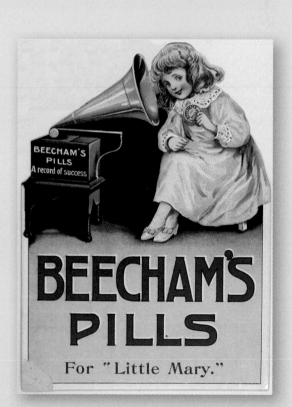

A 19th-century advert for Beecham's Pills, one of the most popular patent medicines, said to be a "wonderful medicine for bilious and nervous disorders."

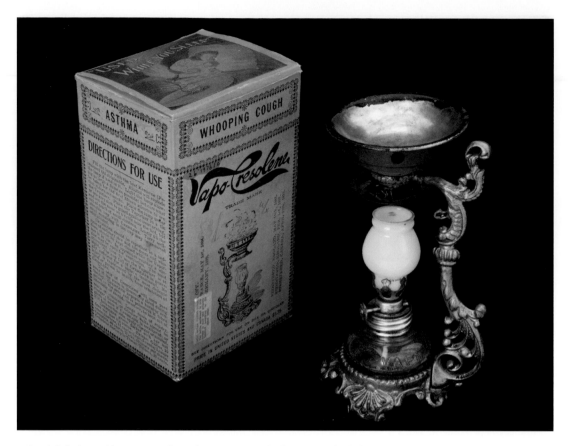

Before inhaled steroid treatments for asthma, patients relied on rest and inhaling opium-based oils delivered through vaporizers at night. This patented US version (1880) used Cresolene, a strong-smelling type of antiseptic, to treat asthma as well as whooping cough and croup.

often from commercial salesmen. The word "patent" (meaning "open") in this context suggests that the discoverer had applied for a patent to seek approval and rights for the medicine from some regulatory body. Patented medicines gained respectability from association with ancient, royal letters patent, granted to give an individual sole manufacturing rights for a unique product. To obtain the patent the ingredients of the remedy had to be declared—at least, that was the idea in principle. The first patent for a medicine in England was for Epsom Salts—a purgative containing magnesium sulphate procured from the waters of Epsom in southern England. The patent was granted to a London physician, Nehemiah Grew, in 1698.

The recipes of proprietary (Latin, *proprius*, "one's own") medicines, on the other hand, were kept secret, and the vendors didn't even have to list the ingredients on the package. They did, however, maintain the sole rights to the profits, which were often very lucrative. In fact, there was considerable blurring in what was a patent medicine and what was proprietary and, for the most part, it became an advantage to cloak their often very ordinary formulae in mystery. They were sold under the cover of colorful names and even more colorful claims.

Many of the patent or proprietary medicines were made by and named after individuals —notable remedies included: Solomon's Balm of Gilead; James Morison's Vegetable Pills; Burgess's Lion Ointment; Clarke's Blood Mixture; Dr Bonker's Celebrated Egyptian Oil; Clark Stanley's Snake Oil Liniment; Holloway's Pills and Ointment; Dr Chamlee's Cancer Specific; Dr D Jayne's Vermifuge ("a sure remedy for worms"); Carter's Little Liver Pills (which turned the urine a brilliant turquoise); Ward's Drops and Ward's Pills (violent purgatives). There were a range of "tonics" or "pick-me-ups" such as Iron Jelloids; Brown's Iron Bitters; Grove's Tasteless Chill Tonic. The "popular" French tonic wine, Vin Mariani, made from Bordeaux wine treated with coca leaves, was said to hasten convalescence after influenza, and was recommended by his Holiness the Pope—with a picture of Pope Leo XIII on the advert. Many of these products contained genuinely active ingredients, albeit now considered harmful or addictive. Dr Collis Browne's "Chlorodyne," for example, was based on a combination of opium, cannabis, and chloroform—small wonder that it became one of the best-selling proprietary medicines.

Extravagant adverts and images accompanied many of these "miraculous" medicines. Bile Beans claimed to "free your system of harmful impurities ... cleanse the bloodstream, tone up the entire system. You feel new life, new vigour, new energy, and your eyes and complexion reflect the radiance of new health this favourite family tonic-laxative has given you." Manufacturers published long lists of testimonials from grateful patients. During the 19th century, an advert for Lydia Pinkham's Vegetable Compound for women stated: "Lydia Pinkham's private letters from ladies in all parts of the world average one hundred per day." Pinkham's hook was that women could take care of issues in their private parts without surgery or having the embarrassment of talking to a male doctor. As well as purchasing these medicines from pharmacists and other outlets, they might also be bought through mail order or sold directly to the customer by traveling salesmen who marketed them at "medicine roadshows," as portrayed in Donizetti's 1831 opera, "The Elixir of Love." Some patent medicines, like Pinkham's Vegetable Compound, made huge fortunes for their owners.

From small-scale chemists to high-street brands

Ready-made brand names or trademarked remedies made up a major part of the pharmacist's stock right through the 19th century and on into the 20th century.

In 1798, John Bell opened his chemist and druggist store in Oxford Street, London—a high-class establishment with its own laboratory on the premises and a full staff of counter assistants, servants, porters, and errand boys. It sold not only to the public, but dispensed medicines from physicians' prescriptions as well as supplying drugs and chemicals to hospitals and dispensaries. Large establishments like John Bell & Co. would supply wooden or metal medicine chests, veterinary supplies, spectacles, leeches, pills, powders, lotions, gargles, and plasters. They often also let blood, lanced boils, drew teeth and treated wounds, abscesses, and ulcers.

Boots the Chemist had its roots in mid-19th-century England when John Boot (1815–1860), an agricultural worker, moved to Nottingham to start a new business. He opened a small herbalist store from which he prepared and sold herbal remedies. His son, Jesse (1850–1931), expanded the range of products to include proprietary medicines and household necessities. He adopted a strategy of buying stock in bulk and selling his goods much cheaper than his competitors, advertising under the slogan "Health for a Shilling." The Boots name quickly became synonymous with quality, value, and service. The store network grew rapidly and by 1915 there were 550 Boots stores throughout Britain. It soon extended

John Bell & Co. would supply wooden or metal medicine chests, veterinary supplies, spectacles, leeches, pills, powders, lotions, gargles, and plasters.

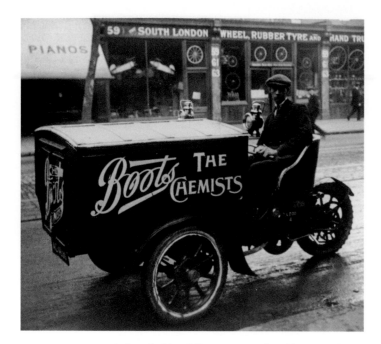

A glum-looking deliveryman sits aboard his Boots the Chemist delivery van in this photo from the 1920s. Boots the Chemist, originating in mid-19th-century England, is now one of the largest chains of retail chemists in Britain.

its manufacturing capacity from medicinal drugs, selling, too, a range of toiletries, convenience foods, and health and beauty products. It remains one of the largest chains of retail chemists in Great Britain.

Walgreens, now the largest drug-retailing chain in the United States, began in 1901 as a neighborhood drugstore in Chicago, owned by Charles R Walgreen, Sr. By 1913, there were four Walgreens drugstores, and by 1929 the total number of stores had reached 525 and Walgreens was quickly becoming the nation's most prominent drugstore chain. It became especially well known not just for their pharmaceuticals and excellent service but also for their magnificent soda fountains. Cold sodas, ice cream, and chocolate malted milkshake were considered important health aids. Walgreens opened its 6,000th store in New Orleans, Louisiana, in 2007.

A few of the more reputable and effective remedies, like Andrews Liver Salts, Phillips' Milk of Magnesia, and Vicks VapoRub, which date from the patent medicine era, are still on the market in high-street chemists and drugstores today.

Adulteration and poisonous medicines

No physician or surgeon should dispense a secret nostrum, whether it be his invention or exclusive property. For if it be of real efficacy, the concealment of it is inconsistent with beneficence and professional liberality. And if mystery alone give it value and importance, such craft implies either disgraceful ignorance, or fraudulent avarice.

Thomas Percival, *Medical Ethics*, 1803

One of the most poisonous substances to creep into medicines and food in the 19th century was arsenic. With no color or taste in its powdered form and easily passed off as sugar or flour, it was the poison of choice for Victorian murderers. It was sold cheaply as rat poison, sheep dip, and fly-papers and was also widely present in green dyes (Scheele's Green, a copper arsenate), used to tint everything from candies to candles and drapes, wallpaper, and clothing. Physicians had for a long time prescribed arsenic for their patients and in 1809 Fowler's Solution, a mixture of potassium arsenite and lavender, was accepted into the *London Pharmacopoeia* and praised as "almost as certain a medicine as we possess throughout the whole range of our *materia medica*."

A recent discovery and analysis of the "Hair of His Late Majesty, King George III," preserved within scraps of paper and found in the vaults of a London museum, turned out to be laden with arsenic. Indeed, the hair contained over 300 times the toxic level, adding further to the mystery of King George's "madness" (see page 83). Further medical detective work discovered that he had been dosed with "James' Powders" containing arsenic, which may have triggered his severe attacks of porphyria.

By the later 19th century, a groundswell of publicity led to deep concerns about the adulteration of foods and medicines. There were few laws regulating their contents and sales, although there had been attempts in the past in a number of countries to inspect and regulate apothecaries and the manufacture of drugs. However, with an increasing number of patent and propriety medicines on the market, standards had slipped. In England various Acts were passed such as the Food, Drink and Drugs Acts of 1872 and 1875; followed by further legislation in 1906 and the Poisons and Pharmacy Act of 1908.

Medications could contain up to 80 percent alcohol, "soothing syrups" for crying babies would contain morphine and cocaine, and advertisers claimed their remedies could cure anything from deafness to cancer. A key campaigner against adulteration was the US chemist Harvey Washington Wiley (1844–1930), who argued for reform. Under the auspices of the US Department of Agriculture's Division of Chemistry (later Bureau of Chemistry), investigations into the purity of medications were carried out. One example that came under scrutiny for misbranding was "Liquozone" with its claim of curing asthma, bowel troubles, consumption, cancer, dandruff, anemia, gallstones, gout, malaria, rheumatism, ulcers, and more. It was discovered to be totally fraudulent, having a chemical composition of 0.9 percent sulfuric acid, 0.3 percent sulfurous acid, and 98.8 percent water.

Concern about adulterated and misbranded drugs culminated in the publication of eleven articles by Samuel Hopkins Adams in *Collier's Weekly* in 1905 entitled, "The Great American Fraud" in which he exposed many of the false claims made about patent medicines. In 1906, President Theodore Roosevelt signed into law the Pure Food and Drug Act, also known as the "Wiley Act" after its chief advocate. It was estimated at this time that there were approximately 50,000 patent medicines being made and sold in the USA. Tighter regulations were included in a 1938 Act, following the formation of the Food and Drug Administration (FDA) in 1930. Though the 1938 Act was extensively amended in subsequent years, it remains the central foundation of the FDA regulatory authority in the USA to the present day.

PUNCH, OR THE LONDON CHARIVARI.—November 20, 1858.

THE GREAT LOZENGE-MAKER.

A Hint to Paterfamilias.

Adulteration of medicines and foods was notorious in the 19th century. This cartoon from *Punch* followed a scandal of mass poisoning in Bradford, England, in 1858, when a lozenge-maker had intended to adulterate his lozenges with plaster of Paris but had added arsenic by mistake.

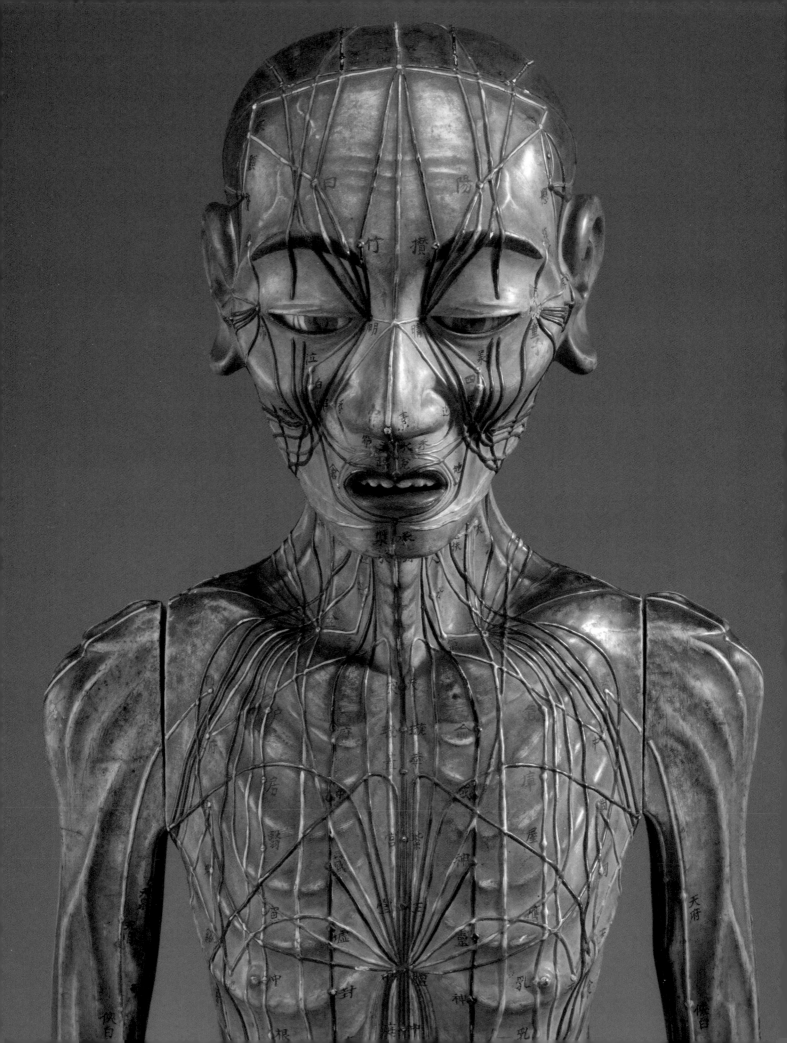

Complementary and Alternative Medicine

Chinese medicine is a great treasure house and should be diligently explored and improved upon.

Mao Zedong, 1958

Acupuncture is the use of therapeutic needle puncturing, to different depths beneath the skin, at specific points on the body's surface. Originating in China, this healing technique has been used for at least 2,000 years. Acupuncture was first introduced into Europe in the 17th century and has become increasingly popular worldwide over the past few decades. Various other forms of healing—now often described in the West as "alternative" or "complementary" to mainstream biomedicin—include homeopathy, osteopathy and chiropractic. These were first developed in Europe and North America in the 18th and 19th centuries, and continue to flourish today. Herbal remedies have a long history and form the basis of traditional medicines in many parts of the world today. The global exchange of medical traditions and practices over the past centuries is a significant aspect of the history of medicine.

Acupuncture and moxibustion

One of the oldest healing techniques that originated in ancient China and is still widely practiced today is acupuncture. According to classical acupuncture theory, health is controlled by the harmonizing of two complementary principles—the *yin* and *yang*—mediated by *qi*, a life process or flow of "vital force." Acupuncture, today, usually involves the shallow insertion of fine, sterile needles into specific points on the body, known as acupoints. These points are determined by meridians, channels through which *qi* flows through the body. The aim is to correct the imbalance or blockage of *qi* energy in the meridians that can lead to illness. Acupuncture is often accompanied by moxibustion using the dried and ground leaves of the herb moxa, or mugwort (*Artemisia vulgaris*), to warm regions and acupuncture points. There are several methods of moxibustion. For example, Chinese medical practitioners may burn mugwort on the end of metal needles through the medium of cigar-shaped rolls or cones to stimulate particular points or painful parts of the body.

OPPOSITE A 17th-century Asian wooden acupuncture model of the upper torso and head. Acupuncture is one of the oldest healing techniques, originating in ancient China and still widely practiced today.

An acupuncturist will also ask for a full case history, take the pulse of a patient's energy flow and decide which points to work on. From early times, a large number of pulse types were distinguished, such as floating, superficial, sunken, or hesitant, and this became the preeminent method of diagnosis for elite physicians. Pulse diagnosis has evolved into a sophisticated and highly complex part of Chinese medicine to detect blockages of *qi*.

Acupuncture and moxibustion in China probably arose from a synthesis of older medical practices such as petty surgery, massage, bloodletting and, hot stone treatment with new ideas about the nature of the universe that flourished in the late Warring States period (*c*.600–221 BC). Although sharp stone and bone needles and knives survive from Neolithic times, acupuncture and moxibustion were originally linked together with a theory of the channels in Han times (206 BC–AD 220), though the accounts describe procedures that are quite different from the treatments that are used today. Huangfu Mi, a Chinese scholar and physician, compiled the *Canon of Acupuncture and Moxibustion* some time from AD 256–282, which assembled a consistent body of doctrines concerning acupuncture and exercised considerable influence over the acupuncture traditions of China, Korea, and Japan.

Bronze acupuncture figurines were first cast in the 11th century AD for the purposes of teaching and examination. They clearly display the circulation networks and label each acupuncture point. When the model was covered with a layer of yellow wax and filled with water, medical students had to locate the required acupoint exactly with a needle, causing water to gush out of the model through a hole. One of the great Chinese medical classics, the *Great Compendium of Acupuncture and Moxibustion* (*Zhenjiu Dacheng*), was published by the physician Yang Jizhou in the early 17th century during the Ming Dynasty. It synthesized past texts and unwritten traditions and is still the basis for modern acupuncture.

Acupuncture (Latin, *acus*, "needle," + *pungo*, "I prick") and moxibustion (*moxa* combined with combustion, "burning") were introduced into Europe in the 17th century through the published and personal reports of European observers in China, Japan, and the Indonesian archipelago. Moxibustion was accessible and readily assimilated into European practice. It was cheaper than needles and became popular as a treatment for gout—which commonly afflicted affluent middle-aged men. The first elaborate Western treatise on acupuncture, *De Acupunctura*, was published in Latin in the 1680s by a Dutch physician and botanist, Willem ten Rhijne (1647–1700), who had seen the "needling"technique practiced while stationed at a Dutch East India Company trading post in Japan. By the early 19th century, acupuncture had become fashionable in France and Britain, where it was used with European models of human anatomy rather than the "body map" based on Chinese ideas. The French physician Louis-Joseph Berlioz (1776–1848), father of the famous composer, found acupuncture to be beneficial for relieving muscular pain and nervous conditions. It was said to be "a most valuable remedy" by the London surgeon James Morss Churchill (1801–75) in his 1821 English treatise on "acupuncturation": "not only in the Eastern Hemisphere, in France, and in America, but throughout the British dominions, and in our London hospitals … Lumbago and sciatica [for example] frequently disappear as if charmed away." Acupuncture became popular in the USA, which prompted some physicians to conduct tests into its efficacy.

OPPOSITE A Japanese housewife of the Bunsei era (1818–1830) undergoes moxibustion treatment. Various methods involve the burning of the herb mugwort, at or near specific body sites, and may be applied in conjunction with acupuncture. These ancient practices, still used today, aim to be holistic: treating body, mind, and spirit as one.

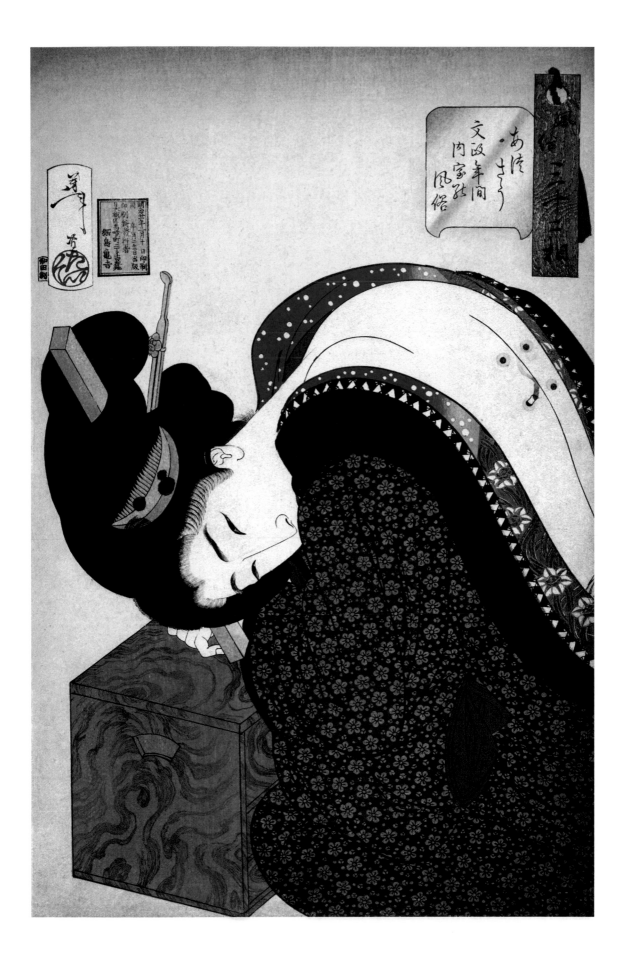

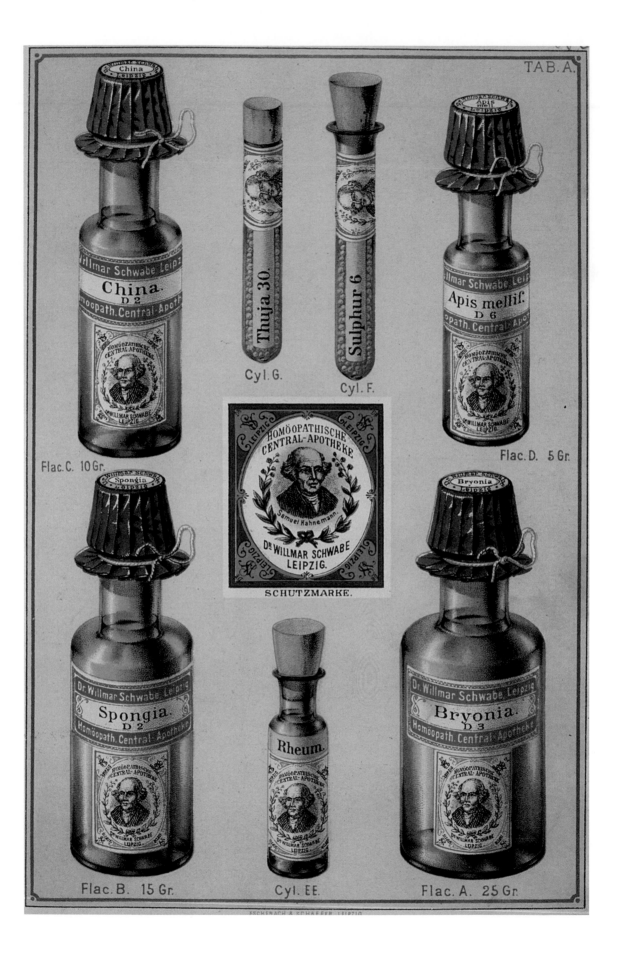

TREATMENTS AND THERAPIES

Over the following century, acupuncture went periodically in and out of fashion both in the East and the West. In 1822, the Imperial Academy in China prohibited the teaching and practice of acupuncture. The reasons for this decline included a dislike of needles among patients, the emergence of gentler therapies such as *tuina* massage, and the preference of elite physicians for herbal medicine. Acupuncture was a manual therapy unsuited for the intellectual scholar-physicians, though the knowledge and skills were retained by rural healers. With China's increasing acceptance of Western medicine, traditional forms of medicine became even less acceptable in the first half of the 20th century. Acupuncture together with a whole system of Traditional Chinese Medicine (TCM) experienced a revival following the establishment of the People's Republic of China in 1949 and acupuncture was "reintroduced" to the West in the 1970s. It is now popular across the world for controlling a range of maladies, from pain to depression. Another ancient practice, cupping, is also sometimes used together with acupuncture and moxibustion. Cupping aims to aid the circulation of stagnant *qi* energy and remove toxins from the body. It is practiced in most Southeast Asian medical traditions, and has recently had a resurgence of popularity in other parts of the world.

> Acupuncture is now popular across the world for controlling a range of maladies, from pain to depression.

Homeopathy and natural powers of healing: Europe and the USA

The homeopathic system, sir, just suits me to a tittle
It proves of physic, anyhow, you cannot take too little.

US journalist, 1848

A number of other practices of medical care and treatment were also developed in Europe and the USA between the 18th and early 20th centuries—especially by physicians who were horrified at such "heroic" practices as bloodletting and the use of toxic drugs and wanted to focus, instead, on using the healing powers of nature (the *vis medicatrix naturae*)—innate in every person. Some, like mesmerism, came under close scrutiny or were ridiculed and others, as, for example, Perkins's "Metallic Tractors," were short-lived crazes. Others, including homeopathy, attracted faithful followers—both practitioners and patients—and continue to flourish to this day.

Homeopathy's founder, German physician Samuel Hahnemann (1755–1843), developed a deep concern with the toxicity of drugs, publishing a book in 1786, *On Poisoning by Arsenic – Its Treatment and Forensic Detection*. He began to look for alternative approaches and introduced the concept of homeopathy in 1796, based on his own personal experiments with Peruvian bark and other botanicals. To heal, the drug must produce in a healthy body symptoms similar to the disease, hence "homeopathy" (Greek *hómoios*- "the same" + *páthos*, "suffering or disease"). He outlined his ideas in such works as the *Materia medica pura* (1811–21), including the concept of the "law of similars": often expressed in Latin as *similia similibus curantur* or "let like be cured with like"; and the "law of infinitesimals" (serial dilution)—the smaller the dose, the more potent the

OPPOSITE Late 19th-century German homeopathic remedies. This "alternative" form of medicine became popular during the 19th century in Britain and the USA but was resisted by "regular" medical practitioners.

medicine. Hahnemann also coined the term "allopathy" ("other than disease") to characterize the work of physicians who used methods either to counteract symptoms or to produce an action unrelated to symptoms, such as purging, bloodletting, or blistering of the skin.

Despite deep-seated animosity and vigilant opposition from "regular" or allopathic medicine, homeopathy spread throughout Europe and North America during the 19th century. Homeopathy was used to treat Napoleon's soldiers during a typhus epidemic following the Battle of Leipzig in 1813 and the world's first homeopathic hospital was opened in Leipzig, Germany, in 1833. In the USA by the mid-19th century there were nearly 2,500 homeopathic physicians. The homeopaths offered pleasant-tasting pills that produced no discomforting side effects. Such medication was particularly suitable for babies and small children, and won the support of large numbers of US women. It was also used during the American Civil War, despite efforts in the Union Army to stamp it out or exclude homeopathic practitioners. Some of the strongest advocates for homeopathy included European royalty and the aristocracy.

During a number of major epidemics, such as cholera in London in 1854, statistics indicated that mortality rates in homeopathic hospitals were lower than those in the conventional medical hospitals, where treatments used at the time were often harmful and did little or nothing to combat the disease. Homeopathy spread to colonial India, gaining in popularity as an "alternative" to heroic Western medicine. It also worked in harmony with the Ayurvedic system of medicine and remains popular today. Mesmerism was also adopted by the British in colonial India in the 1840s, where it was used in surgical anesthesia prior to its replacement by ether and chloroform.

With the rise of modern scientific medicine in the 20th century and the development of new, effective, and lifesaving drugs and vaccines, homeopathy, like other "alternative'" practices, was increasingly considered by the public and the mainstream medical community, as well as by the pharmaceutical industry, to be an unscientific relic of the past. By the 1950s in the USA all the homeopathic colleges that had existed at the turn of the 20th century had either closed or were no longer teaching homeopathy. While it continued in relative obscurity, homeopathy did not completely disappear. Indeed, in Britain, five homeopathic hospitals became part of the newly created National Health Service (NHS) in 1948.

In recent decades homeopathy in many parts of the world has witnessed a renaissance and has become one of the fastest-growing forms of "alternative" medicine. Homeopaths continue to adopt Hahnemann's principles of using extremely diluted preparations of substances to treat symptoms, believing that when a substance in large doses causes certain symptoms in a healthy subject, in infinitesimally small doses it can alleviate those same symptoms in a sick one. Homeopathy's lasting appeal (though not without its critics today) has stemmed from its emphasis on purity and the positive idea of the body striving naturally to cure itself.

Another approach based on natural healing without drugs was the practice of osteopathy, started in the United States in the 1870s by a Kansas doctor, Andrew Taylor Still (1828–1917). He opened the first American School of Osteopathy (now A T Still University of the Health Sciences) in 1892 in Kirksville, Missouri. His philosophy was based on the idea that most diseases were caused by the mechanical interference of nerves and blood flow, and were curable by manipulation of "deranged, displaced bones, nerves, muscles – removing all obstructions – thereby setting the machinery of life moving." Osteopathy (the name was coined from the Greek roots for "bone" and "disease") remains a field of health care that

Mesmerism

The German physician Franz Anton Mesmer (1734–1815) believed that he could cure virtually any disease by manipulating a patient's "animal magnetism" (or natural healing power), claiming: "nature offers in Magnetism a universal means of healing and protecting people." Methods included the laying on of hands or gazing into the patient's eyes (hence the expression "mesmerizing"). Following a scandalous case when attempting to treat the blindness of a woman in Vienna in 1777, Mesmer fled to Paris to promote his concepts, only to be challenged there by a Royal Commission, convened by King Louis XVI in 1784, to examine this practice. Mesmer's disciple, Charles d'Elson, acted as the magnetizer for a large number of experiments. At the end of the trial, the commissioners concluded that the cause of observed responses was not "animal magnetism" but human imagination, abetted by hope.

Mesmeric therapy in France *c.* 1780s. Mesmer and his patient hold magnetic wands to their eyes for the ophthalmic application of mesmeric fluids.

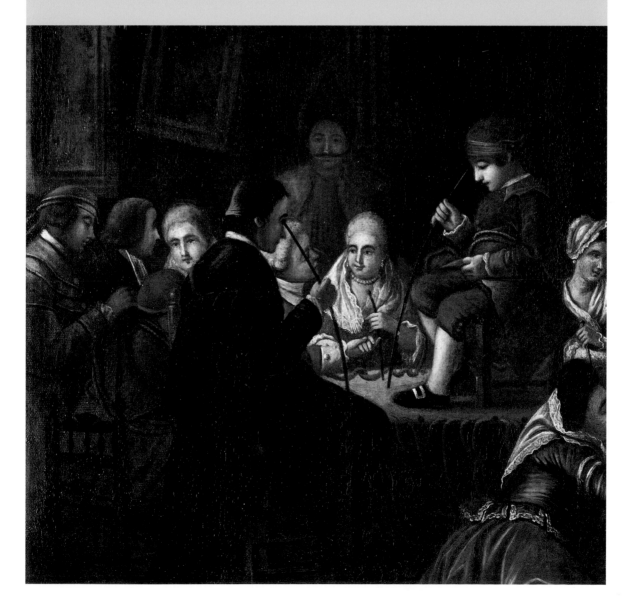

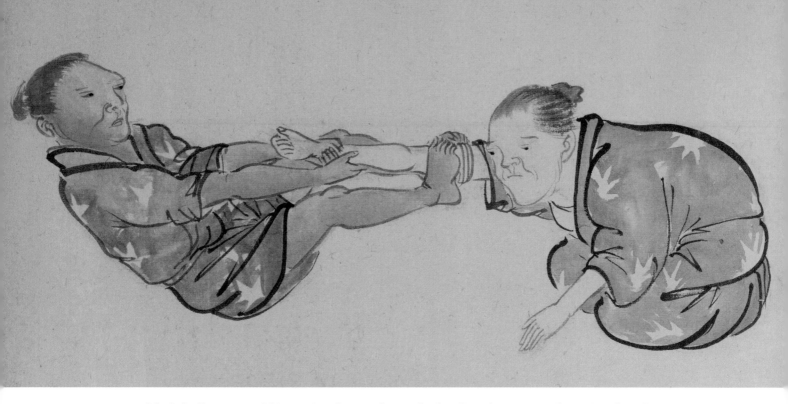

While the healing systems of chiropractic and osteopathy were developed in 19th-century North America, other cultures also practiced various forms of skeletal manipulation, as shown in this 19th-century Japanese watercolor.

emphasizes the role of the musculoskeletal system in the prevention and treatment of health problems, though surgery and drug therapy have been gradually integrated into osteopathy.

Chiropractic (Greek for "done by hand")—another system that still thrives—was founded in 1895 by the Canadian-born grocer and lay-healer David D Palmer (1845–1913), who developed the theory that the misalignment of the spinal vertebrae bones in the body was the basic underlying cause of all "dis-ease" and suggested that physical manipulation of the spine could cure disease. In 1897 he opened the US Palmer School of Chiropractic in Davenport, Iowa, based on a "one cause-one cure" philosophy. Like osteopathy, chiropractic methods have also evolved over the past century to include the adoption of other therapeutic methods.

Among botanical systems of healing from the West that remain widespread and commercially successful today are Bach flower remedies. They were "discovered" and introduced by the British physician and homeopath Edward Bach (1886–1936) in the early 1930s and these flower-based liquid tinctures continue to be recommended by neuropathic healers. Bach's original 38 remedies are directed at specific characteristics and are designed especially to cure emotional imbalances that affect state of health—for instance, *Star of Bethlehem* is advised for those in shock caused by grief or unexpected bad news. The best-known Bach flower remedy is the *Rescue Remedy* combination aimed at treating stress, anxiety, and panic attacks.

Hydrotherapy, naturopathy, reflexology, the Alexander technique, and Pilates were first established as commercial systems by individuals in the 19th and 20th centuries: Sebastian Kneipp (1821–97) and Vincenz Priessnitz (1799–1851) from Central Europe; Benedict Lust (1872–1945) in the USA; William Fitzgerald (1872–1942) in the USA; Frederick Alexander (1869–1955) in Australia; and Joseph Pilates (1883–1967) in Germany, respectively. These systems use nondrug-based therapies, adopting the premise that the body has the power to heal itself.

Traditional herbal remedies—in Eastern and Western medicine

Herbal-based remedies, among all the medicines and practices used since antiquity, continue to be the mainstay of healing in many parts of the world. Practitioners of TCM, Japanese Kampo-yaku, Indian Ayurvedic medicine, traditional Tibetan, and Korean medicine, as well as diverse local healers and herbalists in many parts of the globe, rely on ingredients from plants and other natural products. Plant extracts (from the leaves, roots, flowers, berries, etc.) are selected for their particular beneficial action, and are used to support the healing process of the body. They may be given in the form of a wide variety of teas, tinctures, and tablets. Some of the herbal remedies involve formulae that may range in the number of ingredients from a single herb to complex formulae of over 20 ingredients. A typical Chinese herbal medicine formula, for example, may include between eight and fifteen herbs that are divided into those with the primary therapeutic action (the "Emperor" herbs); those that support this action and address other coexisting patterns (the "Minister" herbs); those that reinforce the primary therapeutic agents and act to counteract any toxic or side effects (the "Assistant" herbs); and finally the "Envoy" herbs that are included in many formulae to ensure all components in the prescription are well absorbed and will help deliver or guide them to a particular part or system of the body.

There are various methods of healing with herbal medicines across cultures, which may appear quite different from modern chemical and pharmaceutical approaches of isolating active ingredients from plants with a view to finding a synthetic equivalent (see New Drugs from Old Remedies). The key to scholarly Chinese herbal medicine, for example, is for the practitioner to choose a medicine, often a combination of plant species, based on the particular symptoms and characteristics of the patient. The prescriptions are also guided by the various theories and philosophies of TCM. More than 11,000 plant species used in over 100,000 compound formulae (or *fufang*) have been recorded in China, and the same plant species can have distinct roles in different formulae. Chinese medicines also contain other ingredients such as animal products, rocks and shells. In order to prescribe

Massage, diet, and exercise

Although heterogeneous, the major complementary and alternative medicine (CAM) systems have many common characteristics, including a focus on individualizing treatments, treating the whole person, promoting self-care and self-healing, and recognizing the spiritual nature of each individual. A number of therapeutic techniques are specifically aimed at eliciting a "relaxation response." The practice of massage, sometimes in conjunction with aromatherapy using essential oils, has a long history. It was practiced thousands of years ago by the Egyptians and Chinese, and was popular in ancient Greek and Roman baths to enhance well-being and physical prowess. The word "massage" comes from the Arabic word meaning to "stroke." It continues to be seen as beneficial for mind, body, and soul. Meditation, reflexology, and yoga can help relieve "stress" —whether manifest in physical or emotional ailments. A balanced diet and a wide range of exercises—from T'ai Chi (Taijiquan) to Pilates— are also recommended to maintain good health or cure aches and pains.

the right formulae, the practitioner will take time to assess a patient's symptoms and needs.

In Japan, some 70 to 80 percent of registered physicians prescribe Kampo botanical medicines and, unlike many parts of the world, the formulae and manufacture of these are strictly regulated and standardized according to pharmaceutical standards set and approved by the Ministry of Health, Labor, and Welfare, the Japanese equivalent of the FDA. Two-thirds of the officially registered formulations are covered by national health insurance.

In the Western world, "health food stores" and internet websites attract customers who value the perceived benefits of "natural" remedies—from herbal remedies to minerals, vitamins, fish oil, and other nutritional supplements. It is possible to buy ready formulated (and nonprescription) products such as Echinacea Cold and Flu Capsules, Tea Tree Cream Antiseptic, Arnica Cooling Gel, Ginkgo Leaf Tablets, Evening Primrose Oil, Tiger Balm, St John's Wort, and many others. Products are also purchased for preventing health problems before they arise.

Complementary and alternative medicine

The WHO defines complementary and alternative medicine (CAM) as a broad set of health care practices that are not part of that country's own tradition and are not integrated into the dominant health care system. Acupuncture and herbal remedies may be seen as "alternative" treatments in the West when used instead, or independently, of mainstream medicine and "complementary" when used as supplements to mainstream medicine. They could also be considered "mainstream" within those communities that continue to use such traditional therapies as part of standard contemporary medical practice. As an overview of the history of medicine reminds us, societies in many parts of the world have always had pluralistic medical systems and defining what is "mainstream" and what is "alternative" has shifted over time and across different cultures. The boundaries between CAM and mainstream medicine, as well as among different CAM systems, are often blurred and are constantly changing.

CAM is a huge and active area, not just for practitioners and patients, but also for researchers and providers of health care. Unlike mainstream medicine, CAM often lacks or has only limited experimental and clinical study; however, scientific investigation of CAM is beginning to address this knowledge gap. In the USA, for example, the National Center for Complementary and Alternative Medicine (NCCAM) was established in 1999. This government agency is dedicated to the scientific study of CAM. Of prime importance is to discover and differentiate those therapeutic remedies and systems of healing that can be of proven medical or beneficial value while, simultaneously, preventing the practice of those that are potentially or positively harmful (including side effects caused by herb-drug interactions). Safety, efficacy, and quality control, as in all forms of medicine, are key issues (see Testing Treatments and Clinical Trials). Training, regulation, and licensing or certification of practitioners, as well as registration of herbal products (including whether these are defined as "food supplements" or "medicines" requiring a full product license), are complex issues that are currently being addressed both at national and global levels.

Of significance, too, is the question of who pays the bill. In many of the poorer countries, traditional or local remedies are the only affordable and accessible option for many people. It is estimated that some 80 percent of the world's population, while struggling to afford essential Western medicines, relies on traditional systems of medicine for primary health care,

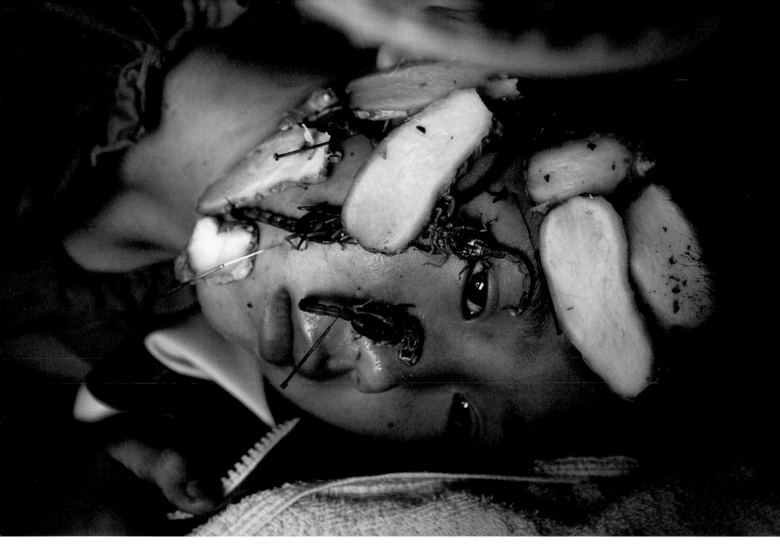

Dead scorpions and ginger flakes are placed on a patient's face during a traditional Chinese medical treatment for curing facial paralysis, at a hospital in Jinan, the capital of eastern China's Shandong province.

with plants and plant extracts forming the dominant components of indigenous medicines. By contrast, the use of various so-called CAM therapies in affluent societies has become a multibillion-dollar industry that is expected to continue its rapid growth, although there is wide variation in whether these are paid for by patients or covered by national health or insurance schemes. There are ongoing studies, for example, based on patient questionnaires, to try and elucidate which CAM practices have high levels of patient demand today and why. Reasons range from disillusionment with "impersonalized" high-tech medicine to the attraction of a more natural, traditional, and holistic approach to health care, especially for chronic conditions, aches and pains, stresses and strains, which cannot easily be remedied by pharmaceutical drugs or surgery (see also "Placebos and the placebo effect," page 204).

While health-conscious patients "shop around" (and this is nothing new), there is an increasing trend for medical practitioners, whether based on Eastern or Western traditions, to offer an integrated or cooperative approach to medicine—advising on different diagnostics and therapies according to the nature of the illness or disability, whether life-threatening, acute, or chronic; physical, mental, or emotional. In South and East Asian countries, State hospitals and clinics may offer acupuncture and herbal therapy alongside conventional biomedicine and surgery, and medical practitioners may have some training in

Systems of health care and therapies

MAJOR DOMAINS OF CAM	EXAMPLES UNDER EACH DOMAIN
Health care systems	Indian Ayurvedic, Unani, and Siddha medicine
	Traditional/Classical Chinese Medicine
	(eg *acupuncture, Chinese herbal medicine*)
	Japanese Kampo
	Latin American-Mexican Curanderismo
	Native American medicine
	(eg *sweat lodge, medicine wheel*)
	Chiropractic
	Osteopathy
	Homeopathic medicine
	Naturopathic medicine
Mind-body Interventions	Meditation
	Hypnosis
	Yoga
	Hydrotherapy
	Visualization imagery
	Dance, music, and art therapy
	Equine, canine, and animal therapy
	Prayer and faith healing
Biological-based therapies	Herbal therapies
	Special diets and nutritional supplements
Therapeutic massage and movement therapies	Massage
	T'ai Chi (*Taijiquan*)
	Alexander technique
	Pilates
Energy therapies	Reiki
	Qigong
	Therapeutic touch
Bioelectromagnetics	Magnet therapy

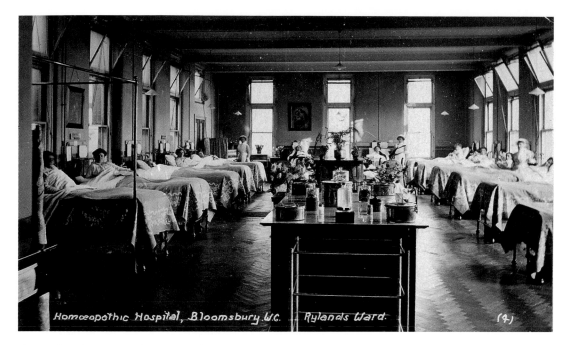

The Royal London Hospital for Integrated Medicine was founded as the London Homoeopathic Hospital in 1849 by Dr Frederick Quin, one of the first doctors to practice homeopathy in Britain. This image shows one of its wards in the early 20th century.

both biomedical and traditional medicine. In the West, a trained and qualified acupuncturist might advise a patient to visit a "regular" doctor if a disease should or can be treated by, say, antibiotics or chemotherapy, while a doctor might advise a patient to visit an acupuncturist for back pain that has not responded to strong prescription painkillers.

An example of this move toward "integrated" medicine in Britain is the Royal London Homeopathic Hospital. It was first established as a homeopathic hospital in 1849 (founded by Frederick Quin) and contains a wealth of archives on practices, patients, and royal patronage—who went there; why, how and by whom they were treated. It was renamed the Royal London Hospital for Integrated Medicine in 2010 to reflect the hospital's changing and broader role over the course of its recent history. It is now the largest public-sector provider of integrated medicine in Europe, offering an innovative, patient-centered service combining or "integrating" the best of conventional and complementary treatments for a wide range of conditions.

There will continue to be challenging developments, as well as controversial and complex tensions, in this area over the coming decades. Meanwhile, exploring the roots and links with the past of many of the CAM therapies, their evolution over time, their exchanges across cultures, and their integration with, or role alongside, modern "conventional" medicine will remain a fascinating topic of study for historians of medicine. A South African saying conveys the ever-changing views on medicine:

2000 BC: *"Here, eat this root."*
1000 BC: *"That root is heathen, here, say this prayer."*
AD 1850: *"That prayer is superstition, here, drink this potion."*
AD 1970: *"That potion is snake oil, here, take this antibiotic."*
AD 2000: *"That antibiotic is artificial, here, eat this root."*

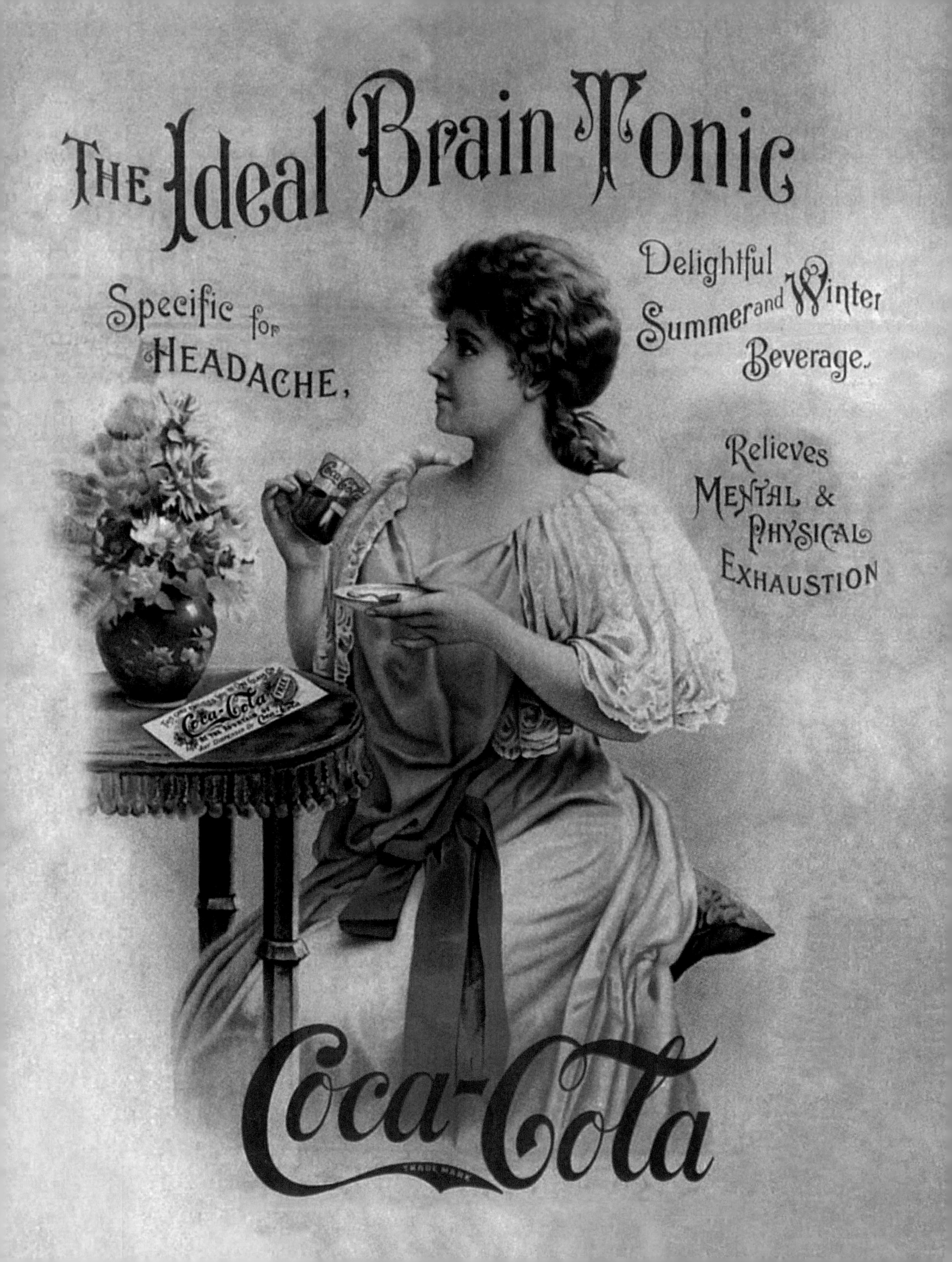
THE Ideal Brain Tonic
Specific for HEADACHE,
Delightful Summer and Winter Beverage.
Relieves MENTAL & PHYSICAL EXHAUSTION
Coca-Cola
TRADE MARK

New Drugs from Old Remedies

Take an ounce of the best Jesuits' bark, Virginian snake-root, and orange-peel, of each half an ounce; bruise them all together, and infuse for five or six days in a bottle of brandy, Holland gin, or any good spirit; afterwards pour off the clear liquor, and take a wine-glass of it twice or thrice a day.

William Buchan, *Domestic Medicine*, 1781—an early recipe for gin and tonic!

In the early 19th century, advances in chemistry enabled scientists to isolate the active principles from a number of plants that had been used for centuries as part of various medicinal remedies. The chemistry laboratory began to replace the physic garden as a source of new medicines, and scientists started to investigate the association between the chemical structure of drugs and the ways in which they act. The first major advance was the isolation of morphine from opium. Morphine was soon introduced into medicine as a powerful painkiller and remains in use today. Other fascinating examples where "old remedies" were found to contain "active" drugs include cocaine from the coca plant and the antimalarial quinine from the bark of the South American cinchona tree. A key development for the pioneering chemical-pharmaceutical industries of the late 19th century was the production of synthetic drugs. Aspirin, launched in 1899 by the German company Bayer, was a particularly important example of the newly discovered synthetic drugs based on the older remedies of the bark of the willow tree and the plant meadowsweet. The impact of discovering and isolating the active principles of plants, and the introduction of synthetic equivalents, has been profound for medicine.

From the coca plant to cocaine

Cocaine, an alkaloid of the coca plant from South America, was isolated in 1860, and, like morphine (see Opium, Morphine, and Heroin), was another drug introduced for a wide variety of medical purposes, including as a nerve tonic, stimulant, painkiller, anesthetic, and antidepressant. It was even used by Sir Arthur Conan Doyle's fictional detective, Sherlock Holmes.

OPPOSITE This 1898 advert promotes the medicinal benefits of Coca-Cola. Originally containing cocaine, it was sold as a patent medicine for five cents a glass at soda fountains. Cocaine, a highly addictive drug, was removed from Coca-Cola in 1903.

Sherlock Holmes took his bottle from the corner of the mantel-piece, and his hypodermic syringe from its neat morocco case. With his long, white, nervous fingers he adjusted the delicate needle, and rolled back his left shirtcuff. For some little time his eyes rested thoughtfully upon the sinewy forearm and wrist all dotted and scarred with innumerable puncture-marks. Finally, he thrust the sharp point home, pressed down the tiny piston, and sank back into the velvet-lined armchair with a long sigh of satisfaction … 'Which is it to-day,' I [Dr Watson] asked, 'morphine or cocaine?' … 'It is cocaine' he said … 'Would you care to try it?'

Arthur Conan Doyle, *The Sign of Four* (1890)

The dried leaves of the coca plant (*Erythroxylum coca*) had been chewed, consumed, and smoked by indigenous peoples in Peru, South America, for centuries as part of religious ceremonies, as a recreational drug, an aphrodisiac, a stimulant, or to ward off fatigue, cold, and hunger. Coca was known to the Europeans with the opening up of the "New World," but, unlike tobacco, it was not widely adopted in Europe. By the mid-19th century, however, botanists began to investigate its medicinal properties. In 1860, the German chemist Albert Niemann (1834–61) extracted cocaine, the main alkaloid contained within the coca leaf, and by the 1880s there was a "craze" for cocaine. And, as with the opium derivative morphine, it could also be injected into the bloodstream using a hypodermic syringe. Robert Louis Stevenson (1850–94) purportedly wrote *The Strange Case of Dr Jekyll and Mr Hyde* (1886) while on a six-day "binge" of cocaine.

The Austrian neurologist and psychoanalyst Sigmund Freud (1856–1939) initially recommended cocaine as an aid for the treatment of both morphine and alcohol addictions. Cocaine also proved beneficial for pain control in surgery and dentistry. Freud began a research project on cocaine that included self-experimentation, while his friend, Carl Koller (1857–1944), demonstrated the effectiveness of cocaine hydrochloride in 1884 as a local anesthetic for eye surgery. Cocaine was soon taken up by other ophthalmologists. The US surgeon William Stewart Halsted (1852–1922) experimented with cocaine to determine whether it could be used for spinal (nerve-block) anesthesia. He himself became addicted to it in the course of his experiments—to shake off his cocaine habit, he was prescribed morphine, supposedly a "cure" for drug dependency! Halsted continued to inject himself twice a day with a high dose of morphine becoming what was then known as a "morphinist."

"Forced March" tablets were a popular branded preparation of cocaine and commonly used by soldiers during the First World War. An elixir of cocaine combined with morphine, alcohol, syrup, and

Coca, cocaine, and Coca-Cola

Coca sherry and coca port became popular with celebrities in 19th-century Europe. In the USA, as the temperance movement gained momentum, druggist and morphine addict John Pemberton removed the alcohol component of his French Wine Coca, a frothy alcoholic drink based on coca and caffeine-loaded kola nuts, and advertised "the virtues of coca without the vices of alcohol." In spring 1886 the renamed Coca-Cola was marketed as "a valuable brain tonic" and "Delicious! Refreshing! Exhilarating! Invigorating!" The cocaine was removed in 1903, replaced with coca flavoring, and Coca-Cola became a best-selling soft drink.

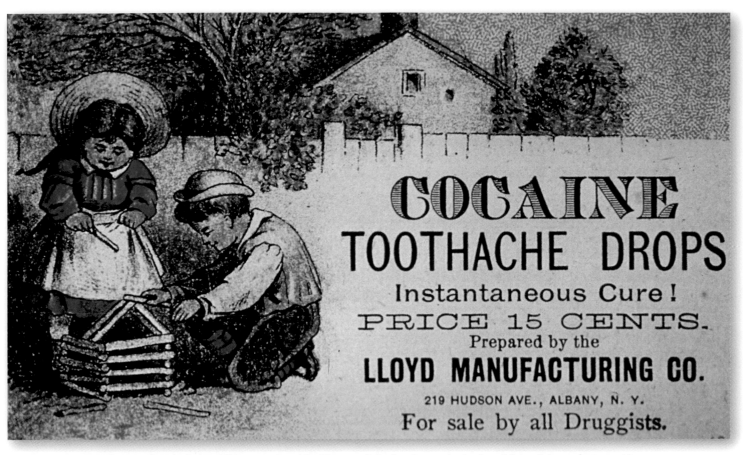

Adverts—often depicting children—such as this 1885 example for "cocaine toothache drops" claimed the products would cure all sorts of illnesses. Procaine ("Novocain"), a synthetic and safer version of cocaine, was first introduced in the early 20th century as a local anesthetic in dentistry.

chloroform water was developed at the Cancer Hospital in Brompton, London (later the Royal Marsden Hospital) in a formulation known as the "Brompton Cocktail." This was prescribed from the 1920s to help relieve the pain of advanced cancer. Cicely Saunders (1918–2005), founder of the modern hospice movement, did much to promote variants of the Brompton Cocktail and especially recommended the opioids for palliative care.

The dangers of addiction to narcotic drugs such as cocaine and heroin, however, became a serious concern in the 20th century. Today, cocaine and heroin are among the most abused of all illicit drugs.

From willow bark to aspirin

In the same fortnight in 1897 that the German drug company Bayer produced heroin (see page 143), now recognized as one of the most dangerous drugs in modern history, they also came up with the formula for one of the most successful painkillers of all times—acetylsalicylic acid (ASA) or aspirin. Bayer finally went into production with "Aspirin" in 1899. The idea for aspirin was based on two old medicinal plant remedies—one was the bark of the willow and the other meadowsweet.

Indeed, the use of these plants as medicines may date back over 5,000 years. There are records from the Sumerian civilization (c.3000 BC), ancient Egypt, the Greek and Roman

Empires, the pre-Columbian Americas, and early modern Europe describing the therapeutic value of extracts from the willow tree. Perhaps the most famous of all people to experiment with the willow tree prior to the development of aspirin was the Reverend Edward Stone (1702–68), rector of Chipping Norton, Oxfordshire, England. Walking home one summer in the mid-18th century, he stopped to rest under some willow trees that had recently been planted along the bank of a stream. Breaking off a piece of the bark and nonchalantly chewing it, he wondered if this bitter-tasting bark might be a cure for feverish agues and rheumatic fevers that were prevalent in the district. It had a similar bitter taste to the Peruvian cinchona bark used for treating fevers.

Stone pursued his idea with scientific rigor, testing and trying out the willow bark in various doses. Initially, he gathered a pound of willow bark, dried it in a bag over a baker's oven for more than three months, pulverized it, and then tried it out on parishioners suffering from agues and intermitting disorders. As he grew "bolder" with it, he increased the dose. He continued to use it as a remedy for five years, administering it to 50 people until he was sufficiently convinced that he had found a local remedy for fevers and chills. He wrote to the Royal Society of London describing his findings in 1763.

Others continued to experiment with the symptom-relieving properties of the bark of the white willow tree (Latin name: *Salix alba*). In 1838, Raffaele Piria (1814–65), an Italian chemist, successfully prepared "salicylic acid" from the bark's active ingredient, "salicin." Another plant, meadowsweet (*Spiraea ulmaria*), incidentally a favorite of Queen Elizabeth I, was also found to contain salicin. Over the second half of the 19th century, various forms of salicylate medicines, including salicin, salicylic acid, and sodium salicylate, became widely used by doctors for the treatment of pain, fever, and inflammation. However, their side effects, particularly gastric irritation, were considerable.

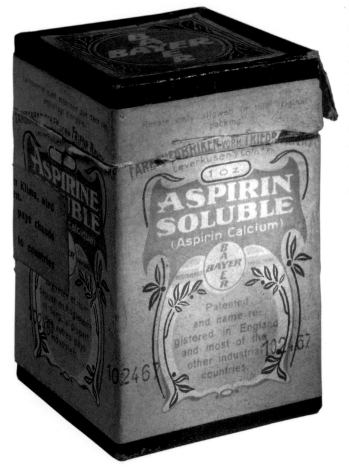

The Bayer pharmacology team wanted to find a substitute for salicylic acid that did not irritate the stomach so much. By adding the acetyl group to the salicylic acid (to become acetylsalicylic acid or ASA), Felix Hoffmann succeeded in creating ASA in a chemically pure and stable form and making a compound that neutralized the chemical element of salicylic acid responsible for its acidity. In fact, Hoffmann was not the first to make ASA. The German chemist Charles Frédéric Gerhardt (1816–56) had actually come up with a formula and published his results in 1853, but did not pursue it. Whether the Bayer team had read his paper we may never know.

A medicine carton containing soluble aspirin powder, shortly after aspirin was launched in 1899 by Bayer in Germany as a relief against pain.

However, when Heinrich Dreser, who was responsible for testing all new products, was given ASA, he rejected it on the grounds that it would "enfeeble the heart." Indignant and determined, head of pharmacology Arthur Eichengrün first tested it on himself and then decided to do his own "discrete" trials. He sent ASA to Bayer's Berlin "rep" who distributed it to a number of Berlin doctors and dentists. The reports of its benefits were glowing. It was also confirmed that this new formula did not have the nasty side effects of salicylic acid. When the reports reached Dreser, he, once again, showed no interest and scribbled in the margin: "The product has no value." Dreser, meanwhile, was swept up in the euphoria of the potential therapeutic and commercial value of heroin.

Fortunately, Carl Duisberg, head of research at Bayer, stepped in and ordered a second full set of trials. The results were again extraordinary and Duisberg put Bayer's weight behind the project. After conducting further "rigorous" evaluations (including trying it out on goldfish), even Dreser recognized its potential. Once given the go-ahead for production, a round-robin was circulated among Bayer's management to come up with a brand name—the winner was "Aspirin"—named after meadowsweet (*Spiraea*) rather than the English willow (*Salix*). Bayer Aspirin was launched in July 1899. The company advertised aspirin's safety by saying that the drug "does not affect the heart." It was also packaged with heroin! By the early 20th century, aspirin was being used all over Europe and the USA and it quickly proved infinitely safer as an analgesic (painkiller) than the habit-forming narcotic equivalents of morphine, heroin, and cocaine.

Aspirin has been a pharmacological triumph. It is estimated that over one trillion aspirin pills have been consumed since it was first launched and it is the best-known and most widely used medicine in the world. Indeed, it has also been used out of this world—as every Space Shuttle carried a small supply.

Aspirin together with other brands and different types of painkillers are now widely available from pharmacists, supermarkets, or on prescription and can help relieve pain from a whole host of conditions—from headaches to backaches. For those suffering from chronic pain or for the terminally ill, the WHO has developed a relatively inexpensive yet effective method of offering a continuum of care, known as the WHO "Pain Relief Ladder." This provides a three-step approach of administering the right analgesic drug in the right dose at the right time—starting with a nonsteroidal anti-inflammatory drug (NSAID), like aspirin, for mild pain; then using a weak opiate, like codeine, for moderate pain; and, when needed, moving onto a strong opiate, such as morphine, for severe pain.

The benefits of low doses of aspirin to reduce blood clots and the risk of stroke, heart disease, and death following a heart attack have also been recognized by medical science in the past few decades, while recent clinical studies have even suggested that aspirin might protect against certain types of cancer. Polypills, which contain a combination of aspirin and other drugs, are now being tried and tested for heart conditions. Regular doses of aspirin should be taken only under medical supervision, as it can cause gastrointestinal bleeding and ulcers in some patients, and Reye's syndrome in children.

Bayer Aspirin was launched in July 1899. The company advertised aspirin's safety by saying that the drug "does not affect the heart." It was also packaged with heroin.

Antimalarials: from the bark of the cinchona tree to quinine

Malaria is an ancient disease with a geographical distribution in past times extending from Archangel in the Russian Arctic to Australia and Argentina in the southern hemisphere. In the 17th century many people in Europe, as well as in the notoriously malarial tropics, suffered from its debilitating and often fatal fevers. At the end of the 19th century, scientists discovered that the malaria parasite was transmitted by the bite of an infective female *Anopheles* mosquito. These tiny insects—not much bigger than an eyelash—have the remarkable power to cause millions of cases of sickness and death every year. With a simple bite, they can ultimately take a life.

Quinine, a drug used to prevent or treat malaria, was first isolated from the bark of the South American cinchona tree in 1820 by the French chemists Pierre Pelletier (1788–1842) and Joseph Caventou (1795–1877). For at least two centuries prior to the production of quinine as a pure chemical compound, Europeans in South America had already discovered the healing powers of the bark of the cinchona tree growing in the high Andes. Jesuit missionaries in South America began to send large amounts of the bark from South America to the major ports of Europe.

A Jesuit in Rome, Pietro Paolo Puccerini, in the 17th century printed one of the first recipes for the bark:

> *This bark comes from the Realm of Peru and is called China or real China of the fevers, which is taken for the quartan and tertian fevers that are accompanied by cold. It should be taken thus: two drachms, finely grounded and sifted, three hours before the fever is due to take hold, should be made in an infusion in a glass of white wine. When the shivering starts, or when the slightest cold is felt, all of the preparation should be taken at once and the patient put to bed ... For four days no other medication whatsoever must be taken. It must be used only on the advice of the physician who may consider whether it is timely to administer it.*

The bark was introduced into England in the 1650s, where the Puritan Lord Protector Oliver Cromwell (1599–1658) called it the "Devil's Powder" because of its association with the Catholic Church. He refused to use it despite suffering badly from malaria, which he probably contracted in the English Fens in Eastern England. Others, however, found the bark to be a valuable remedy for "marsh fevers." Much to the annoyance of elite London physicians, it was a "quack" called Robert Talbor (1642–81) who made his fame and fortune using a "secret remedy" based on the bark to cure European royals and nobility. In the last decade of the 17th century the bark was even introduced to China. During the Kangxi reign (1662–1722), the emperor was suffering from a severe illness—probably malaria—and he was successfully treated by two French Jesuits with the bark.

European botanical explorers trekked across impenetrable terrain, risking lives and limbs, to reach the forests of the eastern slopes of the Andes in order to send seeds or saplings of the bark to Europe—often ending in dismal failure. Malaria, in the 18th century, proved an ever-increasing and intractable burden for many localities of the world. It was an especially major problem for missionaries, explorers, colonists, and the military in many parts of the tropical and subtropical world, where a severe form of malaria (now known as *falciparum* malaria) was life-threatening. West Africa was a region often typified as "White Man's Grave"; for example, almost half the British soldiers stationed in Sierra Leone between 1817 and 1836 died of disease, mostly malaria.

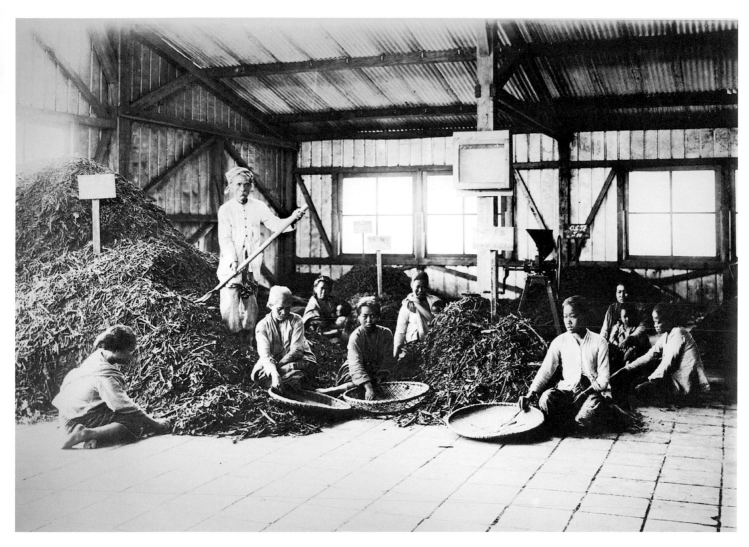

Following the isolation in 1820 of the South American cinchona tree's alkaloid, quinine, as a treatment for malaria, many explorations were undertaken to find and cultivate the best-yielding quinine trees. The Dutch captured the market with the cultivation of cinchona trees in Java. Here we see the dried bark being cleaned.

With the isolation of the alkaloid, quinine (*quina*, Peruvian for bark), in 1820 and its recognition as the most effective active agent within the cinchona bark, this added chemical knowledge led to hope that this new drug would combat malaria. Further expeditions and botanical explorations into the South American interiors were undertaken to find the quinine-yielding cinchona trees with the added aim of establishing plantations in other parts of the world.

One particularly important species—with the highest quinine content—was the *Cinchona calisaya*, a rare Bolivian species. The search for this species led to one of the most tragic episodes in the history of quinine. Charles Ledger, a British merchant, and his faithful servant, Manuel Incra Mamani, a Bolivian *cascarillero* (who made a living stripping the bark from the cinchona trees) played a major role in this story. In the 1840s, Mamani led Ledger to the most magnificent group of *calisayas*. The time was not right, however, to crop the seeds and it would be another 20 or so years before Mamani was able to produce the seeds in their best condition. In April 1865, Mamani walked some thousand miles to deliver the precious seeds to Ledger, who was then in

"Mauve" and "methylene blue"— the birth of synthetic dyes and drugs

The science of synthetic organic chemistry underwent a revolution in the second half of the 19th century, partly in response to the need for new antimalarials. In 1856, an 18-year-old English chemist, William Henry Perkin, set out to synthesize quinine, but failed. However, he did succeed in synthesizing *mauveine* or "mauve" from benzene, a byproduct of the coal-tar industry. Mauve was the first synthetic textile dye and, unlike natural dyes from plants, it did not wash off in water. Mauve became all the rage. Soon the streets of London erupted in what was called "mauve measles" as the new color became fashionable. Queen Victoria (r. 1837–1901) and Empress Eugenie (wife of Napoleon III of France) publicly flaunted mauve dresses and the British issued a postal stamp that became known as the "penny mauve." Perkin's success with mauve sparked the development of a huge synthetic dye industry, especially in Germany.

The new dye industry also led to important advances in medicine. When microbial pathogens were first identified, they were difficult to see under the microscope; synthesized dye stains helped. Paul Ehrlich, the German bacteriologist, noticed that methylene blue was particularly effective in staining malaria parasites. He reasoned that because

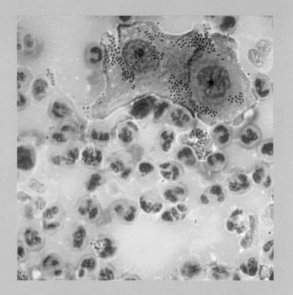

the parasite avidly took up the dye, it might be poisoned by it *in vivo*. In 1891, Ehrlich cured two patients of malaria using methylene blue, the first time a synthetic drug was ever used in humans. Bayer, one of the leading German dye companies, became a major pharmaceutical company in the late 19th century, producing both heroin and aspirin.

Methylene blue, a dye, has been used in scientific research as a way of staining and identifying pathogens, as in this image showing the bacteria responsible for gonorrhea. Methylene blue was also used as a prototype for the development of synthetic antimalarials, including plasmoquine in 1925.

Peru. Ledger dried the seeds and sent half to his brother, George Ledger in London. To the Ledger brothers' utmost surprise, the British government rejected their "prize" offer of this rare and valuable species and, eventually, all George was able to do was to sell one pound of the seeds to the Dutch government for planting in Java for a mere 100 guilders ($31). The rest were sold to an Anglo–Indian, Mr Money, for $79. Both Mamani and Charles Ledger met sad ends. Mamani died after he was thrown into prison for smuggling seeds across the Bolivian border, while Charles Ledger died a pauper in Australia in 1905.

Ironically, it was the Dutch government who, while paying only 100 guilders for the seeds, ended up making one of the best investments in European history. Within a short time the Dutch plantations of Java were producing 97 percent of the world's supply of quinine.

Although the British in India established cinchona plantations, these were of a lower quinine content than those in Java and by the early 20th century, India was receiving most of its quinine from Java.

Quinine proved to be of huge global importance as a treatment for malaria and was one of the few early drugs that could be used not simply to palliate symptoms, such as pain or fever, but specifically to target the underlying cause of a disease (in this case, as it was discovered, the malaria parasites). As William Osler summed it up: "Malaria treatment. This is comprised in three words: quinine, quinine, quinine." It could also be used as a prophylaxis to prevent malaria. When Silas Burroughs and Henry Wellcome started their eponymous pharmaceutical firm in 1880 (see page 199), quinine preparations were among the first that the company manufactured and marketed worldwide. Quinine contributed to a marked reduction in mortality for those going to the malarial tropics and, in the form of quinine sulfate dissolved in sugary lemonade, was administered freely to laborers constructing the Panama Canal in the early 20th century. The American Edwin Wiley Grove (1850–1927) made a fortune from his famous "Grove's Tasteless Chill Tonic" adding a sweet syrup to eliminate the bitter taste of quinine. Often best remembered is the fashion in British colonial India of drinking "Gin and Tonic"—with companies such as Schweppes adding quinine to its Indian Tonic Water.

During the Second World War, Germany captured Dutch quinine reserves in Holland, and the Japanese, occupying Java, seized their overseas plantations along with the bulk of the world's supply of quinine. New antimalarials were desperately needed and one of the most successful outcomes of scientists' endeavors to replace quinine was the development of the synthetic drug chloroquine, which was used widely after 1945. Although by the 1950s malaria had disappeared or been eliminated from most of the temperate world, a global initiative to eradicate malaria in the late 1950s and 1960s—primarily using chloroquine as well as the insecticide DDT—led to hopes that it could be eradicated from the rest of the world. Drug- and insecticide-resistance, however, posed a key problem, and by the 1970s the disease had surged to unprecedented heights, especially in sub-Saharan Africa, where one child died of malaria every 12 seconds.

At a low point in the history of malaria control and research, an antimalarial derived from an ancient Chinese herb—*Artemisia annua*—was "rediscovered" by the Chinese and is another fascinating story of a "new drug" from an "old remedy."

Artemisinin—unlocking the secrets of another remarkable antimalarial

Artemisinin ... is a true gift from old Chinese medicine.

Tu Youyou, *Nature Medicine*, 2011

In 1967 a research program, code-name Project 523, was set up by the People's Republic of China to find a treatment for malaria, especially given the urgent need to replace chloroquine, which was, increasingly, becoming ineffective. The result of this project was the rediscovery of Qing Hao (*Artemisia annua* or sweet wormwood), a plant with antimalarial properties. Particular credit (and a prestigious Lasker Award in the USA in 2011 for "a medical advance that has saved millions of lives across the globe, especially in the developing world") has now been attributed to the Chinese scientist Dr Tu Youyou. Tu was trained in both Traditional Chinese Medicine and modern pharmaceutical sciences. She and her team in Beijing

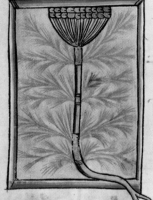

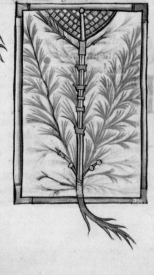

combed numerous ancient texts and folk remedies for possible malaria remedies and tested some 640 Chinese herbs. *Qing Hao* (pronounced *"ching-how"*—meaning "green herb") looked especially promising. A recipe for intermittent fevers in a 4th-century text (*Emergency Prescriptions Kept Up One's Sleeve*) by the physician Ge Hong was a vital lead:

Qing Hao, one bunch, take two sheng [2 x 0.2 litres] of water for soaking it, wring it out, take the juice, ingest it in its entirety.

By drawing on this recipe, in 1971 they extracted what they hoped was the active principle of the plant. To test its safety, Tu and her colleagues tried it out first. It was then found to be effective in laboratory mice and monkeys. They administered it to malaria patients in Hainan Province and slowly it became known internationally by the names of *qinghaosu* or artemisinin.

Extensive trials in China, Vietnam, Thailand, Myanmar, the Gambia, and elsewhere confirmed that artemisinin and its derivatives, artemether and artesunate, were, indeed, safe antimalarials with the ability to reduce parasite levels more rapidly than other drugs. The British scientist Nick White, based in Bangkok, and others recognized that something also had to be done to prevent a buildup of resistance as had happened with previous antimalarial drugs. ACTs (artemisinin-based combination therapies) seemed to be the answer. Chinese scientists registered the first ACT in 1992. This was

This illumination of the herbal artemisia is from a 13th-century manuscript. One variety of this plant, *Artemisia annua*, or sweet wormwood, was used in ancient Chinese medicines. Its antimalarial properties were "rediscovered" in the 1970s in China. Marketed as artemisinin, this "new drug" from an "old remedy" has offered renewed hope for malaria treatment.

the combination of artemether and lumefantrine (another antimalarial) into a single tablet, subsequently manufactured by the Swiss pharmaceutical company Ciba-Geigy (now Novartis) as Coartem. Millions of patients have since been treated with these antimalarials (although the first worrying signs of artemisinin-resistance were detected in western Cambodia in 2006). China and Vietnam provide 70 percent and East Africa 20 percent of the raw plant material and efforts are underway to increase productivity and yields of *Artemisia annua*. New processes for manufacturing synthetic artemisinin-based drugs (using a byproduct, artemisinic acid) are also in the pipeline; this could overcome the costly and lengthy process of relying solely on the natural product.

In 1998 WHO launched its Roll Back Malaria program with the aim of halving the burden of malaria by 2010. Although there is still a long way to go to reach the ultimate goal of "eradication," there have been advances in a number of countries in which the disease is endemic in recent years. A huge amount of international funding (more than US$2 billion in 2011), especially from the Bill & Melinda Gates Foundation, has now been targeted toward solving the malaria crisis. Strategies for prevention, including the distribution and domestic use of long-lasting insecticide-treated bed nets to prevent being bitten by malarial mosquitoes, are also vital and the first clinical trials in Africa of a vaccine are currently underway.

Sweet clover and the discovery of warfarin

The examples of morphine, cocaine, aspirin, and quinine were some of the most important advances for medicine in the 19th century. Other modern treatments derived from plants include digoxin, a heart medicine from the foxglove plant, the antileukemia drug vincristine, found in the Madagascar periwinkle, and the breast cancer agent taxol, first extracted from ancient Yew trees of Japan and the Pacific Northwest.

The discovery of the anticoagulant (blood-thinning drug) warfarin (named after the Wisconsin Alumni Research Foundation, which funded the research) is one of many other intriguing stories. In the 1920s, farmers in Canada and the USA began to observe the painful deaths of their livestock from a strange hemorrhagic condition by which cattle and sheep literally bled to death. Eventually, a connection was made with the ingestion of the plant,

sweet clover, which, when attacked by fungi, had become moldy. Its anticoagulant substance, named dicoumarol, was isolated and in 1948, a synthetic form—warfarin—was launched as a rat poison. The rats ingesting this bait would, like cattle, researchers reasoned, bleed to death. Serendipitously, warfarin was found to be nontoxic to humans and could also have lifesaving possibilities for preventing or treating certain conditions associated with blood clots, notably thrombosis and thromboembolism. In 1955, warfarin was given to US President Dwight Eisenhower following a myocardial infarction. It was said: "What was good for a war hero and the President of the United States must be good for all, despite it being a rat poison!"

The discovery of the healing powers of a myriad of plants represents one of the most significant accomplishments in human medical history. Effective remedies extracted from complex plants continue to challenge scientists to explore other miracle cures lurking in the bushes.

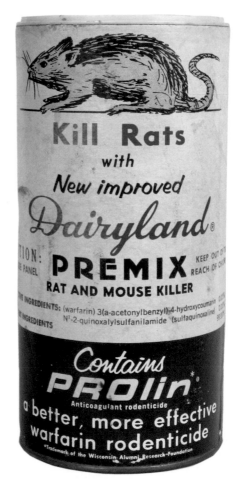

This warfarin-based poison was developed to kill rats but is now also used in medicine for inhibiting blood clotting.

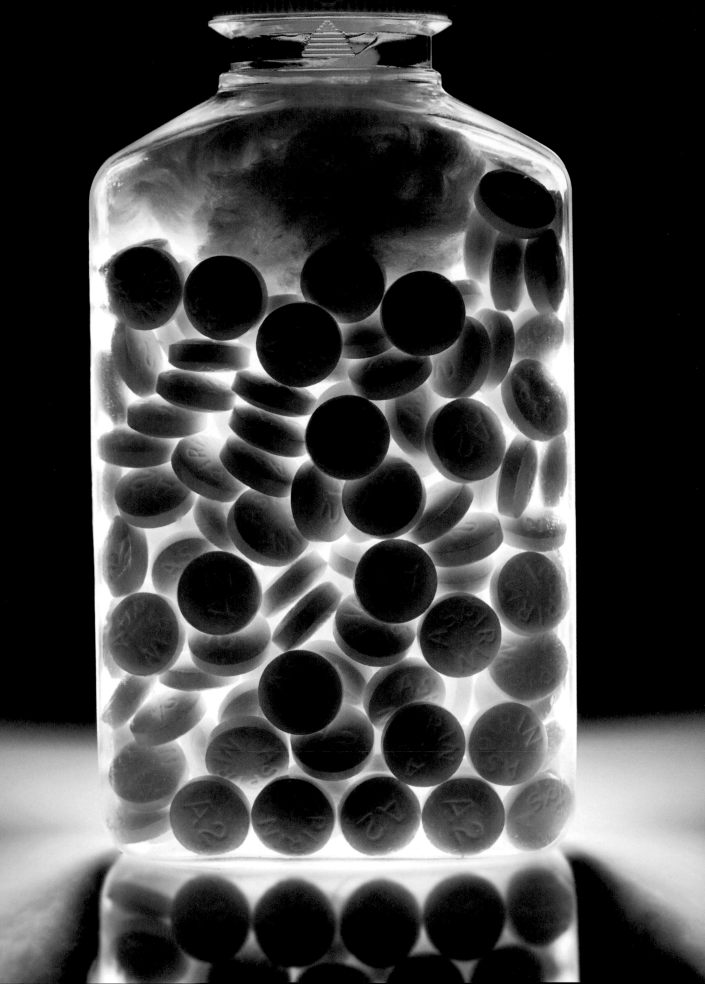

Magic Bullets and Blockbuster Drugs

I will lift up mine eyes unto the pills. Almost everyone takes them, from the humble aspirin to the multi-coloured, king-sized three deckers, which put you to sleep, wake you up, stimulate and soothe you all in one. It is an age of pills.

Malcolm Muggeridge, 1903–90, British journalist, 1962

The first so-called "magic bullet" was Salvarsan, discovered in 1910 to treat syphilis. The term was coined by the German scientist Paul Ehrlich (1854–1915) to describe a chemical agent that would target a specific microorganism in the body without harming healthy cells. Other important breakthroughs in therapy were made in the first half of the 20th century: sulfonamides for certain bacterial infections; insulin for diabetes; cortisone for rheumatoid arthritis; and the first anticancer drugs. The 1950s saw the widespread introduction into clinical medicine of penicillin, followed by other "wonder drugs." Pharmaceutical companies in the second half of the 20th century grew to meet new opportunities for medical cures (and profits). A staggering array of medicines—to treat both infectious and noninfectious diseases —have transformed the landscape of illness in the modern world. Many drugs, such as statins to lower cholesterol levels, are sold in such quantities that they are now termed "blockbuster drugs." The pharmaceutical industry is one of the largest global enterprises, comprising major innovative drug companies, biotechnology firms, and manufacturers of generic medicines. The search goes on for new drugs for diseases ranging from cancers to the common cold.

The first "magic bullets"

Paul Ehrlich was one of a number of scientists who sought cures for disease—or, as he saw it, to search for a chemical compound that would attack and kill a specific microorganism in the body without unduly harming the host's healthy cells. In the first decade of the 20th century, Ehrlich tested numerous compounds against the then recently discovered spirochaete

OPPOSITE A bottle of aspirin tablets. Aspirin has been a pharmacological triumph and is probably the best-known and most widely used medicine in the world.

(*Treponema pallida*) that causes the bacterial disease syphilis. Arsenic was found to kill the spirochaete but also the patient; so Ehrlich and his research team sought to modify arsenic chemically to retain effectiveness with safety. Among a number of arsenical drugs that had been tested for various purposes was one, the 606th of the series tested, that had been set aside in 1907 as being ineffective.

A Japanese scientist, Sahachiro Hata (1873–1938), from the Institute for Infectious Diseases in Tokyo headed by Shibasaburo Kitasato (1852–1931), came to work at Ehrlich's Institute in Frankfurt in 1908. Hata retested Preparation No. 606 on a rabbit experimentally infected with syphilis and found that it was very effective. Once hundreds of animal experiments had repeatedly proved its efficacy against the pathogen, while not being lethal to the animals, its discovery was announced in 1910. It was called arsphenamine and sold under the name "Salvarsan" ("salvation through arsenic"). Salvarsan was marketed by the German pharmaceutical company Hoechst. This first "magic bullet" was initially hailed as a remarkable drug for the treatment of syphilis but it was fairly toxic and had some unpleasant side effects. A modified compound, Neosalvarsan (the 914th arsenical substance), was produced by Ehrlich's team in 1912.

The next breakthrough in the development of drugs for bacterial infections came in 1935 with Sulfanilamide. This discovery came about after a number of experiments with the red-orange textile dye Prontosil. In December 1935 the six-year-old daughter of Gerhard Domagk (1895–1964), research director at Bayer laboratories in Germany, was seriously ill after contracting a streptococcal infection when a needle went into her hand. Domagk administered Prontosil and she recovered. A year later, British physician Leonard Colebrook (1883–1967), at Queen Charlotte's Maternity Hospital, London, demonstrated the dramatic effect of Prontosil on puerperal sepsis—a deadly infection of childbirth. Scientists at the Pasteur Institute in Paris were able to show that Prontosil was broken down in the body and that its active principle was not the dye but the colorless compound p-aminobenzene-sulfonamide (sulfanilamide). New "sulfonamide" or "sulfa" drugs were produced to combat a range of bacterial diseases, including meningococcal meningitis, streptococcal infections, and bacterial pneumonia.

The British pharmaceutical company May & Baker developed one of the most effective of all the sulfonamides (sulfapyridine) in 1938—calling it M & B 693. Winston Churchill, suffering from pneumonia at a critical point in the Second World War, was treated with this drug in December 1943 and made a full recovery. Churchill recalled: "this admirable 'M & B' from which I did not suffer any inconvenience, was used at the earliest moment and after a week's fever the intruders were repulsed."

The story of penicillin

It looks like a miracle.

Howard Florey, 1940

Sulfa drugs were superseded by the next wonder drug—penicillin. On September 3 1928, Alexander Fleming (1881–1955), a 47-year-old Scotsman, returned to his laboratory as the newly appointed Professor of Bacteriology at St Mary's Hospital, London. A stack of his unwashed Petri dishes had been left on the laboratory bench while he was on vacation. He had been culturing the bacterium *Staphylococcus aureus*, an organism responsible for boils, abscesses, and pneumonia. One Petri dish caught his eye.

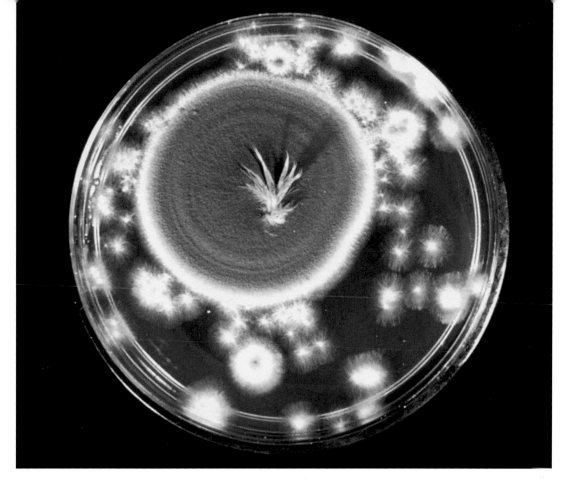

A Petri dish with a culture of *Penicillium notatum*. Alexander Fleming first discovered the antibacterial properties of penicillin (which he initially called "mold juice") in 1928 and its therapeutic value was developed in Oxford during the Second World War.

There was something quite unusual about it. Like many of his specimens, it had become contaminated with colonies of mold. But here there were no staphylococci growing near to a blob of greenish mold. He set about investigating what it was that had inhibited the growth of the bacteria. In 1929 he named the mold penicillin and sent samples to laboratories in Europe and the USA.

However, it was a team of Oxford scientists, including Howard Florey (1898–1968), Ernst Chain (1906–79), and Norman Heatley (1911–2004) at the Sir William Dunn School of Pathology, who first fully realized the clinical significance of penicillin. On Saturday May 25 1940, while the German army advanced on Dunkirk, they conducted a critical experiment.

Eight white mice were given a lethal dose of virulent streptococci bacteria. Four of the mice were then injected with penicillin; four were left untreated. By the following Sunday morning, the four untreated control mice had died, but the four treated with penicillin were alive and healthy. One of the team, Ernst Chain, reportedly jumped up and down with excitement, later recalling:

We knew we had stumbled upon one of those rare drugs which would not only kill bacteria in a test tube, but also in the living animal without harming it. We realized at once that penicillin could play a vital role in war medicine.

Testing it on human patients was next. In February 1941 Albert Alexander, a 43–year-old Oxford policeman, was desperately ill with septicemia following a scratch (from a rose bush)

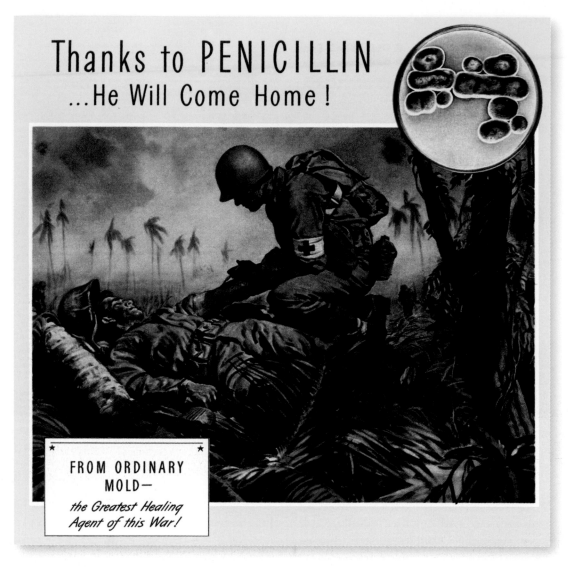

Saving the lives and limbs of injured serviceman. By 1944, laboratories across the USA were stepping up their production of penicillin, in response to wartime demand.

that had turned septic. Initially, the penicillin attacked the streptococci bugs that were destroying his body. Sadly, in spite of ingenious methods of growing and purifying the mold (using bedpans and milk churns) in the Dunn School and recycling any penicillin excreted in Alexander's urine, there was not enough penicillin being produced to keep up the therapy and Alexander died a month later.

The production issue was solved when Heatley, together with researchers at a US agricultural laboratory in Illinois, found a way to use deep fermentation techniques for growing the mold, which produced ten times the yield that the Oxford team had been able to make. Soon a number of pharmaceutical companies began producing penicillin. The first large-scale field trials of penicillin on the battlefield took place in North Africa in 1943. The results were spectacularly successful—soldiers who would have previously lost limbs or died of gangrene survived with the help of penicillin. It was also used to treat cases of venereal disease, enabling men to be returned to the front fit for fighting. By the end of the war there was no doubt that there was, at last, a powerful drug to treat a whole host of life-threatening bacterial infections.

In October 1945, Fleming, Florey, and Chain were jointly awarded the Nobel Prize in Physiology or Medicine for their "discovery of penicillin and its curative effect in various infectious disease." Penicillin soon became the "wonder drug" of the second half of the 20th century and has been hailed as one of the greatest medical milestones of the modern era.

Streptomycin and the age of antibiotics

There was, however, one major global bacterial disease—tuberculosis—that did not respond to penicillin. The soil microbiologist Selman Waksman (1888–1973), who in 1941 used the term "antibiotic" in its medical sense (the Greek, anti-, "against" and biotos, "the means of life"), and his colleagues in Rutgers University in the USA, with the financial support of the drug company Merck, screened thousands of soil microbes in the 1940s in the hope of finding "another" penicillin. One of Waksman's PhD students, Albert Schatz, had a lucky "hit." In 1943 he isolated streptomycin from a mold growing in the throats of chickens that had been reared in a heavily manured field.

Two other drugs—para-amino-salicylic acid (PAS) and isoniazid—were subsequently combined with streptomycin as a way of preventing resistance to any single drug. This triple therapy, developed by John Crofton and his Edinburgh-based team in the 1950s, became known as the Edinburgh method. Combination therapy, based on this model, has since been used for a number of other diseases, including cancer and malaria. Drugs proved spectacularly successful in treating TB and, together with a vaccine, over the following decades saved millions of lives globally.

Following penicillin, another success story for the Oxford team at the Dunn School was cephalosporin. In the mid-1950s, they developed and purified this antibiotic from a fungus found in a sewage outlet in Sardinia. Subsequent generations of cephalosporin proved to be broad-spectrum antibiotics, effective against various bacteria and, together with semisynthetic penicillins, including methicillin, ampicillin, and, later, amoxicillin, the "age of antibiotics" was a period of huge optimism in the history of medicine.

Inevitably, given bacteria's survival skills, resistance would become an issue and Fleming warned of this back in 1945, adding: "moral: if you use penicillin, use enough." The current, much-publicized problem of MRSA (methicillin-resistant *Staphylococcus aureus*)

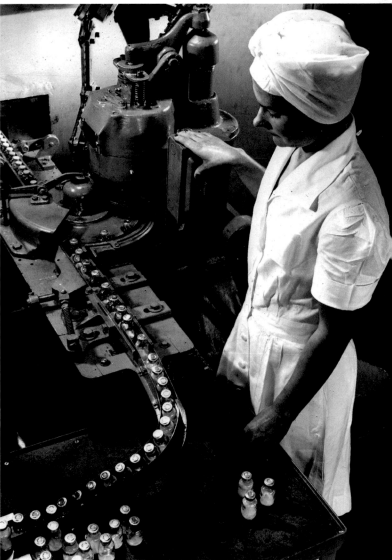

Streptomycin was discovered in 1943, the first antibiotic effective against tuberculosis. By the 1950s, mass production of such new drugs, as in this image, created major pharmaceutical companies, which would ultimately capture a global market.

was first identified in Britain in the early 1960s, soon after the introduction of methicillin. Although this antibiotic is no longer manufactured, the term MRSA continues to be applied for "multidrug-resistant *S. aureus*." We are now also seeing a resurgence of TB in the developing world where antibiotic-resistance to existing regimes is a serious and life-threatening problem.

Replacement therapy—vitamins, insulin, and the "Pill"

While scientists were developing drugs for bacterial infections, others were unraveling the causes and treatments of puzzling noninfectious diseases. In the early 20th century scientists became convinced that the key to poor nutritional health lay in the absence of crucial elements in the diet.

The isolation of vitamin C in citrus fruits provided an explanation for James Lind's trial in the 18th century, showing that oranges and lemons were a "preventive" for scurvy, a disease caused by lack of this vitamin (see pages 201–03). Other vitamins were discovered and found their way into clinical practice for the treatment of dietary deficiency diseases such as rickets, beri-beri, pellagra, and pernicious anemia. Vitamins were also sold commercially and added to some food products.

Another tremendous advance was the discovery of insulin, a pancreatic hormone extract used to control blood glucose levels in the treatment of type 1 diabetes (also known as diabetes mellitus or juvenile diabetes)—a much-feared and usually fatal disease of children and young adults in the past. Hormones, including insulin, are secreted by special endocrine glands, such as the pancreas and adrenal glands, but diabetics are unable to make insulin and need "replacement insulin." Investigations—involving many experiments on dogs—by a research team at the University of Toronto, Canada, led to preparations of insulin from ox pancreas being safely tested on two of the researchers and then clinically in 1922 on a 14-year-old diabetic boy. Leonard Thompson, who before the insulin shots was near death, rapidly regained his strength and appetite as his blood sugar levels fell. Soon afterward, large-scale insulin production using pig pancreas in the USA produced enough insulin by 1923 to supply the entire American continent. Type 1 diabetes in young children was no longer a death sentence. Although insulin was never heralded as a "magic bullet" since it doesn't cure diabetes, its use as a treatment (albeit daily and for life) was a major innovation in early 20th-century medicine.

> "I wish I had my beta-blockers handy."
>
> James Black (1924–2010).

Cortisone was a drug developed out of hormone research in the late 1940s, initially for the treatment of rheumatoid arthritis and, importantly, paving the way for the development of a group of drugs known as steroids, which are effective in a wide variety of different pathological processes, including asthma. Other drug treatments developed from hormone research include the 1960s contraceptive pill (originating from the Mexican yam), after the discovery of the female reproductive hormones estrogen and progesterone, as well as the class of drugs called beta-blockers, crucial in the treatment of heart disease and high blood pressure. One of the first beta-blockers was propranolol, which blocks the stimulant actions of epinephrine on the heart and blood vessels, and became one of the world's best-selling drugs.

A number of scientists have won Nobel Prizes for their contributions to these significant discoveries. When James Black (1924–2010) heard he had won the 1988 Nobel Prize for his contribution to "important principles for drug treatment," he quipped, "I wish I had my beta-blockers handy."

Radiation and cancer chemotherapy

In the late 19th century, cancer was on the rise in many countries and was called by one surgeon, "the emperor of all maladies, the king of terrors." The surgical removal of a solid tumor had varying rates of success for patients who were often by then in advanced stages of cancer.

In 1895 the chance discovery of X-rays by Wilhelm Röntgen changed the outlook for cancer treatment, enabling tumors to be detected and located. It was also noticed that X-rays caused burns and could be used to treat skin problems such as moles and ringworm. The potential for destroying cancerous cells was quickly picked up. In 1898 the radioactive elements polonium and radium were discovered in France by the wife and husband team Marie and Pierre Curie, leading to radiotherapy as a way of treating cancer. In the early days, excessive doses of radiation killed patients. Marie Curie (1867–1934) herself died of leukemia following years of exposure to radiation. Now safer and more effective forms of radiotherapy can reduce inoperable tumors to operable size, and help to stop recurrence after an operation.

The term "chemotherapy" was first used by Ehrlich in a broader context but he also went on to propose that cancerous cells could be destroyed by chemicals without harm to the healthy tissue host. Experimentation stimulated research into cytotoxic drugs—drugs capable of destroying rapidly proliferating cells in tumors.

One of the most fundamental advances in chemotherapy took place in 1948 at the Boston Children's Hospital in the USA. The US physician and pediatric pathologist Sidney Farber (1903–73) used folic acid antagonists (antifolates) for treating acute lymphoblastic leukemia (ALL) in children —demonstrating that antifolates could interfere with and suppress the proliferation of malignant cell growth. Watching children coming into remission, albeit mostly only temporarily, following this early first trial was a remarkable first step. One of Farber's patients was a 12-year-old boy known as "Jimmy." In 1948 a radio show was broadcast from Jimmy's hospital bedside. Americans were moved by his story and donations poured in for a "Jimmy Fund," which continues to this day to help youngsters suffering from cancer. Jimmy (whose real name was Einar Gustafson) recovered from cancer and visited the charity on its 50th anniversary.

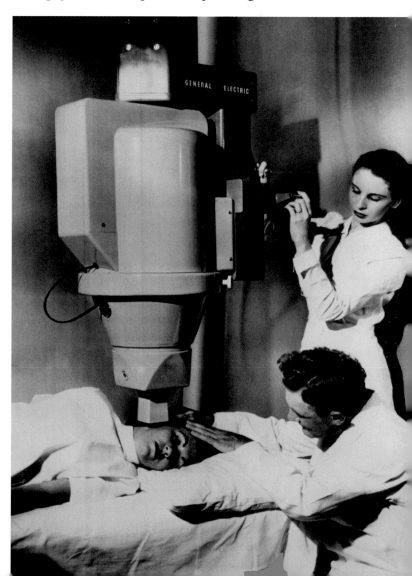

This Cobalt-60 cancer teletherapy unit was first used to treat deep-seated malignancies in London, Ontario, Canada, in 1951. Radiotherapy remains one of the major methods of cancer treatment.

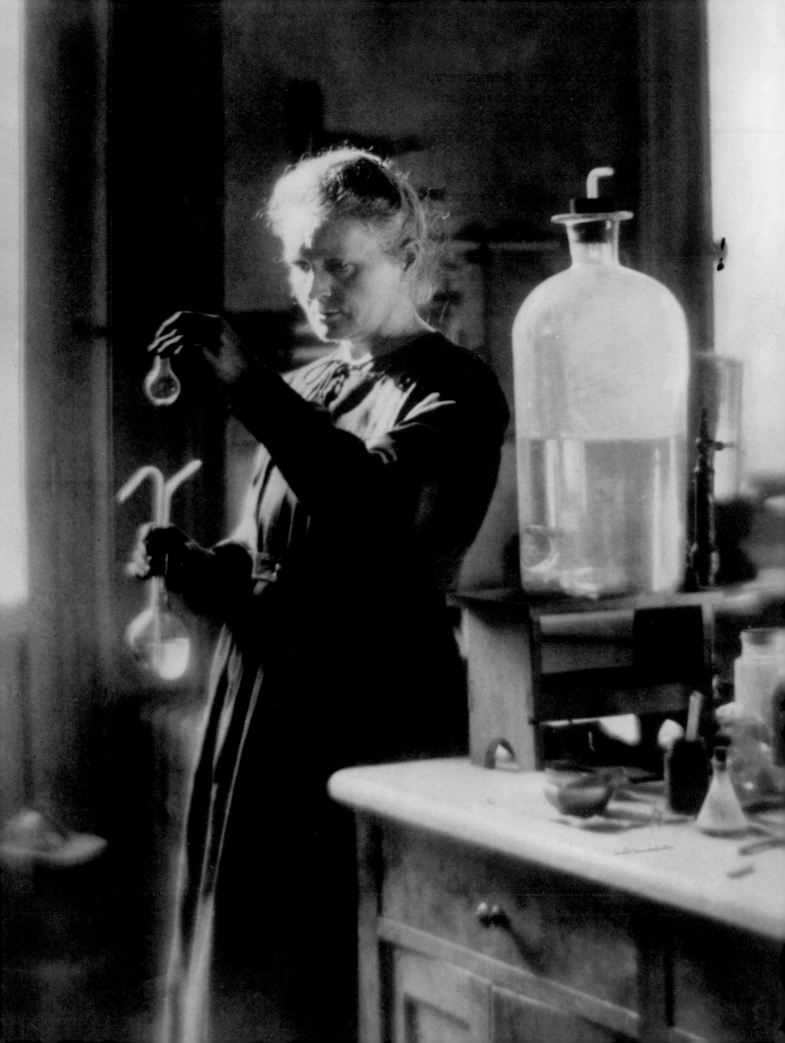

Farber's pioneering work initiated the modern postwar development of a wide variety of anticancer agents, including in the early 1960s the recognition that alkaloids of the Madagascar periwinkle (*Vinca rosea*) blocked proliferation of tumor cells. Vincristine was developed from this finding and by the 1970s the "war against the Big C" led to an increase in commitment, funding, and research to find new treatments for cancer (see page 195).

The therapeutic revolution: from Valium to Ventolin

Alongside the first antibiotics, steroids, and beta-blockers, drugs for cancer, and the contraceptive pill, a few other highlights from the 1950s and 60s include chlorpromazine—the first of a generation of antipsychotic drugs and the greatest single advance in psychiatric care; and diazepam or Valium, a tranquilizer for anxiety and insomnia. Warfarin, initially used as a poison for rats, was developed as an anticoagulant for blood clots. There was also chloroquine for malaria; Promin and dapsone for leprosy; metformin for type 2 diabetes; L-dopa for Parkinson's disease; the bronchodilator Ventolin (salbutamol), for asthma; and a wide range of painkillers. Together with vaccines, these medicines had a major revolutionary impact on people's lives: family physicians could write out prescriptions for a host of ailments while serious diseases could be treated in hospital with increasing confidence of success.

The pharmaceutical industry expanded rapidly in the postwar period, profiting from new discoveries, rising expectations of good health, and a lax regulatory environment. The tragedy of the drug thalidomide, which came to light in the early 1960s, led to the introduction of stronger laws governing the testing and marketing of new drugs, especially in the USA, Britain, and most of Europe. Safety, as well as efficacy, of pharmaceutical products remains of paramount importance today (see Testing Treatments and Clinical Trials).

Antiviral drugs

By comparison with the exciting introduction of antibiotics for bacterial diseases, the search for treatments for viral diseases was much slower. It was, however, the drug acyclovir (Zovirax), an effective antiviral against herpes simplex viruses (which cause cold sores and genital herpes), varicella zoster (chickenpox), and herpes zoster (shingles), which was discovered and developed by scientists at Wellcome Laboratories (UK) and Burroughs Wellcome (USA) in 1977–8, that transformed antiviral chemotherapy.

In 1987 the first antiretroviral drug for HIV/AIDS, AZT (azidothymidine) was approved. AZT was not a magic bullet for this new and alarming pandemic of the late 20th century, but it was a start. Almost a decade later, a "cocktail" of three or more powerful antiretroviral drugs (known as HAART—highly active antiretroviral therapy) was given the go-ahead as a combination therapy, described as the "Lazarus effect." There are now many drugs for the treatment of HIV: they do not cure the disease, but by slowing the progress of the virus, suppressing its replication and preventing it from rapidly destroying the immune system, it can mean that HIV is no longer a death sentence.

OPPOSITE Marie Curie, the Polish-born French physicist, and her husband Pierre discovered the radioactive element radium in 1898, enabling oncologists and surgeons to deliver high doses of radiation to tumors. This iconic image of Marie Curie in the early 20th century symbolized the noble endeavor of science and the hope of curing cancer.

The search for the cure for the common cold

The common cold is a viral disease that has no cure. Ancient Egyptians spread a mixture of lead ore, incense, and honey on their noses; in 1747 John Wesley advised sticking orange rind up each nostril; and more recently, in the mid-20th century, bed rest, cocaine, and forced fluids were the cure of choice. Today we spend a fortune on products that treat only the symptoms of a cold. Researchers at the UK's Common Cold Unit in Salisbury, England, revealed hundreds of different types of cold viruses: rhinoviruses, adenoviruses, and coronaviruses, and subgroups of picornaviruses.

At a time of serious concern about antibiotic drug-resistance (resulting, in part, from overuse and misuse of antibiotics), this poster is a reminder that antibiotics to combat bacterial diseases should not be prescribed for viral infections.

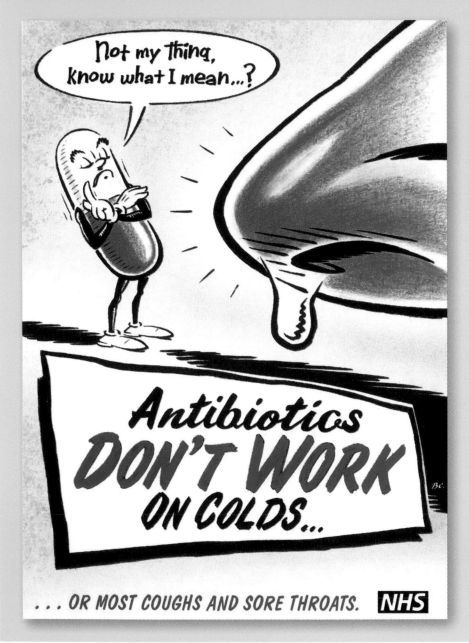

The global threat of influenza—"avian" flu (H5N1) and "swine" flu (H1N1)—has led to the development of new drugs for this viral disease, including zanamivir (Relenza) and oseltamivir (Tamiflu). While vaccines for influenza and a number of serious viral diseases, such as polio, are a first line of defense, the search for more antiviral drugs, even for the common cold, continues.

Advances in cancer chemotherapy

Paclitaxel (Taxol) from the bark of the Pacific Yew tree; tamoxifen (an antagonist of the estrogen receptor in breast tissue); cisplatin, and anticancer drugs based on platinum compounds were some of the drugs to emerge following a huge input of resources for scientific and pharmaceutical research into chemotherapy. Three types of previously incurable cancer— childhood leukemia, Hodgkin's disease (a cancer of the lymph nodes), and testicular cancer— were among the first to respond successfully to various newly discovered drugs. Antiemetics (antinausea) now help overcome some of the unpleasant side effects of chemotherapy. "Adjuvant" and "neo-adjuvant therapy" are terms applied when varying combinations and sequences of surgery, radiotherapy, and chemotherapy are used.

One "targeted therapy" strategy has been to employ large biological molecules known as monoclonal antibodies or Mabs—proteins that can be created to bind to a chosen target with exquisite specificity. These stimulate the patient's immune system to attack the cancer or can prevent tumor growth by blocking key cell receptors. Herceptin (trastuzumab), a Mab to combat breast cancer, was the first bioengineered drug to gain FDA approval in 1998. It works by interfering with a human epidermal growth factor receptor protein (HER2), which regulates cell growth. In certain breast cancers, HER2 is "overexpressed" and this protein has become an important "biomarker" for the disease.

Although Mab research continues apace, a complementary approach is to utilize small synthetic chemicals designed to target specific cancer-causing proteins caused by aberrant genes ("oncogenes"). One such molecule is Gleevec (imatinib mesylate) for such cancers as chronic myeloid leukemia (CML) and gastrointestinal stromal tumor (GIST). Gleevec, the first medicine of its kind to work by inhibiting a particular enzyme that causes cells to proliferate, received FDA approval in 2001 and was featured on the cover of *TIME* magazine as the "magic bullet" to cure cancer.

Another strategy continues to be screening and early diagnosis, and advances in genetics to identify cancer-causing genes have again been key. Well-publicized biomarkers include the BRCA1 or BRCA2 genes, which can be found in women with a high likelihood of developing breast or ovarian cancer and are now easily screened for. Some cancers have been found to be caused by infections, with the hope that antimicrobial drugs and vaccines can be developed to treat or prevent such cancers. An example of this is the recent vaccine for the human papilloma virus (HPV)—a leading cause of cervical cancer. The role and understanding of so-called "lifestyle" risk factors and preventive strategies in cancer control, as well as in other diseases such as heart disease, stroke, and type 2 diabetes, is also of vital importance.

The top 10 most prescribed medicines

1. Antidepressants
2. Lipid regulators
3. Narcotic analgesics
4. Antidiabetics
5. Ace inhibitors
6. Beta-blockers
7. Respiratory agents
8. Antiulcerants
9. Diuretics
10. Antiepileptics

(Top 10 by therapeutic class in the USA, 2011)

"Blockbuster drugs" and biotechnological breakthroughs

The 21st-century pharmaceutical industry is one of the largest global enterprises, comprising major innovative drug companies, biotechnology firms, and manufacturers of generic medicines. As more and more drug discoveries have been made over the past half-century, some began to reach a huge global market—achieving the status of "blockbuster drugs."

Statins, a class of drugs that lower cholesterol levels in the blood, are used to prevent arteriosclerosis when fatty plaques coat the arteries—a major cause of heart disease. It is estimated that they are now given to 40 million patients every day around the world. The rise in popularity of new drugs to treat depression has also been spectacular, with worldwide sales rising from half a billion dollars in 1987 to more than US$40 billion in 2010.

Today, almost all people with insulin-dependent diabetes use a form of recombinant human insulin rather than animal insulin. US start-up Genentech was a leader in the field and became a billion-dollar company, full ownership of which was achieved by Roche in 2009. The Genentech scientists developed a new generation of therapeutics created from genetically engineered copies of naturally occurring molecules. In 1978, they produced the first synthetically manufactured human insulin that could be made in large amounts. The gene for human insulin was inserted into bacterial DNA and expressed using bacteria as miniature "factories." The result was called "recombinant (DNA) insulin," sold under the brand name Humulin.

Many other biotech companies have made key discoveries. Humira (adalimumab), developed by scientists in Britain and the USA and marketed by Abbott Laboratories, is the world's first human monoclonal antibody drug to achieve blockbuster status and is used for a number of conditions including rheumatoid arthritis. Novel approaches such as monoclonal antibodies together with stem cell therapy, gene therapy, immunotherapy, and nanomedicine, are now transforming medicine.

Some of the older drugs have come "off patent," meaning they can be manufactured and sold as cheap "generics." Pfizer's statin drug Lipitor (atorvastatin), for example, the top "blockbuster drug" in 2010, is now off patent, impacting on their profits. China, India, Israel, Brazil, and Thailand all have substantial capacity to produce generic medicines that can be sold at a fraction of the cost of the original drug or vaccine. Cheaper generic drugs are attractive to government health services as a means of limiting the drugs bill. In the USA, generics currently represent 80 percent of dispensed prescriptions. The Israeli company Teva is considered to be the leading generic drugs company globally.

From apothecary stores to "Big Pharmas"

Globalization has led to pharmaceutical and biotech company mergers creating the "Big Pharmas." GlaxoSmithKline (GSK) is one of the world's leading research-based pharmaceutical companies, with headquarters in Britain and a fascinating example of the merging of companies whose origins go back to the 18th and 19th centuries. Glaxo was originally the name given to a powdered baby milk product, and, as a company (first based in New Zealand and later the UK), it started to produce pharmaceuticals in the early 20th century, stimulated by the discovery of vitamin D, which was added to baby food and milk.

Along with other companies, it produced penicillin during the Second World War. Glaxo merged in 1958 with Allen & Hanbury's Ltd (known for its throat pastilles and originally a

London 18th-century apothecary store) and in 1995 with Burroughs Wellcome & Co. Five years later, Glaxo Wellcome then merged with SmithKline Beecham (SmithKline dated back to a 19th-century US drugstore and Beecham to a 19th-century patent medicine maker, Thomas Beecham) to form GlaxoSmithKline—the name "Wellcome" being lost in the merger.

Neglected Tropical Diseases

Many companies and organizations have worked for decades to fight these horrific diseases ...
Today, we pledge to work hand-in-hand to fight these diseases now and in the future.
Andrew Witty, CEO of GSK, The London Declaration, 2012

The World Health Organization (WHO) publishes a list of Essential Medicines that it defines as "those drugs that satisfy the health-care needs of the majority of the population; they should therefore be available at all times in adequate amounts and in appropriate dosage forms, at a price the community can afford."

There has been concern that pharmaceutical and biotech companies have, over recent decades, concentrated on finding cures for the diseases of the West, especially chronic noncommunicable diseases (NCDs) like heart disease and some cancers, which offer the prospect of lucrative profits. HIV/AIDS drugs were developed remarkably quickly once the disease surfaced in the USA and Europe in the 1980s, but the huge cost of the anti-retrovirals proved a significant problem for the developing world, especially sub-Saharan Africa, which was hit hardest by the AIDS pandemic. The Indian drug company Cipla Ltd (founded in 1935 by Indian scientist Khwaja Abdul Hamied) stunned the global health community in the early 21st century when it said that it could produce a cocktail of HIV/AIDS medicines for US$1 per patient per day. The price has since fallen to 20 cents per day and more than 6 million people in the developing world now receive anti-retroviral therapy (ART) with Cipla drugs.

The three big infectious disease killers of the 21st century now attract more attention following the establishment in 2002 of the Global Fund to Fight AIDS, Tuberculosis, and Malaria. However, global

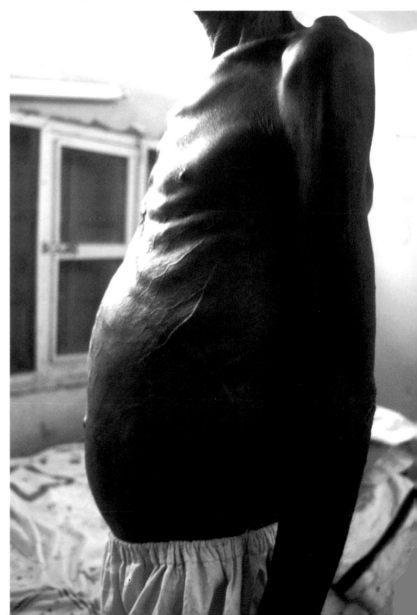

The distended stomach of a Sudanese man suffering from the debilitating ancient worm disease schistosomiasis, one of a number of Neglected Tropical Diseases.

health specialists have been concerned that other serious diseases of the developing world were being overlooked. In 2005, a group of specialists coined the phrase "Neglected Tropical Diseases" (NTDs) to highlight the very real neglect of a number of diseases, mostly those of the tropics and subtropics, that collectively affect over 1.4 billion people, including some 800 million children. Such diseases include onchocerciasis (river blindness), schistosomiasis (snail fever or bilharzia), lymphatic filariasis (elephantiasis), and infestation with intestinal worms (including hookworm).

Some pharmaceutical companies had from the late 1980s initiated programs of freely donating drugs (notably the donations of Merck and GSK of ivermectin and albendazole for onchocerciasis and lymphatic filariasis) followed by the introduction of price-tiering—where rich countries pay the market value for the drug and the poorer countries pay a small fraction of the price. Since the term NTDs was coined there has been considerable collaborative activity from the WHO, philanthropic donors, academic researchers, governments, NGOs, and product development partnerships, as well as from pharmaceutical and generic companies. At an influential meeting in January 2012 at the Royal College of Physicians in London, participants from many organizations from around the world met with representatives of 13 pharmaceutical companies in a new united effort to tackle NTDs, known as the London Declaration. Significant advances have already been made by the global health partnerships, both in supplying treatments and integrating mass drug administration (MDA) programs into broader development strategies, such as improving sanitation, nutrition, and health education—with the long-term aim of eliminating these diseases of poverty.

A key problem area, however, is counterfeit drugs, often sold on the internet or through nonregulated outlets. The FDA estimates counterfeiting accounts for upward of 10 percent of the global medicines marketed and 25 percent of the medicines consumed in poor countries.

The search for "magic bullets" continues

The quest for Ehrlich's "magic bullets" continues, as does the research to understand how drugs work in the human body. As patients, we are familiar with the fact that we might swallow a sugar-coated tablet or drink a liquid medicine, suck a lozenge, rub on a cream, have an injection, inhale vaporized medicines. Some drugs, such as statins, are taken to prevent disease; most, like antibiotics, are to cure disease, while others palliate symptoms. Identifying the "magic receptors" for each drug is a vast and fascinating area.

In spite of the impressive developments in pharmacology and drug development over the past century or so, there are diseases and conditions for which there are, as yet, no effective cures. This includes certain cancers and chronic lung diseases, which are not only leading causes of death and disability in the developed world but are becoming increasingly prominent in the developing world. It is thought that everyone will experience at least one episode of depression during a lifetime. Yet, there is still no magic cure for mental health problems despite the different classes of drugs dating back to the early 1950s and 1960s with the introduction of chlorpromazine (Thorazine) and Valium ("mother's little helper") and, more recently, Prozac in the 1990s. Multiple sclerosis, motor neurone disease, and muscular dystrophy are just a few of the devastatingly debilitating diseases for which modern medicine has to find an effective remedy. With an aging population, some of the neurodegenerative diseases, such as Alzheimer's and Parkinson's, are increasingly a major global problem. As yet, there are no very effective drugs to prevent, halt, or reverse these conditions. At best, only the symptoms can be managed.

Another major global concern is drug-resistance. Overuse and misuse of important treatments such as antibiotics and antimalarials, and the lack of development of new drugs by the pharmaceutical industry, have resulted in some infections now being untreatable. In 2011 the WHO launched a campaign to safeguard antimicrobials for future generations, and scientists are devising new and sophisticated ways to defeat "superbugs."

Personalized medicine and customized pills

Pharmacogenomics, the design and production of drugs tailor-made for an individual's genetic makeup, became a rapidly expanding field following the launch of the Human Genome Project in the 1990s. The aim is to maximize therapeutic effects and avoid adverse drug reactions in certain individuals but also to minimize damage to healthy cells (the dream of Ehrlich with his approach to chemotherapy).

There is a long way to go with this approach but there is tremendous optimism among some scientists that new advances in drug discovery and related treatments, including vaccines, will progressively enable physicians to offer more to each individual in the future. As the scientist G Sykiotis and his colleagues remind us:

> *Twenty-five centuries after Hippocrates, we are at the beginning of an era of individualized, molecular and genomic medicine, where diagnosis, prognosis and treatment will be increasingly based on our understanding of the human organism's genetic and molecular composition.*

Henry Wellcome and the Wellcome Trust, London

I want the work in these laboratories to be done on the highest scientific lines and with such thoroughness and precision that it will stand the test of time and the keenest criticism.
(Henry Wellcome, cofounder of Burroughs Wellcome & Co., 1904)

Henry Wellcome (1853–1936) was a US pharmacist of poor, rural origins. In 1880, with Silas Burroughs (1846–95), they founded Burroughs Wellcome & Co. in London. Combining good science and marketing, the company revolutionized the European pharmaceutical business, becoming known for

their Tabloid Medicine Chests (of compressed tablets), popular with travelers. The early 20th century saw the establishment of the Wellcome Tropical Laboratories in Khartoum, Sudan, with a floating research laboratory on the River Nile. Burroughs Wellcome developed some of the first semisynthetic penicillins and antiviral drugs.

The Wellcome Trust, a British charity set up in 1936 with Henry's legacy, is still at the forefront of biomedical research with a $22.7 billion endowment and an annual charitable expenditure of $1 billion, making it the UK's largest nongovernmental fund for biomedical research.

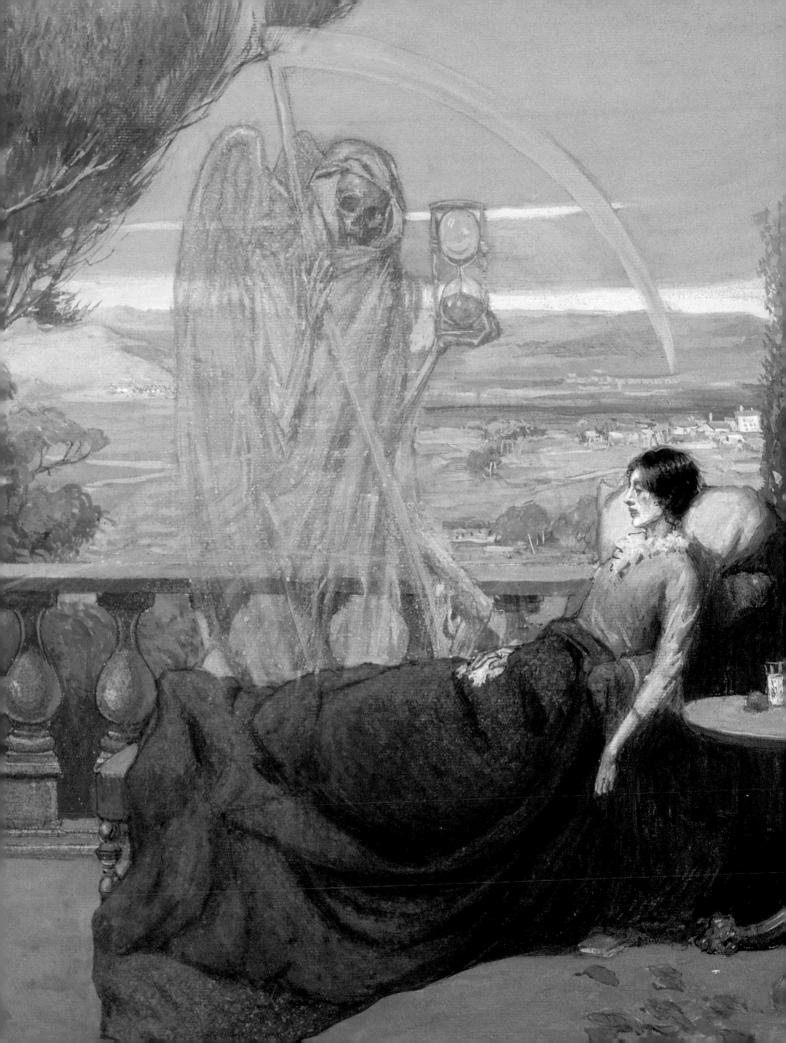

Testing Treatments and Clinical Trials

As to diseases, make a habit of two things–to help,
or at least, to do no harm.

(Hippocratic aphorism)

The first so-called "controlled clinical trial" is attributed to the British naval physician James Lind, who in 1747 methodically compared different treatments on pairs of patients in his search for a cure for scurvy and discovered the value of citrus fruits in preventing this disease. In the centuries that followed, more refined numerical and statistical methods of testing the direct benefits of medical interventions were introduced along with the evaluation of their effectiveness and risks. The first reported modern randomized controlled trial (RCT) of the antibiotic streptomycin as a treatment for pulmonary tuberculosis was conducted in 1947. Thousands of clinical trials of new therapies are currently in progress, and, following strict protocols, can take many years to complete.

James Lind and scurvy

The result of all my experiments was, that oranges and lemons were the most effectual remedies for this distemper at sea.

James Lind, *A Treatise of the Scurvy*, 1753

In the early 1740s, scurvy—the "distemper at sea"—was dramatically highlighted when 997 out of 1,955 sailors died of the disease during a British fleet's voyage to the Pacific. Edinburgh physician James Lind (1716-94) joined the HMS *Salisbury*—then patrolling the English Channel—as surgeon's mate. Surrounded by sailors suffering from scurvy, Lind decided to test some of the theories about possible cures that had been put forward by various physicians and to base his work on "attested facts and observations."

On May 20 1747, he identified 12 men with similar symptoms: "they all in general had

OPPOSITE *An allegory of tuberculosis c.* 1912, by Richard Tennant Cooper. Tuberculosis (TB) was a terrible, and often fatal, disease of young and old. When streptomycin reached Britain in 1947, Austin Bradford Hill conducted one of the first randomized controlled trials to test its effectiveness. Tragically, today TB remains a major killer in the developing world and antibiotic drug-resistance is a serious problem.

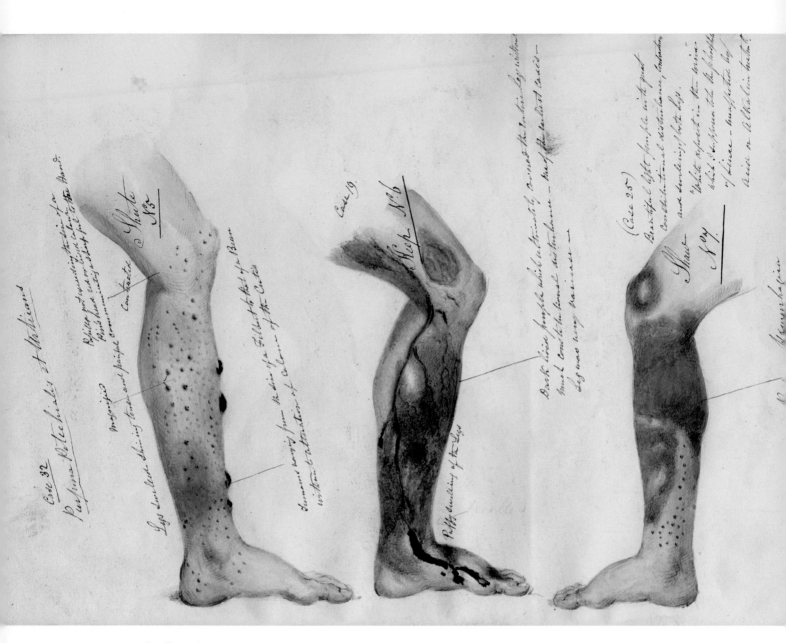

The effects of scurvy, 1840s. British naval physician James Lind (1716–94), in 1747, compared different treatments on pairs of patients in his search for a cure for scurvy and discovered the value of citrus fruits. This is often cited as the first so-called "controlled clinical trial."

putrid gums, the spots and lassitude, with weakness of knees." He sent them down to the ship's sick bay and conducted his now-famous trial. For 14 days each pair of men was to be given an addition to their usual diet:

Pair 1: "a quart of cyder a-day"

Pair 2: "twenty-five gutts of *elixir vitriol* three times a-day"

Pair 3: "two spoonfuls of vinegar three times a-day"

Pair 4: "a course of seawater"

Pair 5: "two oranges and one lemon given them every day"

Pair 6: "nutmeg three times a-day" and "a decoction," which included garlic,
mustard-seed, "balsam of Peru," and "gum myrrh" washed down with barley water

The results were astonishing. The pair receiving two oranges and one lemon daily "which they ate with greediness" recovered rapidly—even before the meagre supply of fruit had run out after six days. Lind had, or so he hoped, found the "remedy" for scurvy—though it took some time before its therapeutic benefits had a wider impact on medical opinion. Eventually, nearly half a century later, lemon juice was issued to the British Navy, and scurvy virtually disappeared from the British fleet. Later, the less effective limes were used, giving rise to the identification of the English abroad as "limeys." It was not, however, until the 20th century, that scurvy was recognized as a vitamin-deficient disease, and scientists were able to show that it was vitamin C that was the key factor in the orange and lemon remedy—the discovery of vitamin C by the Hungarian Albert von Szent-Györgyi (1893–1986) earned him a Nobel Prize in 1937.

The benefits and risks of smallpox inoculation

Physicians increasingly began to collect and collate their own data sets derived from records of patients seen in civilian and military practice- documenting, tabulating, and comparing diseases, possible causes, and treatments. Another fascinating 18th-century example of "testing" medical interventions was the attempt to evaluate the practice and "benefits" and "risks" of the much-debated smallpox inoculation.

To do this, promoters of inoculation, such as John Arbuthnot, Thomas Nettleton, and James Jurin in England, and Zabdiel Boylston and Benjamin Franklin in the USA, began to collate various sets of data. They compared those who had died or survived from smallpox in the "natural way" with those who had died or survived following inoculation. Jurin's analysis, for instance, concluded that the probability of death from inoculation was roughly 1 in 50, while the probability of death from naturally contracted smallpox was 1 in 7 or 8. The early use of mathematical evidence in favor of inoculation over the natural disease influenced he adoption of inoculation, and then the more effective smallpox vaccination from the late 18th century.

Numbers count

Over the course of the 19th and early 20th centuries, compilations of data sets, such as census data and mandatory civil registration of births, marriages, and deaths, were introduced more widely into society, while epidemiology, based on medical statistics compiled and collated from a range of sources, emerged as a valuable field within medicine and public health. For London physician Francis Bisset Hawkins, author of *Elements of Medical Statistics* (1829), and others, "medical statistics affords the most convincing proofs of the efficacy of medicine." In an article on "The applicability of statistics to the practice of medicine," Paris hospital physician Pierre Louis in 1837 stressed the need for "an extensive series of observations, collected with exactness." For Louis, the numerical method—or medical arithmetic—became synonymous with scientific reasoning.

When evaluating treatments and developing the type of experimental "prospective" controlled trial pioneered by Lind's small-scale experiment (that is, introducing a treatment and evaluating its effect on patients over time), physicians and scientists emphasized not only the need for large numbers, but also introduced such concepts as "probability," "placebos," "randomization," and "control groups."

Placebos and the "placebo effect"

The state of the body is linked to the state of the mind.
(Razi, d. c. 925)

In clinical trials, a placebo given to the control group may be a "dummy pill" (a placebo-control trial) or alternatively it may be the "best" available standard treatment (an active-control trial). Placebos are now usually confined to randomized "double-blind" clinical trials, where neither patient nor tester knows who has the placebo.

A different use of the word "placebo" is in the term "placebo effect," where it means more literally "I shall please" from the Latin. Treating a soldier with terrible injuries in the Second World War when morphine supplies were running low, the US anesthetist Henry Beecher (1904–1976) injected saline solution instead. Surprisingly the patient was calm and appeared to feel little pain during the operation, possibly experiencing the "placebo effect." In *The Powerful Placebo* (1955), Beecher described "a high degree of therapeutic effectiveness" in one-third of placebo treatments.

The first randomized controlled trials

In designing experimental trials, one tricky question was always how to decide which group of patients received the treatment and which did not (the "control" group). The early 20th century saw trials on newly discovered drugs and vaccines conducted using a variety of approaches.

The first carefully designed 20th-century randomized controlled trial (RCT) to be reported is attributed to Austin Bradford Hill (1897–1991), Professor of Medical Statistics at the London School of Hygiene and Tropical Medicine and author of the world-renowned book *Principles of Medical Statistics*. When the British Medical Research Council (MRC) wanted to test the newly developed antibiotic streptomycin as a cure for pulmonary tuberculosis in 1947, Bradford Hill had the chance to try out a method of selecting patients for "treatment" or "nontreatment" using the principle of "randomization," without bias, in a clinical trial.

The trial was designed to give a negative or affirmative answer to the question: "Is streptomycin of any value at all in pulmonary tuberculosis?" The patients, unaware of the trial, were randomly allocated into two test groups:

1. Those treated by streptomycin and bed rest.
2. Those treated by bed rest alone (the control group), this being seen as the only alternative standard treatment in this trial.

A set of sealed envelopes, each bearing on the outside only the name of the hospital and a number, was given to the central office of the coordinating centers, concealing the allocation order. The trial, given the limited supply of streptomycin, was conducted on a relatively small number of patients: 55 in the "S" (streptomycin) group and 52 in the "C" (control) group. The patients, in seven participating hospitals, were monitored closely over the course of several months. The results, based on various clinical and radiological changes, were analyzed by staff who did not know whether the patient was an "S" or a "C." The conclusions, published in the *British Medical Journal* in 1948, demonstrated the therapeutic effectiveness of streptomycin in acute forms of pulmonary TB—at least in the short term, though the trial also highlighted concerns about drug-resistance. Bradford Hill's experimental design soon became the gold standard for evaluating new therapies.

Another randomized trial (which had actually commenced before the streptomycin trial but was not published until 1951) investigated a number of whooping cough (pertussis) vaccines versus a "placebo" anticatarrhal vaccine and, in this case, the researchers had asked mothers to give their informed consent before entering their children (aged 6–18 months) in the trial. The results of the follow-up studies showed a significant benefit in the prevention of whooping cough using the pertussis vaccines.

A 1950 MRC trial—the antihistamine common cold study—adopted the principle of using "dummy pills" as "placebos." The control group was given a "dummy" containing phenobarbitone (an early barbiturate), which simulated the effects of "drowsiness" created by the antihistamine being tested. This study, however, showed no proven clinical efficacy of antihistamines for the common cold.

During the decades following these pioneering trials, there was a significant growth in the number of RCTs in both the developed and, more recently, in the developing world. Many of these use large numbers of subjects and controls. These generally adopt the "double-blind" principle of ensuring that neither patients nor investigators know which group is in receipt of the placebo. In some of the most celebrated trials of the late 20th century, more than 130,000 patients from over 20 countries took part in the four ISIS (International Studies of Infarct Survival) randomized trials conducted from Oxford, England, between 1981 and 1993. The ISIS trials were designed to test the efficacy of several drugs in the treatment of acute myocardial infarction (heart attacks) with mortality as the primary outcome. The study showed, for example, that those given a combination of fibrinolytic therapy (to dissolve blood clots) and aspirin (to discourage clots from reforming) had significantly fewer reinfarctions, strokes, and deaths relative to those allocated a matching placebo. The results of such trials can be explored further in a number of online sources.

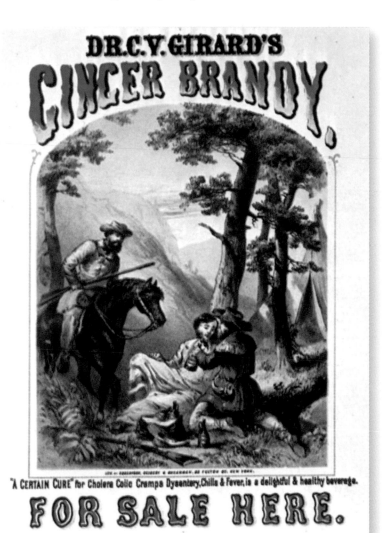

Patent medicines, such as this one for Ginger Brandy in 1860, promised many cures before clinical trials and regulations were introduced to test safety and prevent spurious claims of effectiveness.

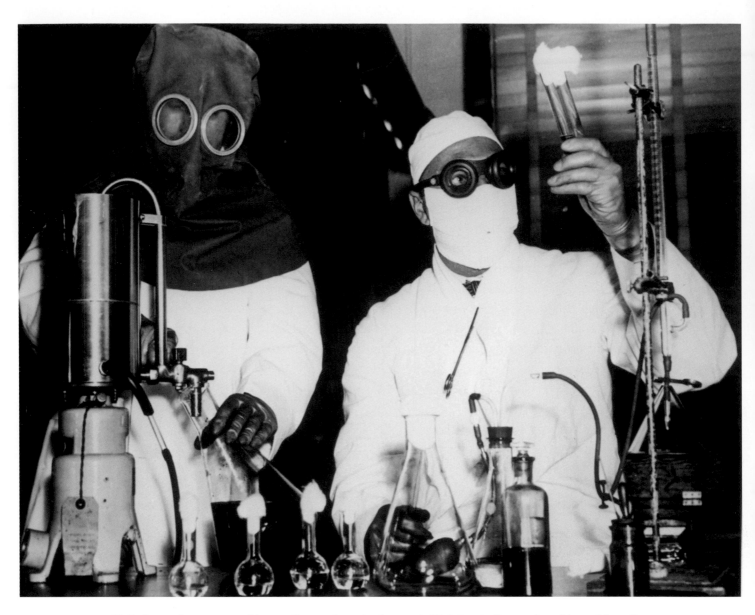

Medical researchers, c. 1925, working on a therapeutic vaccine for encephalitis lethargica (known also as "sleepy sickness"), a mysterious disease that, first observed in 1915, killed or disabled millions across the globe over the following decades .

Testing safety and efficacy of new drugs

While the methodological basis for designing and evaluating RCTs evolved, other aspects of clinical trials came under scrutiny, particularly the ethical and safety concerns of testing treatments on humans. There are currently strict internationally recognized ethical and safety regulations that have to be passed before a clinical trial on humans can be undertaken and a drug, vaccine, or other medical intervention approved for general use. To ensure that the ethical and safety criteria are met, clinical trials are now conducted using a successive progression of monitored and regulated stages.

The preliminary stage is the preclinical phase in which extensive tests are carried out *in vitro* (in the test tube) and *in vivo* (in intact organisms) in the laboratory. For any promising medical interventions, which can take years to discover, the sponsor (often now an innovative pharmaceutical or biotech company) has to submit to a regulatory body and a supervising ethics committee a detailed proposal with sufficient preclinical data, along with a clinical trial protocol that outlines its design and how it will be conducted, to make the case for proceeding with human trials. It is estimated that for every 5,000 new compounds identified in the discovery process, only five or so are considered safe for testing in human volunteers after preclinical evaluations. For new drugs that do pass through this first hurdle, this is then followed by four (or more) sequential phases (a framework introduced in the early 1960s), when testing proceeds to human participants:

The four stages of human drug trials

Phase I *is designed to verify safety, tolerance, and the basic effects of the candidate drug in the body. This is generally conducted on a small number of healthy volunteers.*

Phase II *determines with more accuracy the true efficacy and safety of the treatment. Testing is conducted with several hundred volunteer patients suffering from the condition that the drug in question is designed to treat. It can also be used to study appropriate dosage and formulation. Most Phase II clinical trials are randomized and double-blinded and include "controls" (who may be given a "placebo" or the "best" standard available treatment).*

Phase III *provides expanded and longer studies of Phase II trials with testing for safety and efficacy on much larger groups of patients. Many of these are million-dollar, "mega-trials" using broad patient population groups often in multiregional settings.*

Final approval for marketing a treatment after the end of the Phase III clinical trial is then submitted to the applicable regulatory authority.

Phase IV *or the "post-approval" phase is used to monitor over the short and long term any unforeseen problems, side effects, or adverse drug reactions ("pharmacovigilence"), as well as to test the product in different age or population groups.*

The entire process from drug discovery through drug development and clinical trials to approval for general use may take around ten years and cost millions. Occasionally, where a trial shows at an early stage that the treatment is highly effective, especially for life-threatening conditions, the trial might be stopped prematurely and the treatment fast-tracked through the system. As HIV/AIDS hit the headlines in the early 1980s, a drug was urgently sought and found. This was azidothymidine (AZT), tested previously—unsuccessfully—in the 1960s as a drug for cancer treatment. Following retesting of AZT *in vitro* and in rodents, the first double-blind, placebo-controlled randomized trial of AZT, conducted by Burroughs-Wellcome, showed that it could significantly reduce the replication of the virus in patients, leading to clinical and immunological improvements. The trial had begun in 1985 and was terminated in 1986 enabling AZT to be approved by the FDA's then-new accelerated approval system in March 1987. The time between the first demonstration that AZT was active against HIV in the laboratory and its approval was 25 months, the shortest period of drug development in recent history.

Even when a new treatment has passed all the required safety and efficacy tests and been approved, it might not be prescribed in some countries if it is not considered cost-effective. In the UK, especially since the inception of the "free" National Health Service (NHS) in 1948, it was soon recognized that some form of rationing was needed to ensure cost-effectiveness. In response to this need a rationing body, the National Institute for Health and Clinical Excellence (NICE), was set up in 1999. Using a complex formula to determine the efficacy, efficiency, and clinical cost-effectiveness of interventions, NICE can recommend the conditions under which a treatment can be prescribed to patients at the expense of the NHS. At an international level, the CHOICE (CHOosing Interventions that are Cost-Effective) project was developed by the World Health Organization in 1998. The objective of this initiative is to provide policy-makers with evidence on which to base decisions regarding medical interventions, given the need to provide the best health gains possible with the available resources.

"Guinea pigs," controversy—and tighter regulations

Over the course of history, slaves, condemned criminals, orphan, and children have been used as human "guinea pigs" for testing experimental treatments. Following the Doctors' Trial in 1946–7 of Nazi physicians who had performed medical experiments on concentration camp prisoners during the Second World War, the Nuremberg Code of 1947 laid down ten directives for human experimentation. The famous first principle of the Code was that "the voluntary consent of the human subject is absolutely essential." The World Medical Association drew up the Declaration of Helsinki in 1964, which detailed ethical conduct in medical research involving human subjects, and has been revised continuously over the past five decades.

Breaches of these codes of conduct have occurred, an infamous example in peacetime being the 1932–72 Tuskegee Syphilis Study in Alabama, USA. Here some 400 male black share-croppers with latent syphilis were left untreated to enable the US Public Health Service to monitor the progress of the disease, despite penicillin being available from 1947. When exposed by a journalist in 1972, the outcry led to crucial measures to help protect research subjects in the USA, and in 1997 President Clinton offered a formal apology. "Informed consent" (when participants are told of the aims and risks of the clinical trial and fully understand them before agreeing voluntarily to take part)—consistent with the principles of the Declaration of Helsinki—is seen as especially important in the developing world where an increasing number of clinical trials now take place.

Other shocking high-profile cases have led to radical changes in the way drugs are regulated and tested. The first major example of this in the 20th century that led to tighter controls was the "Elixir Sulfanilamide" disaster of 1937 in the USA. Sulfa drugs were introduced in the 1930s but, with almost nonexistent testing requirements, one product poisoned many patients and caused the deaths of more than a

Sifting through the data and evidence-based medicine

Authoritative online sources such as the James Lind Library and the Cochrane Collaboration Database of Systematic Reviews (named after the influential Scottish physician Archie Cochrane, 1909–88) help condense the vast amount of clinical trial reports. In 1992, a clinical discipline emerged as "Evidence-based Medicine" (EBM). This refers to the "conscientious, explicit, and judicious use of current best evidence in making decisions about the care of individual patients."

hundred people. The public outcry caused by this incident led to the passing in the USA of the Federal Food, Drug, and Cosmetic Act in 1938 to include not only a requirement for disclosure of composition and method of preparation of medicine, but also evidence of a product's safety—a pivotal turning point in the history of pharmacy.

The tragedy of the effects of the drug thalidomide had even wider repercussions on a global scale. Thalidomide was introduced in the late 1950s to relieve morning sickness and act as a sedative. It was hastily marketed and not adequately tested. This was picked up by US FDA official Frances Oldham Kelsey (b. 1914), who prevented it being released in the USA. Meanwhile, thousands of women in more than 40 countries took the drug in pregnancy.

Soon, obstetricians saw a dramatic rise in the number of cases of severely malformed limbs in newborn babies. Doctors, notably Widukind Lenz in Germany and William McBride in Australia, quickly linked these malformations to the use of thalidomide in pregnancy. At the end of 1961, the manufacturers withdrew the drug.

Years later, after public campaigns and legal action, the victims began to receive compensation. But the toll of this tragic

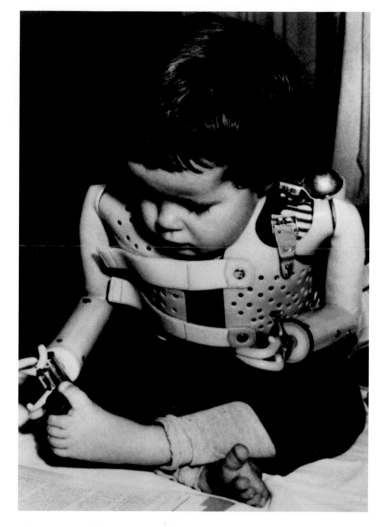

A three-year-old thalidomide toddler in 1965 using power-driven arms. Thalidomide was inadequately tested and caused severe birth defects in babies before it was withdrawn in 1961.

episode was immense—an estimated 8,000–12,000 babies worldwide were affected, with a range of disabilities. It generated widespread public and professional demands for rigorous testing of new drugs and vaccines before allowing them to be marketed. In the USA, the 1962 Kefauver-Harris Drug Amendments to the Federal Food, Drugs, and Cosmetic Act marked the start of the FDA approval process of preclinical and clinical trials in its modern form.

Other later 20th-century developments have included stricter controls in differentiating those medicines that could be prescribed only by a physician from those sold "over-the-counter" in pharmacies. The requirement of safety has, however, necessitated extensive animal pharmacological and toxicological testing in the preclinical phase before a drug could be tested in humans, raising yet another controversial issue of clinical research—the use of animals as "guinea pigs."

From insulin and antibiotics to vaccines and treatments for cancer and HIV, almost every conventional medical treatment that we now rely on rests in part on the study of animals. This practice has not gone unquestioned and has long been a point of tension between

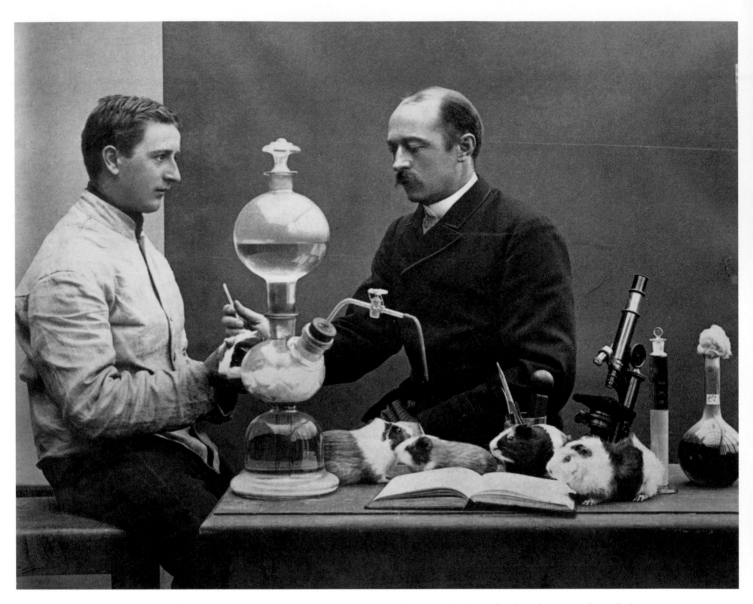

Emil von Behring (1854-1917), German scientist and winner of the first 1901 Nobel Prize for Physiology or Medicine for his pioneering work on serum therapy for diphtheria, uses a syringe to inject a guinea pig held by a lab assistant, *c.* 1890.

scientists and those concerned about the rights and welfare of animals. Victorian Britain saw a rise in those who opposed the use of unanesthetized animals (including guinea pigs, which were introduced in the 17th century for medical research), leading to the passing of a Parliamentary Act in 1876 to regulate animal experimentation. Further legislation in Britain and elsewhere has subsequently been enacted to protect animal welfare.

In 1959 a concept of "3 Rs"—Replacement, Reduction, and Refinement—was introduced by W Russell and R Burch in their book *The Principles of Humane Experimental Technique*, and became pragmatic guidelines for animal testing. Many scientific organizations and funding bodies now have clear guidelines on this issue based on the principles of the 3 Rs—which means that every effort must be made to: replace the use of live animals by nonanimal alternatives; reduce the number of animals used in research to a minimum required for meaningful results; and to refine the procedures so that the degree of suffering is kept to a minimum. As new technologies evolve, alternatives, such as laboratory-grown cells and computer models, are being sought for testing drugs. The safety and efficacy of new drugs for humans, nevertheless, remains of paramount importance for the pharmaceutical industry and other health care providers.

"Wonder drugs" and headline news

Some drugs have been appropriately called "wonder-drugs" inasmuch as one wonders what they will do next.

Samuel Enoch Stumpf, 1918–98

Scientists and physicians have to keep abreast of the latest pharmaceutical products and surgical interventions that prove successful in clinical trials, while newspapers and the media invariably report the "major" success stories (as well as the "scare" stories). Aspirin has been heralded time and again as a "wonder drug"—not just as an analgesic (one of its original claims to fame)—but also as a treatment for heart disease, stroke, and other vascular disorders. In March 2012, many newspapers had front-page headlines about the results of a study showing the "remarkable" effects of aspirin on cancer prevention, treatment, and spread (metastasis). The research, based on data from randomized controlled trials (daily aspirin versus no aspirin), was conducted by a group of international scientists, led by Professor Peter Rothwell of Oxford University, and published in *The Lancet*. Although the trial had been designed to evaluate the effect of aspirin for heart disease and other vascular events, data had also been kept on each patient's outcome of cancer.

One British headline ran: "Aspirin a day cuts cancer risk after just three years," while the BBC reported: "Daily aspirin 'prevents and possibly treats cancer.'" The news was reported widely elsewhere, with US newspapers reminding us of the ancient use of willow bark, which contains the active ingredient of aspirin: "Hippocrates's 3-cent Aspirin Once a Day May Keep Cancer Away." Inevitably, this story has been followed up by such questions as: "If aspirin is a miracle drug, shouldn't we all be taking it?" How should the public read these messages? For aspirin, a nonprescription over-the-counter pill, this is a critical question.

One of the great features of the internet is being able to read online some of the original articles published in medical journals, enabling us to evaluate these results and read more about the caveats, shortcomings, and possible side effects. A contraindication of aspirin, for example, is that it can cause internal bleeding in certain patients and is not suitable for children as it can be associated with Reye's syndrome. An excellent editorial in *The Lancet* (28 April 2012)—"Are we ready to recommend aspirin for cancer prevention?"—provides the reader with a balanced overview. And, more importantly, medical advice is always best.

Testing "traditional" treatments

Aspirin is an interesting example of a drug that was derived from an old herbal remedy, first synthesized in 1897, and quickly marketed as a painkiller by Bayer in Germany. There is also a range of remedies and treatments, some of which date back to ancient times—including other herbal medicines, such as ginkgo biloba, ginseng, and St John's Wort, as well as therapies like acupuncture and moxibustion—that are widely available and are used by many across the world. These often go under the umbrella terms of "traditional medicine" or, in the West,

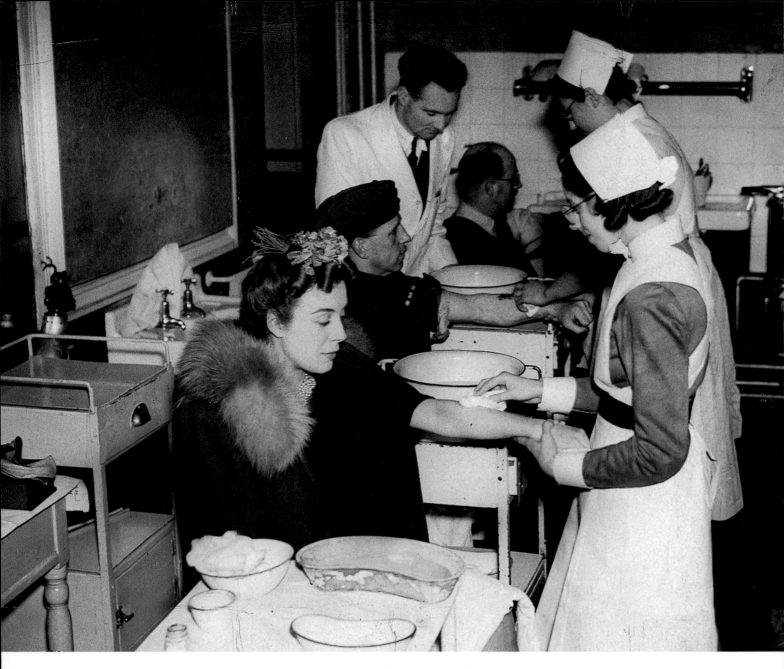

During the Second World War, homeopathic clinicians collaborated with the Ministry of Home Security in Britain in a series of clinical trials on mustard gas at homeopathic hospitals in Glasgow and London in 1941-2. Volunteers were given homeopathic burn treatments (including poison oak and Spanish fly) to test their effects after being blistered by mustard gas solution. The results of these trials, which were carried out before the principles of randomization and "double-blinding" were introduced, are described in the online James Lind Library.

"complementary and alternative medicine (CAM)" (see pages 168–71). In their provocative book *Trick or Treatment: the Undeniable Facts about Alternative Medicine* (2008), authors Simon Singh and Edzard Ernst (the world's first professor of complementary medicine at Exeter University in Britain and a former homeopathic doctor), analyze more than 30 of the most popular treatments with the aim of presenting both their benefits and limits, as well as any possible risks. They stress the current challenges and difficulties of testing the efficacy of certain therapies and suggest that, in some cases, as in biomedicine, positive benefits are due not to the therapy itself, but to the "placebo effect." Singh and Ernst, and others, argue for stricter control and mandatory regulation of *all* such treatments.

Moreover, while there are regulations to register, for example, herbal medicines with the appropriate national regulatory agency, the requirements for approval or licensing vary widely from country to country and in some cases, clinical experience (for instance, the medicine has proven therapeutic effect on the basis of long-standing use and experience) rather than data from clinical trials is acceptable for registration. Experts, including participants of a network of WHO Collaborating Centers for Traditional Medicine and a European consortium for Good-Practice in Traditional Chinese Medicine Research in the Post-genomic Era (GP-TCM), are currently reviewing these disparities as well as developing research methodologies for investigating clinical practices. The hope is that standards of efficacy, safety, and quality control can be harmonized at an international level and, where beneficial, these remedies and traditional methods of healing can be integrated into mainstream global health care systems.

> The safety and efficacy of new drugs for humans, nevertheless, remains of paramount importance for the pharmaceutical industry and other health care providers.

In the coming decades, traditional medicine will, increasingly, come under scrutiny and, where feasible, be the subject of scientific randomized controlled clinical trials. With, for example, 30,000–70,000 plant species being used somewhere in the world as medicines, there is enormous potential for the development of novel pharmaceutical products. The story of the discovery in the 1970s of the Chinese antimalarial, plant-derived artemisinin (see New Drugs from Old Remedies) is just one exceptional example of the value of testing traditional medicines. More difficult to assess is the broader philosophical, cultural, and theoretical basis that guides and underpins much of traditional healing, which cannot easily be evaluated in a conventional way. Also problematic will be how to "measure" the "hidden" benefits, such as the placebo effect and the importance of practitioners spending considerable time with a patient to ensure an individualistic holistic approach to diagnosis and treatment. This latter approach is an essential part of contemporary Traditional Chinese Medicine, Kampo, Unani, Ayurvedic medicine, and other CAM practices, and is one valued by many patients across the world.

The trials and tribulations of testing treatments: assessing safety and efficacy in the 21st century

Developing, testing, and regulating medicines and medical products as they come on the market, whether based on "conventional" or "traditional" medicine, is a hugely complex and, often, highly competitive business. Pharmaceutical companies and regulatory authorities are exposed to constant scrutiny as well as criticism in the media and, sometimes, in the law courts. Mistakes, for example, from contaminated drugs or unanticipated adverse effects, do still occasionally occur. Such events, as recent history shows, have constantly led to tighter controls and rapid withdrawal of dangerous or suspect products.

Taking a broad historical perspective, we can be reassured that massive advances have been made over the past century to measure the "risks" as well as the "benefits" of new treatments, particularly following the efforts of the FDA in the USA, the introduction of international ethical codes in medicine, and the design of rigorous protocols for clinical trials. We have come a long way from the days when arsenic or opium frequently went undetected in medicines, or remedies were advertised to cure anything from cancer to corns.

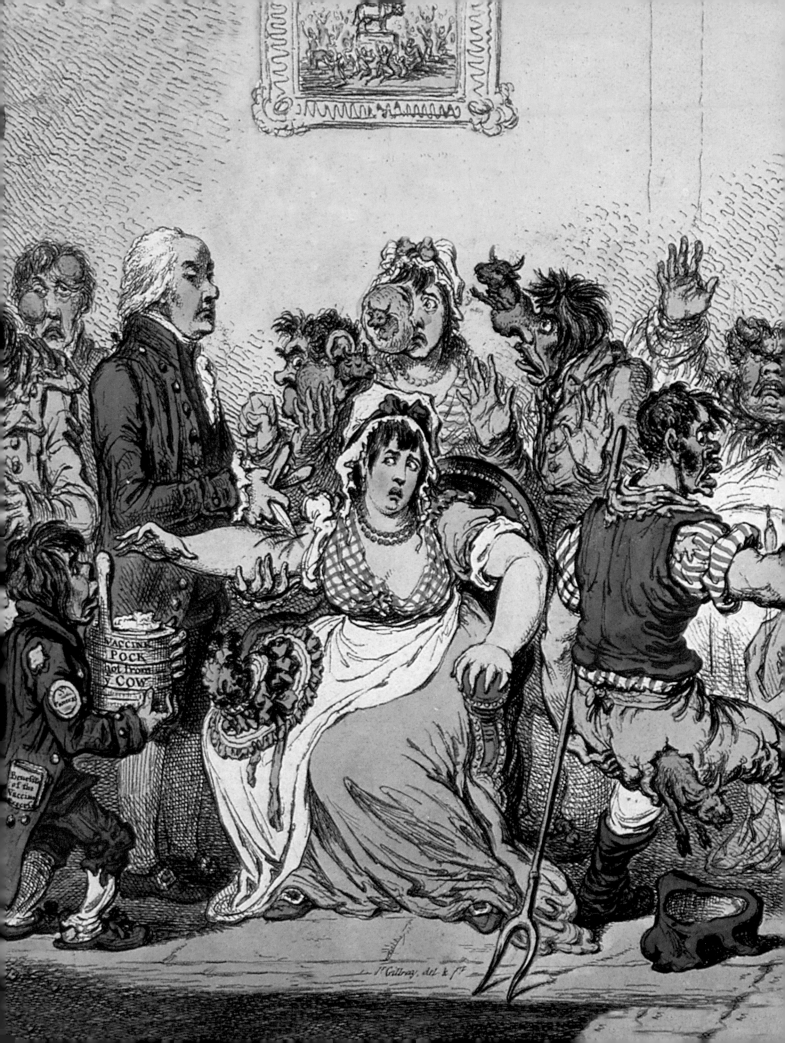

Vaccination and Preventive Medicine

"What renders the Cow-Pox virus so extremely singular is, that the person who has been thus affected is for ever after secure from the infection of the Small-pox."

Edward Jenner, 1798

The use of vaccination to immunize people against infectious diseases is one of the most remarkable stories in the history of medicine. Vaccination was first developed by the English doctor Edward Jenner, who demonstrated in 1796 that scratching some cowpox (an infection of cows) into the skin of humans could prevent smallpox. Nearly a century later, in 1885, a vaccine for rabies was developed by Louis Pasteur. With increasing scientific knowledge in the fields of bacteriology, immunology, and virology, many other vaccines were introduced in the 20th century for diseases such as diphtheria, tuberculosis, and polio. Smallpox was eradicated worldwide by 1980. The search continues for vaccines for some of the world's other major killers, including HIV/AIDS, and the fight is ongoing against variant strains of influenza. Vaccines, along with improvements in sanitation and nutrition and healthy lifestyles, form part of a broad approach to preventive medicine and public health.

The "annihilation of smallpox"

In 1980, the World Health Organization (WHO) declared that smallpox had been completely eradicated from the globe—the only major disease so far eliminated by human intervention and arguably the greatest achievement in the history of medicine. Smallpox was for centuries one of the most dreaded, lethal, and common of all infectious diseases. It was an ancient disease, which became increasingly virulent during the early modern period; in the form *Variola major*, it killed at least 10–20 percent of its victims. Some of the most lethal epidemics of smallpox were in the newly discovered Americas, shortly after the arrival of Columbus in 1492. The pocked and scarred faces of those who survived this horrific viral infection marked them out for life. Queen Elizabeth I of England was seriously ill with smallpox in 1562 but

OPPOSITE The caricaturist James Gillray pokes fun at the "new practice" of cowpox vaccination in this 1802 colored etching showing Edward Jenner vaccinating patients against smallpox.

recovered. She painted her face with white lead and vinegar to cover up her smallpox scars and rumor had it that her refusal to marry arose from an unwillingness to reveal her scars. No cure was ever found for smallpox but the discovery of a vaccine by Edward Jenner (1749–1823) to prevent people contracting the disease led to the final realization of Jenner's goal—"the annihilation of the Small Pox."

How the principle of vaccination (from the Latin *vacca*, a cow) and its earlier counterpart, inoculation, came to be discovered is an extraordinary feat of human intuition and ingenuity.

Smallpox parties and inoculation

While smallpox killed many of its victims, those who survived seemed to be spared from catching the disease again. This observation may have inspired a technique that became known as "inoculation" or "variolation" (after *variola*, the scientific name of smallpox). The idea was to "inoculate" a healthy person with smallpox pustules or pus in the hope that they might get a milder—rather than the full-blown and potentially fatal— form of the disease and would then be subsequently protected (immune). This practice appears to have been used independently in several regions of the world. In the 10th century, the Chinese, for example, removed scabs from the drying pustules of a smallpox patient, pounded them into a powder, and then blew a few grains into the nose of people who had not had the illness—up the right nostril for a boy and the left one for a girl. In other places, pus from the "pocks" of an infected person was inoculated into a scratch in the skin of healthy people.

In the early 18th century, Lady Mary Wortley Montagu, writer and wife of the British ambassador to the Ottoman court, was living in Constantinople (now Istanbul), Turkey. Her stunning beauty had been destroyed by an attack of smallpox, leaving her badly scarred and without eyelashes. In a letter to a friend she described the local "smallpox parties" in which peasant women would routinely perform inoculation:

> I am going to tell you a thing that will make you wish yourself here. The smallpox, so fatal and so general amongst us, is here rendered entirely harmless by the invention of engrafting, which is the term they give it ... an old woman comes with a nutshell full of the matter of the best sort of smallpox, and asks what veins you please to have open'd. She immediately rips open that which you offer her with a large needle (which gives you no more pain than a common scratch) and puts into the vein as much of the venom as can lie on the head of her needle.

Lady Mary had her six-year-old son inoculated by the Embassy surgeon, Charles Maitland, assisted by a Greek woman; the child suffered no complications. In 1721, back in England, her three-year-old daughter was inoculated by Maitland, leading to much publicity. During a severe epidemic of smallpox in Boston, Massachusetts, in the same year, the Reverend Cotton Mather—having read about the news from London—persuaded the medical practitioner Zabdiel Boylston to inoculate those not yet infected. Boylston harvested pus by puncturing with a lancet the pustules of infected patients and then squeezed the fluid into a glass jar. To inoculate the "healthy," he cut a slit into the arm or leg and liberally dabbed on the infected matter.

The experience of smallpox inoculation, which could include three weeks of daily vomiting, purges, and fevers, is described by Peter Thatcher, a 12-year-old Boston boy inoculated on Saturday, 14 April 1764: "Sunday we took a powder in the morning that work'd me nine times ...

Saturday April 21 took a powder which worked me 4 times down and once up. Felt very sick in the Morning and did not get up till 10 o'clock. I have some Pock come out today." On Wednesday, May 2, three weeks after his operation, Thatcher was recovered: "I have been preserved through the Distemper of the Small Pox which formerly was so fatal to many Thousands."

By the late 18th century, inoculation was popular on both sides of the Atlantic, as it became safer, cheaper, and easier. One of the problems, raised by remaining doubters, apart from a 2 to 3 percent risk of death, was that during the mild attack of smallpox people were actually infectious, and needed to be isolated.

Edward Jenner: cowpox to prevent smallpox

Future nations will know by history only that the loathsome smallpox has existed and by you has been extirpated.

US President Thomas Jefferson, in a letter to Edward Jenner, May 14 1806

While the advantages and risks of inoculation were debated in 18th-century medical circles, Edward Jenner, a doctor practicing in Gloucestershire, heard a local story that dairymaids who had contracted the mild cowpox from infected cows' udders appeared to be protected from the much more serious smallpox of humans.

Edward Jenner (1749–1823) vaccinating a boy, shown in this oil painting by Eugène-Ernest Hillemacher, 1884. Jenner's first experiment with vaccination took place in 1796 when he inoculated cowpox from the arm of Sarah Nelmes into the arm of James Phipps.

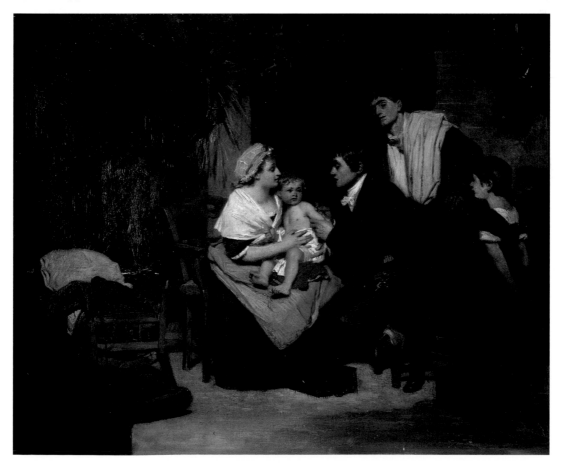

In May 1796, Jenner, acting on a hunch, chose James Phipps, the healthy eight-year-old son of his gardener, and a young dairymaid, Sarah Nelmes, who had contracted cowpox, for an experiment. Jenner transferred infected material from a cowpox pustule on Sarah's hand into a cut on the skin of the young boy. Six weeks later, Jenner inoculated James with smallpox virus taken from a pustule of a smallpox patient. It didn't "take." The boy was, indeed, protected against smallpox. Jenner also successfully "vaccinated" his own son and became convinced that he had found a way of preventing this "most dreadful scourge of the human species," which was far better and safer than inoculation.

The initial reaction of the Royal Society of London in 1797, of which he was a Fellow, was not positive. They rejected his paper, writing that he "ought not to risk his reputation by presenting to the learned body anything which appeared so much at variance with established knowledge, and withal so incredible."

In the end, backed up by further evidence from Jenner, the vaccination was very quickly adopted around the world and he was richly honored and rewarded. By 1801 more than 100,000 people had been vaccinated in England, and by 1811 over 1.7 million in France: Napoleon vaccinated half his army. From 1804–14, 2 million Russians were vaccinated and the Empress named the first vaccinated child Vaccinof. Jennerian vaccination even reached Japan, which was still largely "closed" to the West, and was enthusiastically taken up by its physicians. Dried vaccine on quills and lancets, dried scabs, or cotton threads impregnated with matter from pustules, were just some of the methods used to transport the vaccine around the world. The vaccine was prepared in large quantities in continental Europe by growing the virus on the skins of calves. In some countries mass vaccination centers were set up and over time millions of people were spared the horrors of the disease.

The global eradication of smallpox

Thanks to national vaccination programs, by the 1960s smallpox was no longer endemic in much of the Western world. But 10–15 million people in 43 countries still contracted the disease each year, with about 2 million deaths. In 1966, at a meeting of the World Health Assembly, a decision was taken (albeit by just two votes) to embark on an "Intensified Ten-Year Smallpox Eradication Program."

"Surveillance" and "containment" were key and the aim was to search for active smallpox cases, trace, and vaccinate their contacts, as well as the local population, imposing a "ring" around each outbreak. Messages about the campaign were spread widely and rewards for reporting cases of the disease were offered. In parts of Africa and Asia, health workers battled against great technical, logistical, and cultural challenges. Helped by new technological developments, including a freeze-dried vaccine that remained stable in tropical climates and jet injector guns to vaccinate a thousand people in an hour, the program was, ultimately, a success.

The last cases were recorded in 1975 in the Indian subcontinent (*Variola major*, the most serious form), Somalia in 1977 (*Variola minor*, a milder form) and a lone laboratory-acquired British case in 1978. By 1979 "Target Zero" had been reached and, today, the smallpox pathogen exists only in two high-security laboratories in the USA and in the Russian Federation.

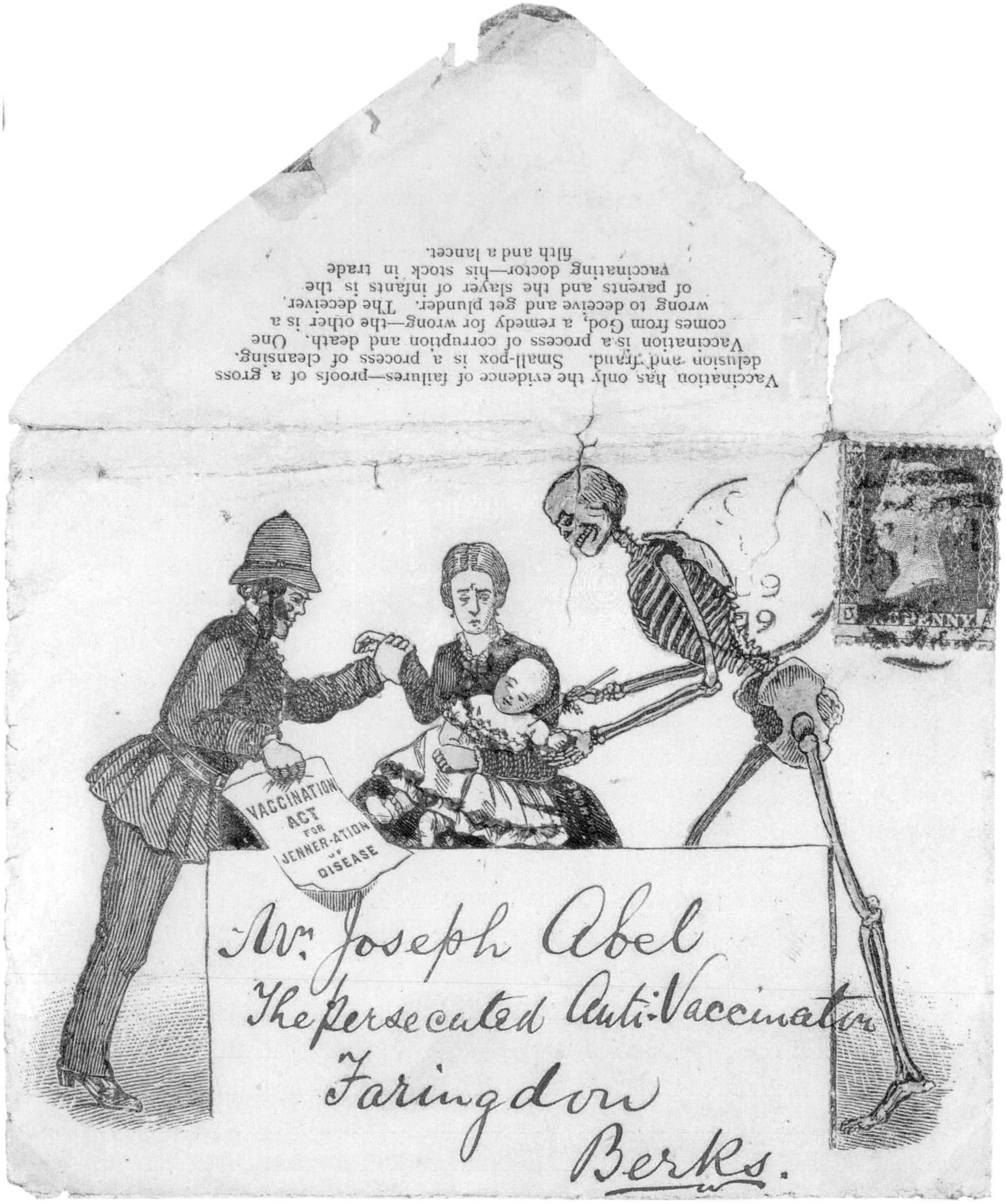

The text within the envelope illustration (printed upside-down) reads:

> Vaccination has only the evidence of failures—proofs of a gross
> delusion and fraud. Small-pox is a process of cleansing.
> Vaccination is a process of corruption and death. One
> comes from God, a remedy for wrong—the other is a
> wrong, to deceive and get plunder. The deceiver,
> of parents and the slayer of infants is the
> vaccinating doctor—his stock in trade
> filth and a lancet.

Handwritten address on envelope:

> Mr. Joseph Abel
> The Persecuted Anti-Vaccinator
> Faringdon
> Berks.

Label on paper held: VACCINATION ACT FOR JENNER-ATION of DISEASE

Antivaccinationists and antivivisectionists in England fought hard to suppress the smallpox vaccine, as shown on this 1899 propaganda envelope.

A mad dog and Louis Pasteur's rabies vaccine

When mediating over a disease, I never think of finding a remedy for it, but, instead, a means of preventing it.

Louis Pasteur, 1884

On July 6 1885 a boy from the French region of Alsace, named Joseph Meister, was brought to the laboratory of the famous French chemist Louis Pasteur (1822–95) by his distraught mother and the owner of a rabid dog that had badly bitten the boy. For centuries, rabies (from the Latin meaning "to rave"), transmitted by the saliva of an infected animal, had been one of the most frightening of all diseases. The word "rabies" conjured up images of "mad" dogs foaming at the mouth and biting people in frenzied attacks, resulting in horrific symptoms and the almost certain death of the victim.

After years of exhaustive work, Pasteur and a team of researchers in Paris, including Émile Roux (1853–1933), had developed a vaccine using the dried spinal cord of rabbits, which they found experimentally to be effective in dogs. But would it work on humans? When Joseph Meister arrived at his laboratory in Paris, Pasteur decided to take the chance. As he later said: "as the death of this child appeared inevitable, I decided [to try] … the procedure which had consistently worked on dogs." The boy was vaccinated and, after another twelve injections over a period of ten days, he survived.

As with Jenner, Pasteur experienced skepticism from his peers in the medical profession. Even Pasteur had to acknowledge that although he suspected the infective agent of rabies to be a "microbe of infinite smallness," he could not actually see the microbe in question using the microscopes then available.

While the smallpox vaccine (like many later vaccines) was administered to prevent people catching the disease, Pasteur's vaccine could be given at an early stage to stop symptoms developing—as rabies has a long incubation period, following the initial bite. In 1886, even after the long train ride to Paris to seek the vaccine, 35 out of 38 Russian peasants mauled by rabid wolves were apparently saved by Pasteur's injections.

Vaccination for humans and domestic animals, combined with strict measures of inspection, quarantine of pets, and the control of stray animals, has successfully eliminated rabies from some countries though it remains a threat in parts of Africa and Asia.

Mad Dog, a caricature of people's fear of a mad dog and of rabies, 1826. Pasteur's rabies vaccine, first used in 1885, was a major advance in controlling this frightening disease.

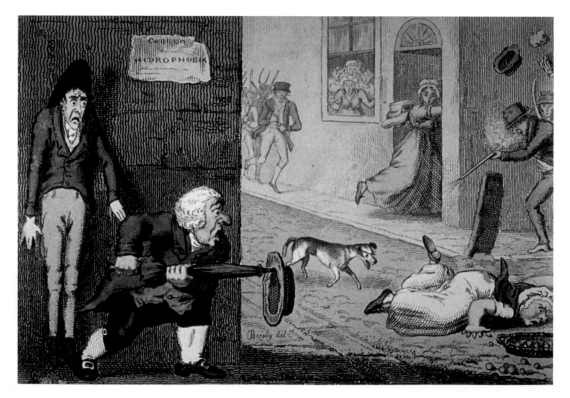

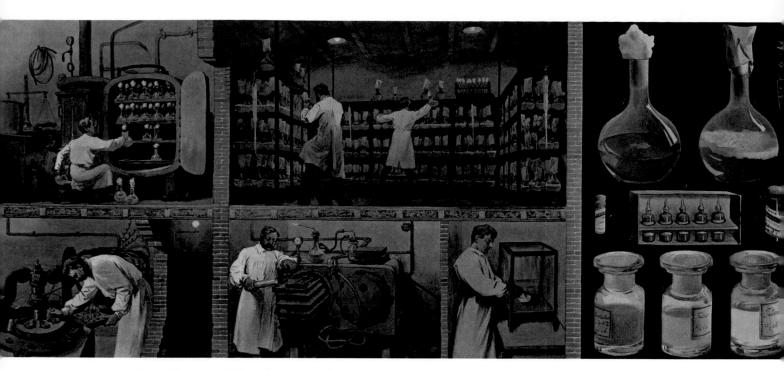

Serum therapy (treatment of disease by injection of serum from immune animals) was a major advance for treating diphtheria in the early 20th century. It was also tried out for tuberculosis (TB), as shown in this 1906 image of its production in Germany. A vaccine was developed in the 1920s to prevent TB, followed by antibiotics to treat it from the 1940s.

Diphtheria and the "Great Race of Mercy" to Nome, Alaska

Another practical therapeutic application to emerge from the scientific fields of bacteriology and immunology in the late 19th and early 20th centuries was the development of "serum therapy" for diphtheria and tetanus; this was followed by vaccines (toxoids) for these life-threatening diseases.

In the 1880s and 1890s, the bacteria causing these two diseases were isolated and it was discovered that it was the secretion of toxins that was responsible for the often fatal symptoms. With this knowledge, antitoxins—to neutralize the dangerous toxins and induce passive immunity—were developed. So-called serum therapy was first used successfully on a young child suffering from severe diphtheria on Christmas Eve, 1891. "Healing-serum factories" were established in the 1890s with horses as "antitoxin producers." The very first Nobel Prize in Physiology or Medicine in 1901 was awarded to the German scientist Emil von Behring (1854–1917) for his contribution to the development of serum therapy and his role of placing "in the hands of the physician a victorious weapon against illness and disease."

One of the most famous outbreaks of diphtheria, a highly contagious respiratory tract illness, and its control using antitoxin was in Nome, Alaska, in the winter of 1925. An urgently needed supply of antitoxin to treat sick children was rushed to the afflicted snowbound town by relays of dogsleds covering 674 miles, and it became known as the "Great Race of Mercy."

Serum therapy was an important advance and led to the development of prophylactic (preventive) diphtheria and tetanus vaccines, which in the late 1940s were combined with a whooping cough (pertussis) vaccine into a single shot. A triple vaccine (DTP or DTaP) is, today, routinely given to infants and children. Diphtheria has been largely eradicated in industrialized nations, though like other childhood diseases it remains serious in unvaccinated populations (and resurged recently in Eastern Europe and the Russian Federation when immunization rates fell). Tetanus is now rare in the West but the neonatal form kills thousands of newborns each year in the developing world, often when unvaccinated mothers give birth in homes without adequate sterile procedures.

Typhoid and typhus vaccines

Typhoid and typhus, spread respectively by contaminated food and water, and by body lice, have long been some of the worst diseases especially during times of war. A strong advocate for preventive medicine, British scientist Almroth Wright (1861–1947) produced one of the first vaccines against typhoid in 1896. During the First World War both the US and British commands officially adopted typhoid immunization as well as better military sanitation. Tetanus antitoxin was available to prevent serious infection in wounded soldiers, and a tetanus vaccine, developed in the 1920s, was widely used along with the typhoid vaccine during the Second World War.

In 1937, Herald R Cox (1907–86) of the US Public Health Service was able to culture the typhus germ in the yolks of hens' eggs—leading to the first effective and commercially viable vaccine for typhus, which proved vital especially for US troops during the Second World War (the introduction of DDT for "delousing" soldiers and civilians in the later stages of the war also became an important measure for controlling typhus).

BCG: a vaccine for tuberculosis

In 1882 German bacteriologist Robert Koch identified the bacterium (*Mycobacterium tuberculosis*) that causes tuberculosis (TB): one of the key discoveries of the bacteriological age (see Germs and Genes). Development of a TB vaccine (based on a weakened strain of *M. bovis*—the bovine form) was eventually achieved in the early 1920s by two French scientists—Albert Calmette (1863–1933) and Camille Guérin (1872–1961)—and called BCG (from Bacillus Calmette–Guérin). This was first tested in humans in 1921 when it was given to a baby at the Charité Hospital in Paris. The baby's mother had died of TB just after the birth. The child was given a dose of BCG orally and did not develop the disease. Further children were vaccinated and the acceptance of BCG grew, particularly in France and Scandinavia.

There was a setback, however, when 250 newborn babies were vaccinated in 1930 in the German city of Lübeck, and over seventy of them died as a result. It was later recognized that this batch was accidentally contaminated with a virulent strain of *M. tuberculosis*. Vaccination with BCG was discontinued in Germany in 1931 and the German Ministry of Health issued detailed guidelines for clinical trials involving children. This tragedy also significantly delayed its introduction to Britain, while concerns over safety, as well as effectiveness, undermined support for BCG in the USA.

The Second World War brought with it a resurgence of TB in Europe and Asia and so the BCG vaccine was used on a massive scale and public confidence in its safety was restored. The WHO, UNICEF, and the Scandinavian Red Cross Societies conducted major BCG campaigns

OPPOSITE At least 3 million people, mainly in Eastern Europe and Russia, died from louse-borne typhus during and after the First World War. This 1919 poster shows the typhus louse shaking hands with Death.

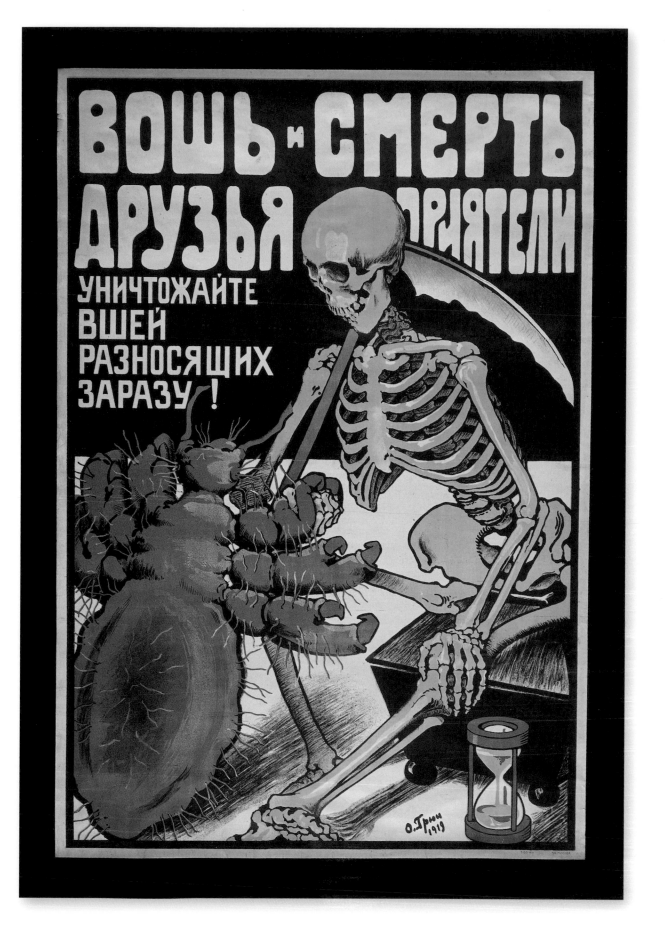

in the 1950s. It is estimated that more than three billion doses of the BCG vaccine have been administered since its introduction. Screening programs using miniature radiography, tuberculin testing, and treatment with antibiotics (see pages 189–90) have also played an important role in the campaigns against TB. Indeed, in the USA, detection of latent infection followed by treatment rather than mass immunization with BCG eventually became the preferred policy.

Polio vaccines—Salk's shot and Sabin's sugar lump

In its severest form, the polio virus invades the nervous system, leading to muscle degeneration, paralysis, and sometimes death by asphyxiation. It was one of the most feared childhood diseases of the first half of the 20th century. US President Franklin Delano Roosevelt (FDR), diagnosed with polio at the age of 39, was paralyzed in both legs—this was always carefully concealed. He backed research into the disease and raised funds through a radio appeal asking everyone to send their spare dimes (10 cents) to the President at the White House. The "March of Dimes" became an annual event and US$630 million was donated from 1938–62. The nation also watched newsreels of children with wasted limbs locked in braces and survivors imprisoned for life in massive "iron lung" respirators to encourage support for the crusade.

Working at the National Foundation for Infantile Paralysis (set up in 1938), Jonas Salk (1914–95) developed a vaccine based on an inactivated or "killed" polio virus administered by injection. In 1955 the first large-scale immunization of over 400,000 children was successfully launched using Salk's vaccine. It had been tested on nearly 1.8 million children (known as "Polio Pioneers") in a double-blind trial, with some receiving the vaccine, some a placebo and the rest acting as controls. It was seen as one of the most exciting medical advances of the 1950s. But the notorious "Cutter incident" of 1955 dampened public confidence in his vaccine. Some 200,000 people injected with the vaccine prepared by the Cutter Laboratories in California became infected; 70,000 developed muscle weakness; 164 children were left severely paralyzed; and ten died. The vaccine had not been prepared properly and contained virulent, nonattenuated polio virus. A storm of controversy led to major reforms in the production and safety of vaccines.

Albert Sabin (1906–93), also supported by the Foundation, went on to develop a live-attenuated vaccine, which was administered orally—usually on a sugar lump—and offered some advantages

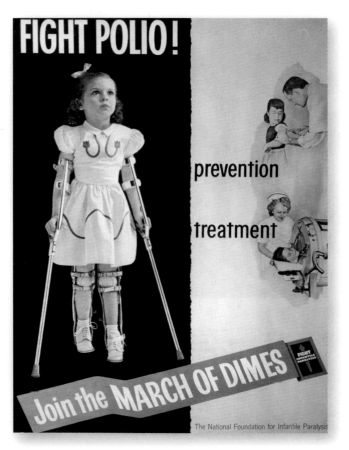

The "March of Dimes" was an annual fundraising event nationwide in the USA from the late 1930s, which included moving posters showing children disabled by polio. The funds raised helped support new research into vaccine developments.

over the Salk vaccine. Sabin conducted his trials on a range of subjects, including his own family and prisoners in federal penitentiaries. This was followed by a large-scale immunization of ten million children in the Soviet Union in collaboration with the Russian scientist Mikhail Chumakov (1909–93). By the early 1960s, Sabin's oral polio vaccine (OPV) became the accepted standard in most countries. On "Sabin Sundays," about 100 million Americans received the vaccine free of charge; now it is routinely given to infants.

In 1988, following the success of smallpox eradication, the WHO, inspired by Rotary International, launched the Global Polio Eradication Initiative and passed a resolution to eradicate polio by the year 2000. At the time, polio was endemic in 125 countries on five continents and more than 350,000 children were paralyzed by the disease. By 2002, three WHO regions (the Americas, Western Pacific, and European Regions) had been certified polio-free, but in Pakistan, Afghanistan, India, and Nigeria (known by the acronym PAIN) the disease remained endemic. The good news is that only 215 cases were reported worldwide in 2012 and India has reported no new cases between January 2011 and January 2013—a truly remarkable achievement. Despite so much progress, political, security, and religious tensions in the last persistent pockets are making the final goal difficult and there is a risk of the virus spreading to neighboring countries, as, for example, when it spread from Pakistan to China in 2011, which had been polio-free for more than a decade.

Measles and the Expanded Programme of Immunization

In the same way that during my Microsoft career I talked about the magic of software,
I now spend my time talking about the magic of vaccines.

Bill Gates, 2011

Measles, a highly infectious viral disease for which, like smallpox and polio, there has never been a "cure," is another vaccine-preventable disease. The US microbiologist and Nobel Laureate John Enders (1897–1985) and his colleague Thomas Peebles (1921–2010) isolated the measles virus in 1954 and developed an effective vaccine against the disease that was licensed in 1963. The US Centers for Disease Control (CDC) quickly began a mass "make measles a memory" immunization program for the elimination of measles, which has left the USA almost measles-free. The measles vaccine is now usually combined with a mumps and rubella vaccine (MMR). With effective childhood immunization programs, most industrialized countries have reduced cases by 99 percent over the past half-century. However, in the developing world, measles, although significantly reduced in recent decades, remains a serious childhood disease, especially in malnourished children.

As vaccine development increased, so too, a picture emerged of inequality worldwide as children in many of the poorer countries remained unvaccinated. The WHO launched the highly successful Expanded Programme on Immunization (EPI) in 1974, covering six common childhood diseases: measles, polio, tuberculosis, diphtheria, tetanus, and whooping cough. A major public-private-philanthropic global health partnership, the Global Alliance for Vaccines and Immunization (GAVI), was established in 2000 backed by the Bill & Melinda Gates Foundation, to extend the coverage of vaccination. The couple, of Microsoft fame and fortune, have pledged over US$10 billion of their personal wealth to research, develop, and deliver vaccines for the world's poorest countries, calling in 2010 for a new "Decade of Vaccines."

Two of the most recently developed childhood vaccines are for the "forgotten killer," pneumococcal disease (caused by *Streptococcus pneumoniae* bacteria, which can lead to pneumonia, meningitis, and other infections) and rotavirus. GAVI is promoting these for inclusion in national immunization programs. Children under five years in low-income countries are at far greater risk of dying from pneumococcal disease (which kills nearly one million children worldwide) than children from high-income countries. Antibiotics are used to treat pneumococcal disease, but some strains of the bacteria have developed resistance.

Rotavirus is the most common cause of severe and fatal diarrhea in children and infants worldwide. It is widely prevalent in areas of poor sanitation. When followed by serious dehydration, it can rapidly lead to death. Globally, rotavirus kills more than half a million children each year, with most deaths occurring in poorer countries. It is estimated that only a third of these children are given solutions made of oral rehydration salts—one of the most cost-effective and lifesaving survival interventions available for diarrheal diseases. Manufacturers, including Merck, Pfizer, and GSK, have offered the vaccines to GAVI-eligible countries at a fraction of their prices in the developed world.

A vaccine (MenAfriVac) for one of the most fatal forms of meningococcal meningitis (serogroup A) in Africa was launched in 2010. It was developed through a partnership between the Meningitis Vaccine Project (MVP), the WHO, GAVI, and the nonprofit organization PATH (Program for Appropriate Technology in Health). It is produced by the Serum Institute of India Ltd and designed specifically for the "African Meningitis Belt," which stretches from Senegal in the west to Ethiopia in the east. This region has periodically experienced serious meningitis epidemics, with fatality rates of 10–50 percent and, to date, around 100 million people have now received the vaccine.

Influenza: seasonal drifts and pandemic shifts

Although the first vaccines for influenza were developed several decades ago, preventing and controlling this highly contagious disease has not been straightforward. Every few years, influenza viruses mutate enough to result in a new strain: a process known as antigenic drift. This is carefully monitored, with new vaccines being produced each year to provide protection against the circulating seasonal strains. Occasionally, a major change in the virus produces a strain so different that humans have little or no preexisting immunity. This process is known as antigenic shift and it can result in pandemics when a new subtype or strain spreads globally. At the time of the deadly 1918–19 pandemic, when more than 50 million people died, there was neither treatment nor an effective vaccine for this killer. Nor were there antibiotics to treat the virulent bacterial infections that sprang up in its wake.

The latest 2009–10 pandemic, which saw over a fifth of the world's population infected and led to over 18,000 deaths, was identified as a novel influenza A virus subtype H1N1, with its origins probably in pigs, giving it the popular name "swine flu." A massive effort to produce a vaccine began shortly after the new virus strain was detected in April 2009, and by September 2009 the FDA had approved four vaccines, though trying to distribute them globally proved challenging, with accusations of inequitable distribution regarding poorer countries. Industry and public health officials are now examining new technologies to increase vaccine availability and distribution and are addressing the challenges posed by the development of vaccines for emergency use in the likelihood of any new future pandemics. An ideal prospect would be to develop a "universal" vaccine that would cover all possible influenza strains.

Vaccines for cancer-causing viruses

Viruses such as hepatitis B (transmitted primarily through infectious blood and bodily fluids, or from mother to newborn) and the human papilloma virus (HPV, the most common sexually transmitted infection) can play a role in a number of conditions, including two forms of cancer—liver and cervical cancer, respectively. There are now vaccines for protection against hepatitis B and some types of HPV prior to exposure. Hepatitis B vaccines, developed in the mid-1980s, were the first vaccines to use recombinant DNA methodology and many countries now routinely vaccinate infants, and high-risk groups, against hepatitis B.

There are two HPV vaccines (Gardasil and Cervarix), first approved in 2006–07, which were shown to prevent potentially precancerous lesions of the cervix; they have proved to be safe and effective and many countries have introduced vaccination programs for young women into their public health systems, though it is important that women continue to seek regular cervical smear or similar screening tests, even after vaccination, to detect abnormal

How do vaccines work?

Vaccines are made using a safe, weakened, inactivated, or partial version of a pathogen, which stimulates our immune system to produce chemicals (antibodies) that will fight a future infection, or, where a few vaccines are combined, that protect against more than one illness. Antibodies are a healthy body's natural response to invading viruses, bacteria, and parasites, but exposure to certain dangerous pathogens for the first time can be deadly. Vaccines serve two related but distinct functions: to protect vaccinated people against infection and severe disease; and to reduce transmission through herd immunity. Since the first smallpox vaccine was introduced in the late 18th century, vaccines have saved the lives of millions of people around the world.

The overall successes of vaccination have sometimes been marred in the past by unforeseen adverse effects, while occasional scares (such as that based on a discredited 1998 report linking the MMR vaccine with autism and bowel disorders) can lead to parental concerns. However, if vaccination rates in a community drop below a certain level, "breakthrough outbreaks" of diseases such as mumps, measles, and whooping cough

occur, which can be life-threatening to the nonimmune. A number of national and global systems ensure safe monitoring of vaccines, for example, the Vaccine Adverse Event Reporting System (VAERS) in the USA.

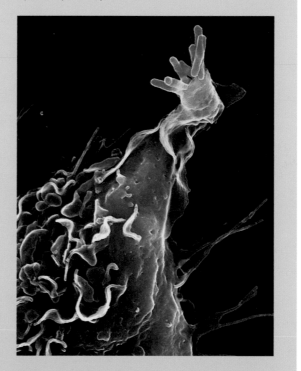

A colored scanning electron micrograph of a white blood cell (green) engulfing a tuberculosis bacterium (orange).

cell changes in the cervix before cancer has had a chance to develop. HPV vaccines have also been approved for males in several countries. It is hoped that the use of HPV vaccines could help reduce cervical cancer deaths (the fourth most deadly cancer in women) by two-thirds around the world. Ongoing research is focused on the development of HPV vaccines that will offer protection against a broader range of HPV subtypes.

"Waiting for a vaccine": The Big Three and the NTDs

In 2002, the Global Fund to Fight AIDS, Tuberculosis and Malaria (GFATM)— the "Big Three"— was established to prevent an annual 5.6 million deaths from these three leading infectious diseases. Over the past decade there have been significant successes in reducing mortality and morbidity from these diseases through such interventions as antiretroviral therapy for HIV/AIDS; the DOTS ("Directly Observed Treatment, Short-course") program of detecting and treating patients with TB; and the use of long-lasting-insecticide-treated bed nets and artemisinin-based combination therapies to prevent and treat malaria.

However, in spite of the impressive advances, they remain major global killers—with the majority of cases occurring in sub-Saharan Africa—and effective vaccines are urgently needed. There are currently an estimated 34 million people living with HIV and 1.7 million AIDS-related deaths annually. One-third of the world's population is infected with latent TB and there are around 8.7 million new active cases and 1.4 million deaths annually. Malaria accounts for over 200 million cases and a reported 660,000 deaths each year—86 percent of these in children under five.

Scientists have searched for a vaccine for HIV/AIDS since the virus was first isolated in 1983–4. HIV (human immunodeficiency virus) mutates much more rapidly than most and has a long dormant period in which the virus kills immune T helper cells called CD4+ cells, which are the coordinators of the human immune system. When HIV kills enough CD4+ cells, it leaves the immune system unable to fight off infections. If the number of CD4+ cells drops below a certain point, a person is considered to have progressed from HIV infection to AIDS (acquired immune deficiency syndrome). By attacking the very cells that a vaccine would, ideally, stimulate to produce immunity, this creates major challenges for HIV vaccine researchers. A glimmer of hope has come following a vaccine trial, known as RV144, which took place in Thailand between 2003 and 2009 with more than 16,000 participants. RV144 showed a modest level of efficacy and lowered the risk of infection by 31 percent; the search for more effective vaccines continues.

The WHO declared TB a global emergency in 1993 as a staggering number of cases were emerging in Africa and Asia, as well as in the former Soviet Union and Eastern Europe. This was partly fueled by the HIV/AIDS pandemic, with 1.1 million new TB cases being coinfected with HIV in 2011, and partly as a result of multidrug-resistant (MDR) and extensively drug-resistant (XDR) strains of TB. Political instability and poverty in parts of the world most affected have added to the difficulties of controlling TB. The BCG vaccine, first used in humans in 1921, is still the only vaccine available for preventing TB. However, its efficacy is variable and its use varies from country to country. Moreover, while it offers some protection against severe forms of pediatric TB, it is unreliable

Malaria accounts for over 200 million cases and a reported 660,000 deaths in 2010—86 percent of these in children under five.

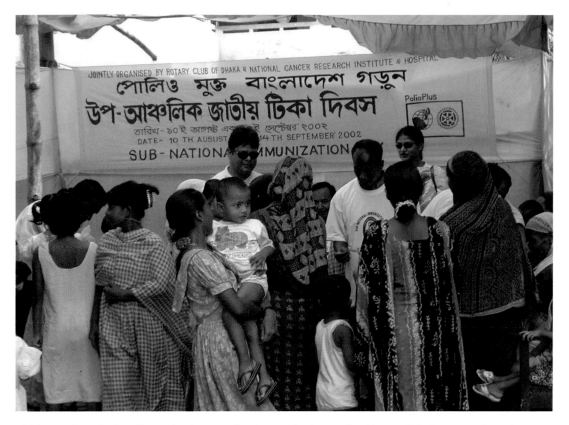

Children are brought for polio vaccination on National Immunization Day (NID) in Bangladesh, 2002. On the 20th anniversary of NID in Bangladesh in 2013, 24 million children were vaccinated in an effort to sustain its polio-free status. The global campaign to eradicate polio has seen tremendous successes, with the goal of a polio-free world by 2018.

against adult pulmonary TB, which accounts for most of the TB burden worldwide. Major international research efforts are underway to improve the existing BCG vaccine or develop new vaccines; several candidates are in early-stage trials.

For malaria, exciting news was published in the *New England Journal of Medicine* in 2011 of the preliminary results of a Phase III clinical trial of a new vaccine, RTS,S (or Mosquirix), designed for children in Africa. The trial vaccine reduced clinical episodes of malaria and severe malaria by approximately one-half in 5–17-month-old children. Eleven African research centers in seven African countries are currently conducting this trial, together with its creators, GSK and the PATH Malaria Vaccine Initiative (MVI), with grant funding from the Gates Foundation. The results of the trial look promising and if recommended for use, GSK and MVI will make it available and affordable to those who need it most. Even a partially effective vaccine for malaria, when used in combination with other preventive and treatment strategies, could greatly reduce the desperate toll on human life.

As yet, however, there are no vaccines for most of the world's 17 so-called Neglected Tropical Diseases (NTDs), which include onchoceriasis (river blindness), trypanosomiasis (sleeping sickness), and blinding trachoma. These diseases cause severe pain and permanent disability to over one billion people living below the World Bank poverty line. The rising costs and complexities of producing new vaccines are combined with the hurdles of delivering them to areas of the world where health service infrastructures for vaccination are poor or nonexistent.

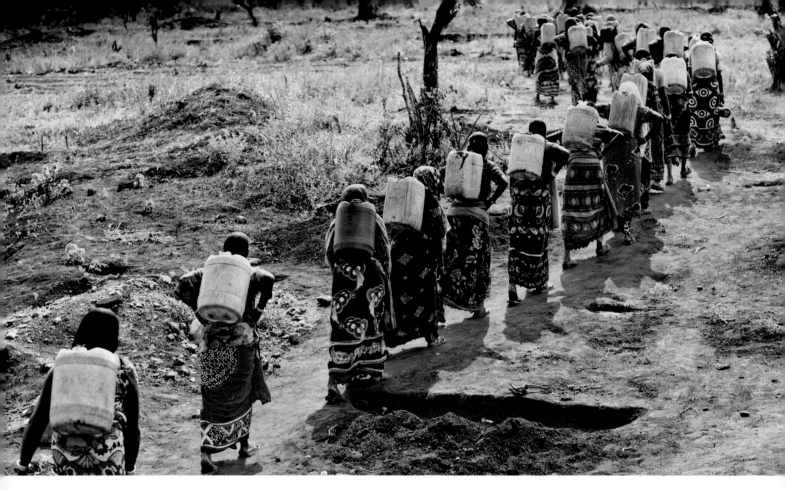

A line of women on their way to collect water in Ethiopia. In many of the poorer parts of the world, even the supply of drinking water and basic sanitation remain huge problems in the 21st century.

Spreading the message: from vaccines to sanitation and "healthy lifestyles"

During the past four decades, unprecedented gains have been achieved with vaccines in saving lives, building from the lessons and experience of the successful smallpox eradication program. The elimination of polio from most of the world is another remarkable achievement. Vaccine safety has increased, and efficacy has been much improved by the development of new "adjuvants"—agents that stimulate the immune response. There are extraordinary opportunities to extend the portfolio of immunizations against viral and bacterial diseases and to pioneer the first vaccines against human parasitic, fungal, and helminthic (worm) infections. The future of vaccinology, also, now lies in the expansion of the targets of vaccines beyond infectious diseases to include autoimmune diseases, allergies, insulin-dependent diabetes, chronic diseases of aging, hypertension, and cancer. This is a challenge that will engage and tax the ingenuity of scientists and vaccine manufacturers.

Many of us in the 21st century owe our lives and health to significant discoveries in science, pharmacy, and medicine—from vaccinations to "magic bullets" and pioneering surgical innovations. We are also reminded by history of the vital significance of broader public health measures, such as water sanitation and sewage systems. Indeed, in a poll of over 11,000 readers of the *British Medical Journal* from around the world in 2007, the introduction of clean water and sewage disposal—the "sanitary revolution"—was voted as the most important medical milestone since 1840, when the journal was first published. Yet, today, more than 780 million people in the developing world are still without safe drinking water sources and 2.5 billion people lack access to improved sanitation. The importance of recognizing the need for clean water has led to the near elimination of dracunculiasis, or Guinea worm disease, which is transmitted through drinking water contaminated with parasite-infected fleas. Eradication efforts have been based on health education and behavior change, such as teaching people to filter all drinking water. From an estimated 3.5 million cases in the mid-1980s, only 542 cases were reported in 2012. This has been achieved despite there being no cure or vaccine.

Health education also plays a prominent role in preventive strategies for many of the noncommunicable diseases (NCDs), such as cardiovascular diseases, chronic respiratory diseases, cancers, and diabetes. Cardiovascular diseases are the leading cause of death in the world, with around 17.3 million deaths annually, 30 percent of all global deaths. Cancers account for 7.6 million deaths annually; respiratory diseases, 4.2 million; and diabetes, 1.3 million. Although these are highly complex diseases, epidemiologists have identified key "risk factors," including obesity resulting from unhealthy diets and lack of physical exercise, smoking, and alcohol. While public health initiatives and preventive measures, including banning smoking in public places, disease screening, and persuasive media messages encouraging "healthy lifestyles," are making an impact in the developed world, 70–80 percent of deaths from NCDs now occur in low- and middle-income countries, where much remains to be done to control the growing burden of "lifestyle" risk factors. Road traffic injuries are the leading cause of death among people aged 15–29 years, with 90 percent of the world's fatalities on the roads occurring in low- and middle-income countries. Simple road safety campaigns could save lives.

The Millennium Development Goals, 2000–2015

Advances in social and economic development, as well as targeted public health measures such as sanitation and slum clearance, have played a crucial part in contributing to rising life expectancies in the wealthy countries of the world. Yet, inequities across the globe remain stark. From the plight of people living on US$1.25 a day in rural Africa, to urban dwellers in shanty towns in low- and middle-income countries, and the social gradient of health in high-income countries, life chances differ greatly depending on where people are born and raised. The UN launched the Millennium Development Goals (MDGs) in 2000 to address the underlying social determinants of health as well as specific disease priorities, and to identify eight goals to achieve by the year 2015:

1. Eradicate extreme poverty and hunger
2. Achieve universal primary education
3. Promote gender equality and empower women
4. Reduce child mortality
5. Improve maternal health
6. Combat HIV/AIDS, malaria, and other diseases
7. Ensure environmental sustainability
8. Develop a global partnership for development

Meeting these goals is challenging, but global health leaders are increasingly focusing on the need to address the problems faced by the world's poorest and most vulnerable, and, ultimately, it is hoped their endeavors and commitment will make a major impact on the future of global health in the coming decades.

Timeline

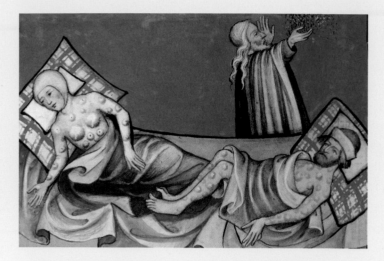

c.1800–1300 BC Egyptian papyri
These ancient papyri include some of the world's oldest written medical documents, such as the Ebers papyrus and the Edwin Smith papyrus

5th century BC Hippocrates
Greek physician, known as "the father of medicine," and his followers write the Hippocratic Corpus and the Hippocratic Oath

c.1st century BC Sushruta
Indian surgeon writes the *Sushruta Samhitā*, a classic text of Ayurvedic medicine and surgery

1st century AD Dioscorides
Greek physician produces his *De materia medica* describing over 300 medicinal plants including the opium poppy

2nd century AD Galen
Greco-Roman physician becomes the most celebrated and influential physician in the Roman Empire; Galen's many works include his ideas about the humoral theory, anatomy, and bloodletting

c.8th–13th century Islamic medicine
Greek medicine spreads into the Islamic world through the work of Arabic translators of medical texts

c.1315/16 Dissection
First recorded public dissection of a human body in Christendom takes place in Bologna, Italy

1347–53 The Black Death
One of the most deadly plague pandemics in human history spreads from Asia to the Middle East, North Africa, and Europe. Over 25 million people die (possibly as many as one-third of Europe's population)

1495 Syphilis
A "new" disease erupts in Europe following the French siege of Naples

1500s Smallpox and measles
Infectious diseases reach the "New World" with devastating consequences

1543 Human anatomy
Flemish anatomist Andreas Vesalius publishes *De humani corporis fabrica,* with illustrations of the structure of the human body based on dissection of human corpses

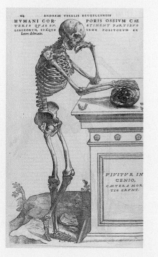

1590s Chinese medicine
Li Shi-Zhen writes *Bencao Gangmu,* his influential compendium of medicinal herbs

1628 Circulation of the blood
William Harvey publishes his treatise proposing that the heart is a pump that circulates the blood around the body

1630s–50s Cinchona bark
European explorers bring this early remedy for malaria back from South America; in 1820 it is found to contain quinine

1721 Smallpox inoculation
Lady Mary Wortley Montagu introduces the Turkish practice of smallpox inoculation to England

1747 Clinical trials
James Lind conducts a clinical trial that shows the benefits of oranges and lemons in preventing scurvy

1796 Vaccination
Edward Jenner first tries out a cowpox vaccine to prevent smallpox. His treatise describing vaccination is published in 1798

1796 Homeopathy
Samuel Hahnemann establishes a new system of medical healing called homeopathy—still used today

1816 Stethoscope
Invented by René Laënnec, this diagnostic tool enables physicians to listen to a patient's lungs and heart

c.1826–37 Cholera
This frightening disease spreads from Asia, North Africa, and Europe, reaching England in 1831 and the Americas in 1832

1828 Body snatchers
Burke and Hare in Edinburgh, Scotland, are arrested for murdering victims to send to the anatomy school; Burke is hanged and his body dissected

1842 Public health
Edwin Chadwick publishes his *Report of an Inquiry on the Sanitary Conditions of the Labouring Population of Great Britain,* recommending improvements in sewerage, water supply, and drainage

1846 Hand-washing
Ignaz Semmelweis investigates high mortality rates from puerperal (childbed) fever in hospitals, concluding that hand-washing is vital to prevent infection

1846 Anesthesia
William Morton administers ether to a patient undergoing surgery at the Massachusetts General Hospital, Boston

1849 Women in medicine
Elizabeth Blackwell is the first female doctor to gain a medical degree in the USA

1851 Quarantine
Following major cholera pandemics, the first International Sanitary Conference is held with the aim of making quarantine an international cooperative effort for disease control and prevention

1854 Preventing cholera
John Snow has the handle of the Broad Street pump in London removed to prove that cholera is transmitted through drinking water contaminated with raw sewage

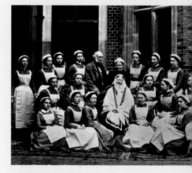

1854–6 Nurses in the Crimean War
Florence Nightingale and Mary Seacole, independently, assist with nursing wounded and sick soldiers. Nightingale subsequently plays a major role in the development of nursing as a profession

1856 From dyes to drugs
William Henry Perkins synthesizes mauveine, marking the beginnings of the organic chemical industry; this later leads to the development of synthetic drugs

1858 Cells
Rudolf Virchow—in *Die Cellularpathologie*—proposes that the cell is the smallest unit of life and that every cell is generated from another cell

1865 Antisepsis
Joseph Lister uses carbolic acid in surgery, beginning the practice of antisepsis

1877 Tropical medicine
Patrick Manson establishes a link between bloodsucking mosquitoes and the tropical disease lymphatic filariasis (elephantiasis)

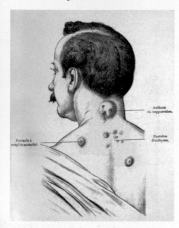

1878 Germ theory
Louis Pasteur reads a paper before the French Academy of Sciences entitled "Germ Theory and Its Applications to Medicine and Surgery"

1882 Identifying the cause of TB
Robert Koch identifies the bacterium, *Mycobacterium tuberculosis*, responsible for tuberculosis (TB)

1885 Rabies vaccine
Pasteur successfully vaccinates a boy who has been bitten by a rabid dog

1894 Bubonic plague
Alexandre Yersin identifies the bacterium responsible for bubonic plague; the role of the black rat and the rat flea in transmitting bubonic plague is discovered a few years later

1895 X-rays
Discovered by Wilhelm Röntgen, X-rays enable physicians to screen for diseases such as TB and cancers, as well as aiding surgery and early developments in radiotherapy

1897 Mosquitoes and malaria
In India, Ronald Ross discovers malaria parasites in mosquitoes; the following year he elucidates the life cycle of malaria in birds

1898 Radium
Marie and Pierre Curie discover the radioactive elements polonium and radium—the latter used for treating deep cancers

1899 Aspirin
Bayer launches the new aspirin pain-relief drug and sells it in a double package with heroin

1901 Serum therapy
The first Nobel Prize in Physiology or Medicine is awarded to Emil von Behring for his work on serum therapy, especially its application against diphtheria

1910 First "magic bullet"
Paul Ehrlich and Sahachiro Hata discover Salvarsan to treat syphilis

1918–19 Influenza
The so-called "Spanish flu" circulates the globe, killing an estimated 50 million people—the most devastating pandemic in modern history

1920s TB vaccine
The BCG vaccine for tuberculosis is introduced

1922 Insulin
Scientists in Toronto, Canada, first use insulin from ox pancreas to treat diabetes

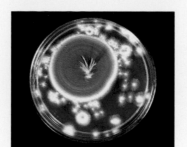

1928 Penicillin
Alexander Fleming in London discovers a mold with antibacterial properties, which he names penicillin

1930 The FDA
The US Food and Drug Administration (FDA) is named as a government agency to regulate the content and safety of consumer foods and drugs

1935–6 Sulfonamides
These drugs are found to be effective against certain bacteria and used to treat puerperal or "childbirth" fever and other infections

Early 1940s Antibiotics
Howard Florey, Ernst Chain, and Norman Heatley at Oxford University, England, develop penicillin as the first highly effective antibiotic for previously fatal bacterial infections

1943 Streptomycin
Albert Schatz working with Selman Waksman discovers streptomycin, the first effective antibiotic against TB

1944 DNA
Scientists first show that DNA is the carrier of genetic information

1948 RCTs
The first reported randomized controlled trial (RCT)—to test the efficacy of streptomycin as a treatment for pulmonary tuberculosis—is published

1948 WHO
The World Health Organization (WHO) is set up as an agency of the United Nations with its headquarters in Geneva, Switzerland

1948 The NHS
The National Health Service is launched, nationalizing the health service and providing "free care for all" in Britain

1953 The double helix of DNA
The molecular structure of DNA is first described by James Watson and Francis Crick, based also on the experimental work of Maurice Wilkins and Rosalind Franklin

1954 Organ transplant
First successful kidney transplant is performed between identical twins in Boston, USA

1955–62 Polio vaccine
The first vaccines for polio are introduced leading to its near eradication by the early 21st century

Early 1960s The Pill
The first oral contraceptive pill is introduced

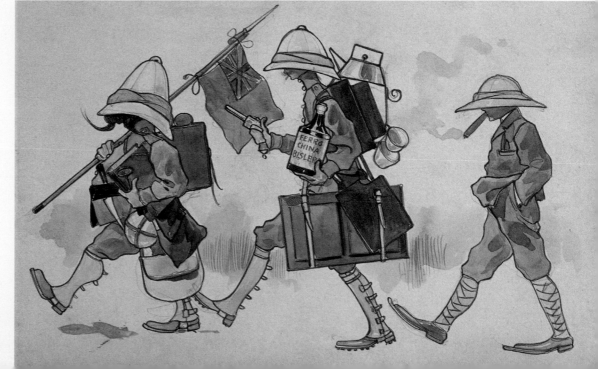

Early 1960s MRSA
The first cases of MRSA (methicillin-resistant *Staphylococcus aureus*) are identified in a British hospital

1964 Medical ethics
The Declaration of Helsinki details ethical conduct in medical research involving human subjects and is a landmark in medical ethics

1967 Heart transplant
Christiaan Barnard in Cape Town, South Africa, performs the first heart transplant

1970s
Recombinant DNA technology
The field of modern biotechnology begins with tremendous potential for genetically engineered drugs and vaccines

1970s Medical imaging
New technologies such as MRI (magnetic resonance imaging) are developed, enabling the body to be scanned to detect and diagnose disease

1970s A "new" antimalarial
Chinese researchers "rediscover" the ancient herbal remedy *Artemisia annua* and develop an antimalarial drug called artemisinin

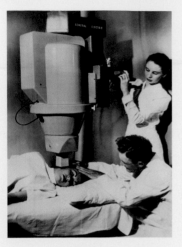

1971 Chemotherapy
The National Cancer Act is passed in the USA with the aim of increasing research to find a cure for cancer

1975 Monoclonal antibodies
Scientists, including César Milstein, discover the principle for the production of monoclonal antibodies, leading to their use as powerful therapeutics

1979 Smallpox eradication
The WHO announces the global eradication of smallpox and in 1980 it is officially removed from the list of world diseases

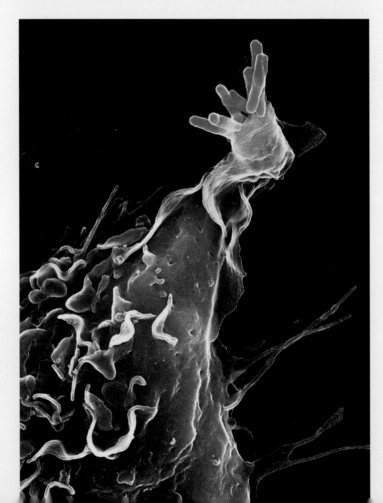

1980s Cyclosporin
An immunosuppressive drug is introduced to prevent organ transplant rejection

1982
Genetically engineered insulin
The first biosynthetic human insulin becomes commercially available under the brand name Humulin

1982 A new infectious agent
Stanley Prusiner describes a new kind of infectious agent, which he calls a "prion"; prion-related diseases include BSE ("mad cow disease") in cattle and vCJD ("variant" Creutzfeldt-Jakob disease) in humans

1983–4 HIV/AIDS
The causative virus (later called HIV or the human immunodeficiency virus) for AIDS (acquired immune deficiency syndrome) is identified soon after the first cases of AIDS are detected

1986
Genetically engineered vaccines
The first genetically engineered vaccine for Hepatitis B is approved

1990 Human Genome Project
This is launched with the goal of identifying all human genes and sequencing the 3 billion bases of a composite human genome; it is completed in 2003, two years ahead of schedule, at a cost of nearly US$3 billion

1996 Bird flu
A highly pathogenic new strain of influenza, H_5N_1, is first detected in some geese in China, later raising fears of a major human pandemic, but so far its spread from human to human has been limited

2000 Philanthropy
The Bill & Melinda Gates Foundation is formally established to fund programs to enhance global health and reduce extreme poverty

2000 MDGs
The United Nations Millennium Development Goals (MDGs) are introduced, setting targets for 2015 to eliminate extreme poverty and hunger and combat major global diseases

2001
Telesurgery and robotic surgery
The first major transatlantic surgical procedure is performed between surgeons in New York City, USA, and a patient in Strasbourg, France, with a separation of nearly 7,000 km (4,350 miles), using telerobotic-assisted surgery

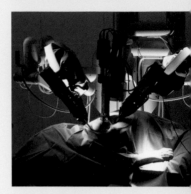

2003 SARS
A "new" mysterious disease named SARS (severe acute respiratory syndrome) spreads around the world; it is identified as a coronavirus

2008 Poverty and disease
The WHO publishes its influential report: "Closing the Gap in a Generation: Health Equity Through Action on the Social Determinants of Health"

2009 Swine flu
The first cases of a new type of influenza, H1N1, are reported

2010
Antibiotic-resistance initiative
The Infectious Disease Society of America (IDSA) launches its "10 X 20 Initiative" to pursue a global commitment to develop ten new antibacterial drugs by 2020

2012 Neglected Tropical Diseases
Global health partners sign the "London Declaration," pledging new levels of collaborative effort to fight these diseases of poverty

2012 Stem cells
The Nobel Prize in Physiology or Medicine is awarded jointly to John Gurdon and Shinya Yamanaka for their researches paving the way for stem cell therapy, regenerative medicine, and drug discovery

Further reading

In undertaking the challenge of researching and writing *The Story of Medicine: From Bloodletting to Biotechnology*, I would like to thank Josephine Hill, who helped me find and collate a vast range of material from libraries and online medical and historical journals. Inevitably, I have had to generalize, simplify, and touch only briefly on some of the fascinating themes that span over 3,000 years of global history. For those who want to explore the rich history of medicine further there are many excellent sources in libraries and archives around the world, as well as on the internet. The Wellcome Library in London, for example, is one of the world's major resources for the study of medical history, as well as housing a growing collection of material relating to contemporary medicine and biomedical science in society. The Wellcome also has a wonderful collection of images, some of which are included in this book: others can be viewed on their website.

General and accessible books that cover the field in diverse ways include: Robert E Adler, *Medical Firsts* (John Wiley & Sons, 2004); William Bynum and Helen Bynum (eds), *Great Discoveries in Medicine* (Thames & Hudson, 2011); Jacalyn Duffin, *History of Medicine* (University of Toronto Press, 2010); Irvine Loudon (ed.), *Western Medicine: An Illustrated History* (Oxford University Press, 1997); Michael T Kennedy, *A Brief History of Disease, Science and Medicine* (Asklepliad Press, 2004); Clifford A Pickover, *The Medical Book* (Sterling, 2012); Roy Porter (ed.), *The Cambridge Illustrated History of Medicine* (Cambridge University Press, 1996); Anne Rooney, *The Story of Medicine* (Arcturus, 2009); and David Weatherall, *Science and the Quiet Art* (Oxford University Press, 1995).

William Bynum's *The History of Medicine: A Very Short Introduction* (Oxford University Press, 2008) is an informative "short" synopsis of the subject and there are others in this series, including Leslie Iversen's *Drugs* (2011) and Tony Hope's *Medical Ethics* (2004), which are excellent guides to a range of topics.

Any of the stimulating books by the late Roy Porter, including *The Greatest Benefit to Mankind: A Medical History of Humanity from Antiquity to the Present* (Harper Collins, 1997) and *Blood and Guts: A Short History of Medicine* (Penguin, 2003), are well worth reading. For entertainment on this subject, the UK's BBC Radio 4 program *The Making of Modern Medicine* (BBC Audiobooks, 2007), written and narrated by Andrew Cunningham, is an enthralling six-hour listen. The five-volume *Dictionary of Medical Biography* edited by William Bynum and Helen Bynum (Greenwood Press, 2007) is a valuable source of reference for discovering more about history's greatest doctors and scientists. Chapters by international scholars in Mark Jackson (ed.), *The Oxford Handbook of the History of Medicine* (Oxford University Press, 2011) highlight recent historical and academic debates in many of the subfields of the subject.

I have also learned much from wide-ranging books on specialist topics, including Harold Ellis, *The Cambridge Illustrated History of Surgery* (Cambridge University Press, 2009); Anne Hardy, *The Epidemic Streets* (Oxford University Press, 1993); Peter Hotez, *Forgotten People, Forgotten Diseases* (ASM Press, 2008); Margaret Humphreys, *Malaria: Poverty, Race and Public Health in the United States* (Johns Hopkins University Press, 2001); Guenter B Risse, *Mending Bodies, Saving Souls: A History of Hospitals* (Oxford University Press, 1999); and many others.

There are some great classics in the history of medicine, from Daniel Defoe's semifictional *A Journal of the Plague Year* (1722) and Paul de Kruif's best-selling book *Microbe Hunters* (1926) to Hans Zinsser's popular study *Rats, Lice and History* (1935). Two of my favorite autobiographies are Arthur E Hertzler, *The Horse and Buggy Doctor* (University of Nebraska Press, 1938), and Lewis Thomas, *The Youngest Science: Notes of a Medicine-Watcher* (Penguin, 1983).

Medicine, today, moves at an ever-increasing pace. The international medical journals *The Lancet* and *Nature Medicine* are excellent sources for keeping abreast of the latest developments, while the World Health Organization (www.who.int) provides up-to-date information on the incidence, prevalence, and outbreaks of major diseases.

Index

Page numbers in *italics* denote an illustration/caption

Author acknowledgments

The Story of Medicine was commissioned by Quercus as a companion volume to my book *Disease: the extraordinary stories behind history's deadliest killers* (Quercus, 2007). I would like to thank the past and present editorial and production teams at Quercus, including Richard Milbank and Slav Todorov, Kerry Enzor, Kate Fox, Richard Green, Emma Heyworth-Dunn, Katharine Reeve, Nick Clark, and Andrew Barron who have worked so hard and enthusiastically on the publication of *The Story of Medicine*.

I am most grateful to the Author's Foundation of The Society of Authors, which generously gave me a grant to enable me to conduct a number of aspects of the research for this book. Josephine Hill, who acted as my research assistant in the early stages of the project, was outstanding, and I am immensely appreciative of all her help. St John's College, Cambridge, has provided me with a stimulating and supportive intellectual environment in which to write.

My sincerest gratitude also goes to Anne Hardy, Maureen Malowany, and Bill Tyrrell who, as friends and colleagues, have played a major role in this book. Our exchanges have been many, as well as both fun and fascinating, and their expertise, ideas, and knowledge have helped to shape *The Story of Medicine*.

I would like, too, to express my thanks to William Bynum and Margaret Humphreys, who read drafts of the entire book, and to other scholars who have also meticulously read, contributed to and commented on sections and chapters of this book at its various stages, including Virginia Berridge, Roberta Bivins, Mary Crawford, Marguerite Dupree, Guy Edwards, Lev Efraim, Philip van der Eijk, Harold Ellis, Kevin Esplin, John Henderson, Salima Ikram, Leslie Iversen, Colin Jones, Vivienne Lo, Piers Mitchell, Alfredo Morabia, Jehane Regai, Guenter Risse, Martin Roland, Emilie Savage-Smith, Andrea Tanner, Oliver Thomas, and Martin Worthington. Their generous input and rapid responses have been invaluable. If I have not been able to incorporate all suggestions and changes into the final version—my apologies. And, of course, all remaining mistakes are mine alone.

Finally, I would like to add a very special tribute to my husband, Christopher, and our sons, Richard and William, who have been such a fantastic support to me throughout my career and have contributed to this book in more ways than I could mention. I dedicate this book to my family—with my love and thanks.

Picture acknowledgments

The Advertising Archives: 4 bottom right, 116, 172, 188, 205; **akg-images:** 2, 37, 70, 162, 221, /R. u S. Michaud 77, 146; **Alamy:** /World History Archive/Image Asset Management 42, 223 center; **The Art Archive:** /Private Collection/Eileen Tweedy 219, /The Tate Gallery, London/Eileen Tweedy 68, /University Library, Istanbul, Gianni Dagli Orit 144; **The Bridgeman Art Library:** /Forbes Magazine Collection, New York 56, /L'hôpital de la Salpêtrière/Archives Charmet 84, /Musée de l'Assistance Publique, Hôpitaux de Paris/Archives Charmet 72, /Musée Rolin, Autn 151, /Whitford & Hughes, London 141; **Cambridge University Library:** /By permission of the Syndics of Cambridge University Library/T-S Ar.34.239: 149; **Corbis:** 28, 75, 136, 232 top, /The Art Archive/ Alfredo Dagli Orti 17, /Asian Art & Archaeology Inc 161, /Bettmann 80, 97, /Christie's Images 26, /Hulton-Deutsch 115, /Francis G Mayer 98, /Ocean 184, /Reuters 169, /George Steinmetz 103; **Deutsches Medizinhistorisches Museum:** 106; **Getty Images:** /Hulton Archive 4 top right, 192, 206, /Science & Society Picture Library 4 bottom left, 32, 65, 176, /Stock Montage/Archive Photos 210; **Mary Evans Picture Library:** 156, /Everett Collection 191, 234 top; **Courtesy of the National Library of Medicine:** 175, 194, 220; **Panos Pictures:** /Mikkel Ostergaard 230; **Rex Features:** /Daily Mail/Anthony Wallace 212, /Roger Viollet/Jacques Boyer 189; **Photo Scala Florence:** /Heritage Images 157; **Science Photo Library:** 30, 227, 234 bottom, /A. Barrington Brown 52, /Jean-Loup Charmet 40, /A Crump. TDR, WHO 197, /Mehau Kulyk 93, /Peter Menzel 102, 234 center, /NYPL 224, /Omikron 209; **TopFoto:** /Granger Collection 23, 182, /National Archives/Heritage Images 153, 202; **University of Manchester/Dr Jacky Finch/Museum of Cairo:** 88; **Wellcome Images:** 187, 233 top, /Mark de Fraeye 123, /Rafiqul Islam 229, /Science Museum, London 69, 86, 111, 143, 154, 158, /St Bartholomew's Hospital Archives & Museum 108; **Wellcome Library, London:** 1, 4 top left, 8, 10, 13, 14, 18–19, 20, 29, 38, 44, 46, 47, 48, 50, 55, 59, 60, 62, 66, 78, 90, 94, 101, 104, 112, 118, 120, 122, 124, 126, 131, 132, 135, 138, 139, 165, 166, 171, 179, 180, 200, 214, 217, 223, 232 center & bottom, 233 bottom; **Wisconsin Historical Society:** 183.

Quercus

New York · London

Any member of educational institutions wishing to photocopy part or all of the work for classroom use or anthology should send inquiries to Permissions c/o Quercus Publishing Inc., 31 West 57th Street, 6th Floor, New York, NY 10019, or to permissions@quercus.com.

ISBN 978-1-62365-058-2

Library of Congress Control Number: 2013937927

Distributed in the United States and Canada by Random House Publishing Services c/o Random House, 1745 Broadway New York, NY 10019

Manufactured in China

2 4 6 8 10 9 7 5 3 1

www.quercus.com